Madness in the City
of Magnificent Intentions

Madness in the City of Magnificent Intentions

A History of Race and Mental Illness in the Nation's Capital

MARTIN SUMMERS

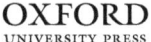

OXFORD
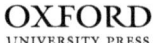

Oxford University Press is a department of the University of Oxford. It furthers
the University's objective of excellence in research, scholarship, and education
by publishing worldwide. Oxford is a registered trade mark of Oxford University
Press in the UK and certain other countries.

Published in the United States of America by Oxford University Press
198 Madison Avenue, New York, NY 10016, United States of America.

© Oxford University Press 2019

All rights reserved. No part of this publication may be reproduced, stored in
a retrieval system, or transmitted, in any form or by any means, without the
prior permission in writing of Oxford University Press, or as expressly permitted
by law, by license, or under terms agreed with the appropriate reproduction
rights organization. Inquiries concerning reproduction outside the scope of the
above should be sent to the Rights Department, Oxford University Press, at the
address above.

You must not circulate this work in any other form
and you must impose this same condition on any acquirer.

CIP data is on file at the Library of Congress
ISBN 978–0–19–085264–1

CONTENTS

Acknowledgments ix

Introduction 1

1. "Humanity Requires All the Relief Which Can Be Afforded": The Birth of the Federal Asylum 13

2. The Paradox of Enlightened Care: Saint Elizabeths in the Era of Moral Treatment, 1855–1877 39

3. "From Slave to Citizen": Race, Insanity, and Institutionalization in Post-Reconstruction Washington, DC, 1877–1900 71

4. Care and the Color Line: Race, Rights, and the Therapeutic Experience, 1877–1900 95

5. "Mechanisms of the Negro Mind": Race and Dynamic Psychiatry at Saint Elizabeths, 1903–1937 125

6. "He Is Psychotic and Always Will Be": Racial Ambivalence and the Limits of Therapeutic Optimism, 1903–1937 153

7. Mental Hygiene and the Limits of Reform: Saint Elizabeths in the Community, 1903–1937 190

8. "An Example for the Rest of the Nation": Challenging Racial Injustice at Saint Elizabeths, 1910–1955 217

9. Whither the Negro Psyche: Integration and Its Aftermath, 1945–1970   247

10. From Model to Emblem: Community Mental Health and Deinstitutionalization, 1963–1987   277

Conclusion   309

Notes   315
Selected Bibliography   369
Index   377

For Karl

ACKNOWLEDGMENTS

This is not the book that I set out to write. Trained as a cultural historian of the nineteenth- and twentieth-century United States, with particular interests in race, gender, and sexuality, I intended to write a book about black masculinity, institutions, and the state when I began my research in 2001. A chance encounter in the National Archives with a dusty, brittle admissions book of a federal insane asylum that summer set me on the path to writing this history of race and mental illness in the nation's capital. Over these past eighteen years, I have learned a great deal about the field of medical history and even more about myself as a historian. Along the way, I have accumulated many debts which I am grateful that I now have the opportunity to acknowledge.

My largest intellectual debt is owed to scholars who showed a great deal of enthusiasm, encouragement, and support for my project in its earliest stages. As someone who was excited yet tentative about entering a field in which I had no graduate training, my initial trepidation was alleviated by the early positive responses from James Mohr, Ellen Herman, and Laura Briggs. Jim and Ellen, my colleagues at the University of Oregon, were some of my most ardent champions and wisest counsels. I thank them for the years of advice and friendship that they have given me, as well as for all of the letters they have written on my behalf. Laura was a commenter on a paper that I gave early in the research process, and her engagement with the work and thoughtful remarks helped shape the scope of the project and the kinds of questions that I ended up pursuing. She has remained a steadfast source of support over the past dozen years, and I am deeply appreciative.

My growth as a scholar has been made possible by the relationships that I have developed and the conversations that I have had over the past several years with other scholars who are doing important work on the history of race and medicine. I thank Dennis Doyle, Sharla Fett, Susan Reverby, Samuel Roberts, and Keith Wailoo for the interest they have shown in my work, for their camaraderie, and for modeling the kind of scholarship that I aspire to produce. I am also grateful to Laurie Green and John Mckiernan-González, my former colleagues at the University of Texas at Austin and collaborators, for the many hours-long discussions that we have had over kitchen tables, in hotel lobbies, and on the phone over the past several years. Even though working on our coedited collection delayed progress on this monograph, it was a rewarding experience and greatly contributed to my maturation as a scholar. I thank them for their constant companionship on this journey.

Writing a 132-year history of a single institution and its relationship to the surrounding community has required a great deal of archival, research, and financial assistance. I want to thank the staffs at the American Antiquarian Society, DC Public Library (Washingtoniana Division), George Washington University's Special Collections Research Center, Harvard University's Houghton Library, Institute of Pennsylvania Hospital Archives, Library of Congress, National Archives, National Archives II, National Library of Medicine, and Saint Elizabeths Hospital Archives. I especially want to thank Saint Elizabeths' former librarian, Velora Jernigan-Pedrick, for her indispensable assistance in working through an un-inventoried collection. Matthew Gambino, who was working on a dissertation on Saint Elizabeths, graciously put me in contact with Ms. Jernigan-Pedrick, and I am grateful to him for it. Clinical staff members and historical enthusiasts Suryabala Kanhouwa and Jogues R. Prandoni generously shared their knowledge about Saint Elizabeths and their published research with me. The enthusiastic reception and support of Patrick Canavan, Saint Elizabeths' CEO in the mid-2000s, for my project was particularly welcome, as was the advice and offers of assistance by Marc Shaw, the lead architect of Saint Elizabeths' new state-of-the-art hospital.

This monograph could not have been completed without the timely and professional assistance of the interdisciplinary services staffs at the University of Oregon, the University of Texas at Austin, and Boston College. I am also particularly indebted to the library staff at the National Humanities Center—Jean Houston, Eliza Roberts, Brooke Andrade, and Sarah Harris—who ran an incredibly well-oiled machine and tracked down obscure material with alacrity and good cheer. I wish to thank Holly Reed and Kaitlyn Crain Enriquez of the National Archives Still Pictures Division for their last-minute assistance in obtaining images for the book. I have also benefited from the excellent and meticulous research skills of graduate students and undergraduate students alike, including Elizabeth Medford, Juandrea Bates, Wangui Muigai, Adam Rathge, Andrew Schneider, and Emily Sloan.

Financial support from a number of universities, research centers, and foundations was indispensable. New Faculty and Summer Research Awards from the University of Oregon in 2001 and 2003, respectively, funded the very early stages of this project, as did research monies associated with the university's Underrepresented Minority Recruitment Program. A Dean's Fellowship from UT-Austin in 2006 provided further research support. An American Council of Learned Societies Frederick Burkhardt Fellowship allowed me to spend a year at the Radcliffe Institute for Advanced Study. In addition to the ACLS, I would like to extend my gratitude to Barbara Grosz, then dean of Radcliffe; Judith Vichniac, director of the fellowship program; and the Radcliffe staff, especially Melissa Synott. I want to thank the Office of the Provost of Boston College for a sabbatical fellowship in the spring of 2011 that enabled me to begin writing. The provost also provided supplemental funding for a National Humanities Center fellowship in 2013–14. I would like to acknowledge the wonderful leadership and staff of the NHC—Geoffrey Harpham, Elizabeth "Cassie" Mansfield, and Lois Whittington in particular—as well as the generous support of Ruth W. and A. Morris Williams Jr. I would not have been able to complete this book without them. Karen Carroll's editorial assistance while I was an NHC fellow improved the manuscript's clarity and sharpness. Finally, I want to thank all of those people who have kindly given their time to write letters of recommendations over the years—for more unsuccessful fellowship proposals than I care to admit. In addition to Jim Mohr and Ellen Herman, these generous folks include Laura Briggs, King Davis, Glenda Gilmore, and Robert Self.

 I have profited enormously from the support and friendship of amazing colleagues at a number of institutions. At the University of Oregon, Ellen Herman, Shari Huhndorf, Jeff Ostler, and the late Peggy Pascoe were ideal senior colleagues and invaluable friends. Jafari Allen, Tiffany Gill, Frank Guridy, Jim Sidbury, and James Wilson made UT-Austin a welcoming place and an invigorating, if all too brief, intellectual sojourn. I have benefited from the leadership in the Department of History at Boston College, including past and present chairs Lynn Johnson, Jim Cronin, Robin Fleming, Kevin Kenny, and Sarah Ross. I have also enjoyed a collegial environment and especially the friendship of Robin Fleming, Kevin Kenny, Lynn Johnson, Priya Lal, Patrick Maney, Karen Miller, Arissa Oh, Prasannan Parthasarathi, Sarah Ross, Dana Sajdi, Franziska Seraphim, and Deborah Levenson, my stalwart and star-crossed Spanish tutor. I am indebted to my current and former colleagues in the African and African Diaspora Studies Program, especially Richard Paul, Régine Jean-Charles, Cynthia Young, and Rhonda Frederick for their friendship and support.

 In the course of writing this book, I have had the good fortune of receiving excellent and challenging feedback from friends, colleagues, and strangers. The following folks have contributed to the final shape of this book either through reading drafts of chapters or the entire manuscript or just through questions and comments delivered in informal or formal conversations: Heidi Ardizzone, Elizabeth Alexander, Elizabeth Armstrong, Nancy Bercaw, Susanna Blumenthal,

Julian Bourg, Joel Braslow, Lundy Braun, Erika Bsumek, Simone Caron, Sylvia Chong, Nancy Cott, Dennis Doyle, Matthew Gambino, Tiffany Gill, Janet Golden, Jennifer Gunn, Mark Hauser, Rana Hogarth, Lynn Johnson, Stephen Kenny, Elizabeth Krause, Regina Kunzel, Toni Lester, Deborah Levenson, David Levering Lewis, Jacqueline Malone, Michelle Moran, Rebecca Nedostup, Deirdre Cooper Owens, Anne Parsons, Naomi Rogers, Tim Rood, Jonathan Sadowsky, Dana Sajdi, Londa Schiebinger, Robert Self, Suman Seth, Karen Sotiropoulos, Melissa Stein, Melissa Stuckey, Megan Sweeney, Emma Teng, and Rhonda Y. Williams. The process of writing this book was also enormously enriched by the many discussions that I had with a phenomenal array of scholars at the National Humanities Center—in hallways, over glasses of wine during happy hour, and over delectable meals, especially Tuesdays' grits! For their intellectual camaraderie, I would particularly like to acknowledge the members of the History, Race, and the State Seminar, especially Julie Greene, Luis Cárcamo-Huechante, Sylvia Chong, Tim Marr, Elizabeth Krause, Martha Jones, Evelyn Brooks Higginbotham, and Marixa Lasso; and members of the Knowledge and Context Seminar, especially Andy Jewett, Lynn Festa, Chad Heap, and Charlie McGovern. Various versions of chapters were presented at a number of conferences and public lectures. For their generous engagement with my work, I would especially like to thank the organizers of and audiences at the University of Notre Dame's Henkels Lecture in April 2007; the University of Mississippi's Porter L. Fortune, Jr. Symposium in March 2012; the University of Oregon's Peggy Pascoe Memorial Lecture Series in November 2013; the University of Minnesota's Dorothy Bernstein Lecture in the History of Psychiatry in September 2014; and the History Department at Brown University in March 2016. The anonymous readers for Oxford University Press also provided invaluable feedback, and I thank them for it.

At Oxford University Press, I have benefited from Nancy Toff's support, editorial diligence, and low tolerance for language that obfuscates rather than clarifies. I also want to thank Nancy's assistant, Elizabeth Vaziri; Marie Felina, the book's project manager; and Judith Hoover, the copy editor.

It gives me extraordinary pleasure to be able to acknowledge my friends and family, whose steadfast support means the world to me. Unfortunately, two of my friends and mentors did not live long enough to see this book's publication. Peggy Pascoe and Clement Alexander Price taught me a great deal about being a good historian, a good teacher, and a good soul. I'm still trying to live up to the standard they set.

I have had the good fortune of having Franklin Parrish in my life for more than half of it. We both keep getting better with age, I like to think. I met Erika Bsumek in my first year of graduate school, and she has been a dear friend ever since. I thank her for all of the encouragement and support she has given me over the years and for all of the wonderful times and life events that we have been able to share. I also want to thank the Fujiwara-Morozumi clan, our West Coast family. Lynn, Steve, Kyra, Joanna, and Martin have enriched my life in more ways than I can count, and I am so grateful to them for it.

I thank my father, Charles Summers, and my brother, Scott Summers, for modeling for me what it is to live a life of integrity and purpose. Although I did not end up working with the same kind of student population, my late mother Loretta Summers' passion for teaching, along with the way that she led her life, continues to inspire me. I also thank my father's partner, Kay Henry; my sister-in-law, Wendy Summers; my niece and nephew, Lauren and Christian Summers; my aunt, Barbara Mead; my godsister Nikitea Vaughn; and my godson, Liam Hannon, for their love and support. And words cannot express how much I love and miss my sister, Carla Summers, who taught me so much about life, music, and food. I think about her every day.

And, finally, I am so happy to be able to acknowledge Karl Mundt. He has had to endure more closed study doors over the past decade than a husband should have to, and he has never once complained. His love and support as a partner and a friend are beyond measure. Whenever an academic asks me if my husband is an academic as well, his or her eyes light up when I respond, "No, he is a choreographer and a dance teacher." I don't know what that says about our respective career choices. But I do know that I could not have made a better choice for a life partner.

Introduction

For most of its history, Saint Elizabeths Hospital was considered by nearly everyone who had a relationship to it to be an exceptional institution. Founded in 1855 in Washington, DC, the insane asylum was envisioned by Congress and Presidents Millard Fillmore and Franklin Pierce as providing "the most humane care and enlightened curative treatment" to the soldiers and sailors of the nation as well as the residents of the nation's capital. While considering an offer to become its first superintendent, Dr. Charles H. Nichols expressed the desire to his friend, the reformer Dorothea Lynde Dix, that he be given the resources and latitude to build a "model hospital." Dr. William Alanson White, who directed the hospital for nearly the first four decades of the twentieth century, often spoke of the institution's unique position as a research and teaching hospital. Its location in the nation's capital, its funding from the federal government, its proximity to elite medical schools, and its special patient population made White's assessment of Saint Elizabeths' singularity one that was shared by his colleagues in the psychiatric profession. Even as the paradigm of mental health care was transitioning from the large public hospital to the decentralized community center model in the post–World War II era, government and hospital officials hoped that Saint Elizabeths would "provide an example for the Nation" in how to make the transformation seamlessly.[1]

Saint Elizabeths' exceptionalism—both presumed and real—was due in no small part to its status as a federal institution in a federal district. For roughly a century, during which the care of the mentally ill fell primarily to state and local governments, Saint Elizabeths was one of the few mental hospitals that was largely funded by Congress and that served patients who were considered wards of the federal government.[2] In some ways, when Nichols aspired to make Saint Elizabeths a model hospital, he was expressing his belief that he and his staff could make it the pacesetter for the rest of the nation's asylums. But he and those who followed him as superintendent also maintained a certain investment in the notion that Saint Elizabeths' exceptionalism exceeded national borders. As it was, effectively, the national asylum, Saint Elizabeths carried the burden of representing the virtues of the American medical profession's approach to treating mental illness. Those associated with the hospital often interpreted this burden not as an unwanted responsibility but as an opportunity to demonstrate the American capacity to keep pace with the advances in the treatment of mental illness made by the British, French, and German medical professions and to trumpet the values that were specific to American culture and society. As Nichols's successor, Dr. William Whitney Godding, expressed in 1878, shortly after assuming leadership of the hospital, Saint Elizabeths "should be in a position to show to other nations the liberal provision that America makes for her defenders when they become insane."[3]

In the very early days of its operation, the hospital's Board of Visitors articulated this particular strain of exceptionalism when it reported on the construction of a lodge for African American patients. "The erection and occupancy of a lodge for colored insane," the board boasted, "possessing most of the provisions of an independent hospital, inaugurates, we believe, the first and only special provision for the suitable care of the African when afflicted with insanity, which has yet been made in any part of the world, and is particularly becoming to the Government of a country embracing a larger population of blacks than can be found in any other civilized state."[4] While the board pointed to the lodge as a testament to the liberal humanitarianism, scientific and medical advancement, and racial magnanimity of the United States, the segregation of black and white patients was befitting an institution located in a city in which the slave trade had been banned only six years earlier and in which slavery would be legal for another six years.

The coexistence of these seemingly contradictory features of Washington, DC—the rhetoric of freedom and equality and the reality of slavery and racism—was reflected in the label Charles Dickens gave the capital after his visit in the early 1840s. The "City of Magnificent Intentions" referred directly to the grandness of the capital's design and architecture and the relative emptiness of the city itself. But when he wrote of slave traders in Washington as "hunters engaged in the Pursuit of Happiness," Dickens was also critiquing the emptiness of the grand ideals of American democracy.[5]

The need to construct separate facilities for a racial group that, despite occupying an ambiguous position in the psychiatric imagination, would constitute a significant portion of its patient population was further indicative of the exceptionalism of Saint Elizabeths. From its very beginning, in fact, Saint Elizabeths admitted African American patients. Some were soldiers and sailors, but the majority of African Americans committed were civilian residents of the District of Columbia who were medically diagnosed as insane and legally determined to be too poor to afford private care. Although they did not always come close to matching their percentage of the total population of the District, the substantial numbers of African Americans in Saint Elizabeths made it one of the few insane asylums in the United States with a significant racially heterogeneous patient population before the mid-twentieth century. As such, the hospital is an ideal site in which to examine the coexistence of racialist thought and scientific objectivity, medical altruism and racist treatment, and institutional power and individual agency.

This book is a history of the relationship between Washington, DC's African American community and Saint Elizabeths Hospital from its founding in 1855 to the deinstitutionalization of the District's mentally ill population in the 1970s and 1980s. It is at once a cultural history of medicine that acknowledges the real materiality of disease while also taking into account the socially constructed nature of illness; an institutional history that situates both the admirable and the less than noble efforts of medical professionals within an ever evolving field of psychiatric knowledge and the more mundane arenas of bureaucracy and politics; and a social history of African American patients and the communities that cared for, loved, feared, and abandoned them.[6] In weaving these various strands together, the book reveals the connections among ideas of racial difference, moral and medical understandings of mental disease, the institutional disciplining of "deviant" bodies, the myriad ways in which those who were diagnosed as insane bore their illness, and their own attempts as well as those of their families and friends to manage their therapeutic experience.

Racializing Disease, Racializing the Sufferer

Race—as both ideology and lived experience—figured prominently in how hospital officials understood the mission of the institution and subsequently designed and operated it, in how hospital officials conceptualized categories of mental disease and consequently developed therapeutic regimes to address them, and in how patients experienced their confinement in Saint Elizabeths. Ideas of racial difference functioned in the hospital's clinical settings and wards in more complex ways than the segregation of patients that was customary in medical institutions prior to the mid-twentieth century, or the racial animosity that some white doctors, nurses, and attendants, immersed in a racist culture, would have inevitably exhibited toward their black patients. Ideas of racial difference were foundational to the production and deployment of psychiatric knowledge from the mid-nineteenth to the mid-twentieth century. Indeed, what a history of Saint Elizabeths reveals is the ways in which the American psychiatric profession engaged in an (often) unarticulated project that conceptualized the white psyche as the norm. This not only meant that the white sufferer of mental illness occupied center stage in the psychiatric profession's consciousness, even though this was rarely explicitly expressed. It also meant that the psychiatric profession's routine manufacturing of racial difference constructed the black psyche as alien and fundamentally abnormal. This belief in distinctive racial psyches contributed to the persistent marginalization of mentally ill African Americans over the course of the development and evolution of American psychiatry, from the era of moral treatment in the mid-nineteenth century to the rise of neurology in the late nineteenth and the hegemony of dynamic psychiatry in the mid-twentieth.

A history of Saint Elizabeths and its relationship to the District's African American community encourages a fundamental reassessment of how race and racism operated in the asylum and larger psychiatric profession. The historiography of mental illness and mental institutions in the United States is several decades old and has produced numerous interpretive schools: from asylums as manifestations of benevolent reform to asylums as mechanisms of social control.[7] As robust as this historiographic tradition has been, however, few scholars have situated race at the center of their examinations of the asylum. Until recently, few of the works that have dealt with the presence of African Americans in mental institutions have used race as a category of analysis, instead merely documenting the discriminatory treatment to which they were subjected. In other words, they largely assumed that race relations within the asylum simply mirrored the relationships between blacks and whites that existed in the larger culture.[8] While this was certainly the case in many respects, more recent work has begun to explore the manner in which ideas of racial difference were embedded in the very ways that psychiatrists thought about mental health and mental illness and how they subsequently treated and managed patients.[9] The important challenge of current historical scholarship on mental illness and psychiatry in the United States is to unearth the complex, subtle, and explicit ways that psychiatrists and experts in cognate fields produced and reproduced the "truth" of racial difference as they incorporated these preconceptions into their approaches to insane whites and people of color.[10]

Psychiatrists' positing of the reality of distinctive racial psyches and their prioritizing the white sufferer of mental illness began before Saint Elizabeths opened its doors in 1855 and continued to shape much of the institution's ethos. In situating the hospital in a part of the District considered to be a healthy environment for whites, and by justifying the racial segregation of patients on the principle of therapeutic efficacy, for instance, Superintendent Nichols placed the restoration of reason and the preservation of sanity for white Americans at the center of his medical mission. Some six decades later, with the enthusiastic support of Superintendent White, many of Saint Elizabeths' psychiatrists, capitalizing on their access to large numbers of African American patients, undertook clinical research aimed at developing comparative profiles of the black and white psyche. In doing so, they theorized the existence of a normatively primitive black psyche, which, similar to the psyche of a child, might serve as a window into understanding the abnormal psychology of the white sufferer of mental illness.

The presumption of a primitive, or child-like, black psyche, moreover, inhibited the development of intensive psychotherapeutic engagements between white psychiatrists and African American patients. At a point in the early twentieth century when mental illness was beginning to be understood as a product of an individual's maladjustment to his or her environment, the dynamic psychiatric approach of plumbing the depths of a person's unconscious through psychotherapy was rarely applied to African Americans. Indeed, the extent to which psychotherapy was used on African American patients at Saint Elizabeths prior to World War II was shaped, in the main, by the acute need to address the surface manifestations of their psychoses and a desire to transform them into tractable laborers. Although there were certainly some black patients who underwent the kind of intensive psychotherapy aimed at unearthing the complexes that underlay their mental illness, they were hardly the typical patients to receive this particular type of intervention. Saint Elizabeths' psychiatrists were doing more than just privileging white sufferers of mental illness, however; they were also constructing a paradigmatic black madness that aligned with both the profession's prevailing knowledge about mental illness and their own assumptions about the racial character of people of African descent. As the history of Saint Elizabeths illustrates, psychiatrists' struggle with the existence of a group of people considered to possess a distinctive and inferior psyche led to a great deal of ambiguity, ambivalence, and antipathy when it came to treating mentally ill African Americans.

The ambiguous nature of the mad Negro had its very origins in the early nineteenth century, when physicians began characterizing insanity as a disease that was associated with the advent of modernity. Rapid economic development, educational advancement, and democratization, particularly, created an environment in which individuals were constantly exposed to phenomena that might result in physical and mental enervation, emotional stress, or heightened passions. The counterpart to civilization-induced insanity was the presumed mental health of those races situated lower on the evolutionary scale or those people who were caught in cultural stasis, including Africans and people of African descent, Native Americans, and indigenous peoples in Australia, New Zealand, and the South Pacific. Physicians based their explanations of so-called primitive people's alleged immunity to mental illness on both biological and cultural postulates, indicating the intimate relationship between body and mind in nineteenth-century medical thought.

The constitutional imperviousness to insanity was attributed to both cerebral underdevelopment and the physical robustness of the primitive body. Culture also factored in in important ways. The fact that primitive peoples led relatively stress-free agrarian lives, physicians believed, accounted for the low prevalence of insanity among them. In the case of African Americans, the paternalism that characterized the slave-master relationship served to blunt the forces that might trigger mental illness in most individuals. The stern hand of the master prevented enslaved people from engaging in the kinds of vice that constituted both predisposing and precipitating causes of insanity, such as intemperance and "reading vile books." Additionally, the benevolent care with which slaveholders treated their bondspeople, this logic went, removed from their lives those sources of emotional stress—"fear of poverty," "disappointment in ambition," "excitement in politics," and so forth—that might serve as the catalyst of mental derangement.[11] In effect, the salubrious nature of slavery's labor-discipline regime bolstered the innate biological protection from mental disease that African Americans possessed. Despite this medical consensus, however, Saint Elizabeths counted African Americans among the very first patients who crossed its threshold in 1855.

The indeterminate relationship between biology and culture continued to shape psychiatric thought about black insanity in the late nineteenth and early twentieth centuries. By the 1880s, a new medical consensus—one that was subscribed to by William Godding, who directed Saint Elizabeths from 1877 to 1899—emerged. It explained an apparent rise in the number of African Americans being institutionalized by attributing it to emancipation. Ill-equipped either biologically or culturally to withstand the pressures of living in a modern civilization as free people, African Americans were purportedly succumbing to diseases against which they had held immunity during slavery, including tuberculosis, syphilis, and insanity. On the one hand, the failure of their nervous systems to evolve, combined with their unnaturally overdeveloped sexual organs, made African Americans more susceptible to madness, sexual or otherwise. The location of the etiology of black madness in the Negro's biology fit well with an ethnological paradigm of race, the ascendancy of hereditarianism, and the development of neurology, a field of medicine that was based largely on a somatic understanding of insanity. On the other hand, the increasing propensity to become insane could be attributed to the lack of cultural development or the evolutionary proximity between African Americans and Africans. In either sense, emancipation had precipitated a degeneration of sorts, and the epidemic of somatic and mental diseases augured the race's extinction.[12]

This postemancipation narrative of the atavistic Negro—the newly freed slave who was incapable of adjusting to his new status as citizen and was rapidly devolving back to his ancestral savage past—contributed to the patient management strategies at Saint Elizabeths. Prone to diagnose mentally ill African Americans as being afflicted with mania and to characterize them more often than whites as dangerous and vicious, from the late nineteenth century to the 1930s hospital officials could make an easy decision to house African American male patients, regardless of their specific disorder or their civil status, in the same complex as insane prisoners and the criminally insane. And yet Saint Elizabeths staff members were just as likely to traffic in old, threadbare portraits of the docile, good-natured Negro whose institutionalization may have been more attributable to the race's normal mental underdevelopment than an actual disease entity such as acute mania or chronic dementia. These ambiguous characterizations of African Americans were further complicated by the disconcerting acknowledgment by Saint Elizabeths' psychiatrists that what they had been prepared to diagnose as mental illness in their white patients may have in fact been a manifestation of the Negro's natural psychological makeup.[13]

The reduction of black madness to a state of mind that was not only antithetical to mental health but also different from white madness persisted well into the twentieth century. Paradoxically, the tendency to think about insane African Americans as flattened caricatures that were informed by larger racist cultural discourses contradicted dynamic psychiatry's emphasis on the individual nature of mental illness. Rather than equating the natural histories of mental disorders with those of somatic diseases, which were considered to have generalizable symptoms and predictable outcomes, dynamic psychiatrists—whether they subscribed to Freudian psychoanalysis, Carl Jung's analytical psychology, or Adolf Meyer's psychobiology—advocated for the necessity of exploring the entire "life history" of the mentally ill person, a history that was rooted in and shaped by specific relationships and unique experiences.[14] There was certainly room for considering the role of corporate identity in the etiology of mental illness, evident in Sigmund Freud's concept of phylogenetic prehistory and Jung's theory of the collective unconscious. Acknowledging the influence of the accretion of ancestral worldviews, cultural practices, and experiences allowed Saint Elizabeths' psychiatrists in the early twentieth century to develop a comprehensive understanding of an individual's mental disease, on the one hand, while holding onto the belief in the inherent distinctiveness of the black and white psyche, on the other. Their research in comparative psychology, however, ultimately failed to yield any concrete empirical data on racial differences in the etiology or symptomatology of mental illness. In this sense, racial difference remained a problematic concept in psychiatric thought. As much as psychiatrists attempted to reify race as a scientific category of human variation, they ended up relying on vernacular understandings of racial distinctiveness—their own as well as those of their white patients and white society more generally—to make sense of black insanity and to manage their black patients.

This commonplace belief in racial difference, along with the ambiguity of black madness, resulted in therapeutic encounters between white psychiatrists and their African American patients that were marked by overt racism and, more often than not, racial ambivalence. To be sure, these psychiatrists' motivations for entering into the profession and their commitment to medical humanitarianism should not be questioned. There can be no doubt that in most cases psychiatrists and nurses were driven by a desire to at least understand their patients' maladies, even if their efforts to heal them were hampered by high patient-staff ratios, lack of resources and time, and so forth—although this claim deserves less confidence in the case of attendants. That desire, however, was too often burdened by a stubborn belief in racial difference. Placing the white sufferer at the center of their vision produced a therapeutic regime at the hospital in which African American patients occupied a marginal sphere. Their relegation was often framed as a necessary component of their treatment, moreover, whether it was sequestration in segregated and inferior wards or coerced labor in the hospital's laundries and kitchens. In this sense, the therapeutic encounter between white staff and African American patients should not be considered extrinsic to or incompatible with the preservation of a particular racial order within and outside the hospital. Rather, it was emblematic of both the social reproduction of that racial order and the privileging of the white sufferer within psychiatric thought and practice. Racialist thought and racist practices, in other words, cannot be disentangled from the medical care that African American patients experienced at Saint Elizabeths.[15]

By the mid-twentieth century, there was a significant turn within the psychiatric profession toward a universalist understanding of the psyche, a turn that accompanied the growing skepticism of the reality of race—as a biologically determined and deterministic category of human difference—within academic and public policy circles. But even as the decline in theories of racial distinctiveness, accompanied by the psychopharmacological revolution, paved the way for a race-neutral approach to mental illness, African American patients at Saint Elizabeths still had to deal with the legacy of the profession's prioritization of the white sufferer.

It was also in the mid-twentieth century that the demographics of Saint Elizabeths began to change. As African Americans increasingly constituted a larger part of the patient population in the postwar period, the institution experienced a decline in its stature as a preeminent research and teaching hospital. This relationship is more correlative than causative, but it is an important one nonetheless. Saint Elizabeths had enjoyed a reputation as being a leader in the field of asylum medicine and institutional psychiatry from the mid-nineteenth century to World War II, when the population it served was predominantly military and it practiced racial segregation. In the postwar period, as the army and navy stopped sending its active-duty service personnel to the hospital and veterans began transferring into the Veterans Administration system, Saint Elizabeths' patient population became increasingly civilian and older. With the continued in-migration of African Americans and white flight in the 1950s and 1960s, the patient population also became blacker. Gradually Saint Elizabeths went from being *the* asylum for the nation to merely "a state institution for a stateless population."[16]

Mental Illness and Claims-Making in the Nation's Capital

Although by the 1970s and 1980s Saint Elizabeths became increasingly defined—both in policy circles and in the popular imagination—by the services it delivered to an inner-city population, those African Americans whom it served were hardly powerless people acted on by large institutional forces. Rather, African Americans, both patients and ordinary citizens, demonstrated a significant amount of agency in their interactions with Saint Elizabeths. Exploring the history of the hospital's relationship to the black community from within a few years of emancipation to the post–civil rights era provides a fruitful opportunity to examine the role that the government played in the lives of African Americans and the role that African Americans believed the government should play in their lives. In the case of black patients, this book documents myriad examples of people whose actions illustrated their determination to shape the conditions of their existence at Saint Elizabeths. The agency of patients was matched by that of their friends and family, who frequently engaged with the hospital as a way of making claims on the state for equal treatment.

In fact, another aspect of Saint Elizabeths' exceptionalism figured prominently in how African Americans would interact with it as an institution of the state. For most of Saint Elizabeths' existence as a federal asylum, Washington, DC did not enjoy home rule and the city's residents were excluded from the formal arenas of citizenship. After a brief period of limited sovereignty with a territorial government between 1871 and 1878, the District reverted to direct rule by Congress and the executive branch. For the next ninety-plus years, Washington would be governed by a Board of Commissioners, whose members were appointed by the president. Half of the city's budget would be funded by Congress, in compensation for not being able to tax federal property, and the citizens would have no representation in Congress. District residents would not even be able to vote for the office of president or vice president until 1961. Elite Washingtonians, for the most part white, were still able to influence public policy through the Washington Board of Trade, and racially exclusive neighborhood-based citizens' associations also provided white residents some access to the levers of local government. Formally disfranchised along with their white neighbors, black Washingtonians sought to assert their citizenship and equality before the law in a variety of arenas, including their relationship to Saint Elizabeths.[17]

Occasionally, this assertion of citizenship and equality before the law was a collective endeavor. For instance, black neighborhood civic associations advocated for a federal investigation into the conditions at Saint Elizabeths after the murder of an African American patient by white attendants in the mid-1920s. In the 1950s the local chapter of the National Association for the Advancement of Colored People and the predominantly black Medico-Chirurgical Society pressed for the integration of the hospital's wards. Grass-roots organizations sought to collaborate with Saint Elizabeths to establish mental health counseling centers in public housing projects in the late 1960s, and in the 1970s local residents demanded representation on community mental health center advisory boards and input into decisions regarding the transfer of the hospital from the federal government to the District. Just as hospital and government officials invoked the exceptionalist nature of Saint Elizabeths to tout the nation's values, African Americans involved in these collective endeavors also deployed the language of exceptionalism. In their case, however, they emphasized the contradictions of the existence of racism in the capital of the world's leading democracy as a way of furthering their own civil rights claims. Access to and equal treatment within medical services became an important aspect of citizenship for African Americans in the postemancipation period and continued to be so through the twentieth century.[18]

But equally important, black Washingtonians asserted their citizenship in more individualized and quotidian ways. Just by drawing on Saint Elizabeths as an asset to deal with a problem that was internal to their family or community was an important declaration that they were entitled to the same access to government resources as whites. Moreover, by collaborating with the staff to manage—and in some instances endeavoring to control—the inpatient, outpatient, and postinstitutional experiences of their loved ones, black Washingtonians made it clear that instead of submitting to the medical and governmental authority wielded by the hospital, they would play an important role in the therapeutic condition of their family members. Of course, some patients' family members abandoned them, and certainly some African American residents of the District perceived the institution to be an overbearing instrument of government power. But just as many interacted with Saint Elizabeths as a deliberate act of making claims on the state that reinforced their status as citizens who were equal before the law. In this regard, African Americans' engagements with the hospital reveal the existence of "rights consciousness," what one historian describes as the enactment of equal status through "less explicit declarations of rights."[19] It was the expression of this rights consciousness—by both patients and their advocates—that makes the history of the relationship between African Americans and Saint Elizabeths Hospital so much more than one that can be reduced to medical racism or social control. Rather, the history of the relationship between Saint Elizabeths and black Washingtonians is a story of health care professionals, national and local government officials, and patients and their communities contending with one another over the important role of race in understanding mental illness and in providing care for those who were afflicted by it.

A Note on Names and Language

In writing a social and cultural history of race and mental illness in the nation's capital, I have relied on the case files of patients at Saint Elizabeths. The case files are stored at the National Archives and, while access to the more recent files is governed by the Health Insurance Portability and Accountability Act of 1996, the ones that I have used are open to the public. Nonetheless I have decided to shield the identity of patients unless their commitment to Saint Elizabeths is clearly indicated elsewhere in the public record, such as a newspaper article or a transcript of a congressional hearing. In an attempt to protect their privacy, I have not changed their first name but have used only the first initial of their last name. When referring to or citing a relative of a patient who has the same last name, I have used the same method. In cases where the identity of a patient might be revealed by using the real name of a friend or a family member who has a different surname, I have assigned a pseudonym to the latter. I clearly indicate in the notes when I have done so.

The hospital that is the subject of this study began its career with the title Government Hospital for the Insane. Almost immediately, inmates, their families, and the staff itself began using the name Saint Elizabeths—in reference to the name of the tract of land on which the hospital sat—in an effort to strip commitment to the hospital of any stigma. The name of the hospital was not officially changed to Saint Elizabeths until 1916. Nonetheless I have chosen to use this name throughout the book. I occasionally use Government Hospital for the Insane—especially in the early chapters—when to do otherwise would change the context of a particular reference. For those intimately connected to the hospital, it has always been Saint Elizabeths, with no apostrophe, even though journalists, editors, and ordinary folks want to turn it into a possessive. The hospital's name is often written as Saint Elizabeth's or Saint Elizabeth. I have chosen not to use the intrusive *sic* when quoting or referencing a misspelling of the name.

And finally, while I am attentive to the power of language to debase and dehumanize, and to the importance of evolving terms in larger quests for dignity and empowerment, I have decided not to use presentist language exclusively in referring to social groups in historical contexts. The terms *African American* and *black* appear regularly throughout the book, but I have decided to use *Negro* and *negro* (with implicit scare quotes) occasionally to convey the classifying, hierarchical, and racist intent behind their use. So, for instance, when referring to psychiatrists' belief in a distinctive black psyche in the nineteenth and early twentieth centuries, I will sometimes use small-n *negro*. African Americans during this time considered whites' refusal to capitalize *Negro* to be one more way in which they sought to dehumanize them. By the mid-twentieth century, *Negro* was in common usage by both whites and blacks, and my occasional use of this term in the latter half of the book reflects the turn toward the acceptance of a universal psyche in the psychiatric profession. Similarly, although I use the term *sufferer of mental illness* throughout the book, I have also made the decision to occasionally use words that are now considered outdated and derogatory, such as *lunatic* and *mental patient* (again, with implicit scare quotes), to properly historicize the psychiatric profession's thoughts about people who were diagnosed with mental disease. To borrow from disability studies scholar Susan Schweik—who grapples with the use of language in her history of ugly laws—I find it "inefficient and historically inaccurate to substitute more palatable contemporary terms for the hard language" employed in the past.[20]

1

"Humanity Requires All the Relief Which Can Be Afforded"

The Birth of the Federal Asylum

In the heady months following the opening of the Government Hospital for the Insane in 1855, the institution's Board of Visitors issued its first annual report. Like others who saw themselves engaged in the humanitarian enterprise of reforming how the nation dealt with the mentally ill, members of the board were exceedingly optimistic and confident about the capabilities of the institution. The board's self-assurance lay mainly in its conviction that the administrative and therapeutic regimes of the hospital were in line with prevailing mid-nineteenth-century medical thought about the importance of providing inmates with the proper custodial and convalescent environments. They also suggested that there were certain features of the hospital that gave it advantages over other asylums. One was its location in a relatively undeveloped area southeast of the capitol, although this was overstated since most asylums were somewhat removed from congested urban areas. The other feature was the federal nature of the hospital and the fact that its primary patients were members of the US Army and US Navy. Coming out of authoritarian organizations, these individuals would be more amenable to the rigid environment demanded of the dominant treatment model of the time, thereby increasing the probability that they would be cured. "That the soldier and sailor are habituated to obedience and order, are all circumstances, which, taken together," the report declared, "are calculated to give us a more complete and easy control of the time and habits of our patients, than has hitherto been practicable in any American Hospital for the Insane."[1]

As was the case with most people who were responsible for administering and overseeing mental hospitals, as well as with the psychiatric profession in general, the Government Hospital's superintendent and board adhered to an ethos of paternalism. They envisioned the institution and the dynamics within it as approximating the familial relationship, with the superintendent serving as the loving yet stern father, the staff as his subordinate helpmates, and the patients as the wayward children in need of firm guidance. As the fifth annual report stated, "Hospital life seems as *normal*, so to speak, to the insane, as the institution of the family is to the social life of the sane."[2]

The board's paternalism was enhanced by the hospital's unique mission: to tend primarily to those who served the nation in a military capacity. The emphasis the military placed on subordination of the individual to the group, duty, and hierarchical ordering of social relations complemented the doctor-patient relationship and institutional lifestyle that was necessary for recovery. The federal responsibilities of the Government Hospital, moreover, placed it in the hugely important position of serving as a symbol of national ingenuity in the arena of mental illness treatment. The hospital, according to Charles H. Nichols, its first superintendent, would be a beacon of progress not only for other American asylums but for the international community as well. As "an exponent of American knowledge and philanthropy," Nichols averred, the hospital would "have some influence upon the character of the other similar institutions, of the country, and that influence ought, in time, to be large and good." Additionally, a well-functioning hospital would "also affect the judgment that the citizens or subjects of other countries and governments, traveling or sojourning in this country, will form in respect to the character of American institutions, and the practical merits of [the] American form of government."[3]

One particular point of pride for Nichols and the board was the existence of a structure on the hospital's grounds that was dedicated exclusively for African American patients. Because of the substantial black population in the District of Columbia in the 1850s and the absence of a county or municipal public asylum, it was clear to government officials early on that the hospital was going to have to admit African Americans—both those in the military and those among the civilian population. Other hospitals admitted mentally ill African Americans in the antebellum period, but none did so with the foresight and constancy of the Government Hospital. Established in 1773, Virginia's Eastern Lunatic Asylum admitted free blacks from the very beginning, but it did not begin admitting enslaved African Americans until 1846 and did so for only ten years. For decades, free black and white patients occupied the same wards, but the asylum began segregating on the basis of race in 1841. When Worcester State Lunatic Hospital in Massachusetts began admitting African American patients in 1833, it had to initially confine them to the brick shop in order to avoid interaction between "Africans" and "other female patients." Although the South Carolina Lunatic Asylum opened in 1828, the state legislature did not authorize the admission of African American patients until 1848, and then only as a preemptive move to blunt abolitionist criticism. Ten years later, the asylum's regents released the African American male patients and decided not to admit any more until appropriate lodgings could be constructed for them. It continued to admit mentally ill black women.[4]

At the Government Hospital, by contrast, ideas of racial difference were not an afterthought or a byproduct but were central to its institutional identity and original organization. Race figured prominently in how the superintendent and Board of Visitors understood the mission of the Government Hospital and, subsequently, designed and operated it. Since there was no question as to whether the federal institution would open its doors to African American soldiers, sailors, veterans, federal prisoners, and civilian residents of the District of Columbia, the administrative staff had to grapple with how to reconcile the medical imperative of caring for the insane with larger cultural assumptions about racial difference. Yet the humanitarian impulse behind the establishment of an inclusive public hospital operated by the federal government did not accordingly produce a liberal racial regime within its walls. Rather, segregationist expectations held by local and federal officials—and the medical profession's prioritizing of the white sufferer of mental disease—ensured that such a regime would not develop, even as the asylum staff recognized the necessity of addressing mental illness within the African American community.

Managing Insanity in the New Nation's Capital

The federal government entered into the business of providing institutional care for the insane rather late. By the time Congress approved the initial appropriation for the Government Hospital in 1852, there were already close to thirty public and private insane asylums throughout the United States, the majority in northern and midwestern states.[5] Although a handful of these hospitals were established in the colonial and early national eras, the bulk of them emerged during a period of reform in the 1830s and 1840s, in which county and state governments responded affirmatively to calls for more humane and efficient care of the insane.

Prior to this period, those individuals who were thought to be insane were primarily the concern of local authorities. Throughout the seventeenth and eighteenth centuries, the measures taken by colonies to deal with the mentally ill—as well as "idiots," orphans, and other individuals who were incapable of caring for themselves—were based on England's poor laws. Colonial statutes generally regulated the management of the estates of individuals considered to be non compos mentis, provided them with relief from creditors, and appointed guardians to be responsible for their daily care. This care was offered within private homes and paid for by any revenue generated from the estate of the mentally ill individual. If he or she owned no property, the cost of care was assumed by the local community. Only the mad considered dangerous were sequestered within county jails or almshouses, although the practice of placing the insane within poorhouses became more common by the mid-eighteenth century.[6]

When Congress established the District of Columbia—with its constituent localities of Georgetown, Washington City, and Washington County in Maryland and Alexandria County in Virginia—in 1800, the states from which the national capital was formed had already begun to implement policies that addressed mental illness on a statewide basis. Virginia was the first, and it began to do so during the colonial period. In 1769, in response to concerns that "several persons of insane and disordered minds have been frequently found wandering in different parts of this colony," the General Assembly authorized the establishment of a public hospital in Williamsburg. The act empowered magistrates in any county, city, or borough in the colony to declare an individual insane—given that sufficient evidence and testimony had been provided—and to order his or her admission to the hospital. The act also mandated compensation to authorities who were responsible for transporting the insane to the hospital and required that the colonial treasury pay for the expenses associated with maintaining propertyless inmates, "any sum not exceeding twenty-five pounds per annum." The Eastern Lunatic Asylum opened in 1773 and admitted men and women, black and white, and Virginians of all ranks, except slaves. On the eve of Washington's incorporation, the hospital was already at complete capacity, with thirty inmates, and prospective admissions were regularly turned away.[7]

Maryland lagged behind Virginia in its efforts to cope with its mentally ill population. Insane people who were not boarded out to private households were housed in county jails and almshouses through the end of the colonial period. In 1797 the state's General Assembly passed An Act to Encourage the Establishing of a Hospital for the Relief of Indigent Sick Persons, and for the Reception and Care of Lunatics. The law authorized the establishment of a state hospital in or near Baltimore. Prior to the construction of the hospital, the state also empowered chancery courts to order trustees of insane individuals to admit them in an asylum in Philadelphia, in situations when their "going at large is dangerous or improper." The hospital eventually opened in 1801, and it would serve the federal government as much as it did the state of Maryland or the county of Baltimore.[8]

Like individual states, and the colonies before them, Washington, DC, responded to the problem of insanity primarily within the context of its efforts to address poverty. Although Washington never became the manufacturing or commercial center that its initial leaders envisioned—remaining instead a sleepy town servicing the federal government for most of the nineteenth century—the problem of poverty, and particularly the transient poor, was no less acute there than elsewhere. As part of a larger campaign to improve public health, the city council passed legislation in 1802 that created a position of overseer of the poor, established a larger committee of trustees to supervise public relief, and obligated the mayor to employ the services of a physician to attend to the medical needs of indigent residents. Poor relief consumed a significant portion of the city's budget, amounting to more than 40 percent in 1802. In subsequent years, the percentage of the city's revenues spent on poor relief declined, leveling out at between 15 and 17 percent by 1806. It was in this year that the city council specifically dedicated a set amount of the public dole to taking care of the insane.[9]

Poor relief itself was a combination of aid distribution—in the form of clothing, food, firewood, and money—to needy families and the boarding out of individuals to private homes, the Washington County almshouse, or the Washington Infirmary in Washington City. Established in 1806 and opened in 1809, the infirmary was the District's public hospital, although, like most hospitals of the era, it functioned primarily as a poorhouse. Six years later the city council merged the infirmary with the District's workhouse, creating the Washington Asylum. The new asylum combined the reformatory function of the workhouse and almshouse with the medical charity role of the infirmary.[10] Through the early 1840s, people identified as of unsound mind who were either considered dangerous or who had no family members who were capable of caring for them were confined to the county jail or the Washington Asylum's workhouse. Moreover, little money was spent on either the outdoor relief or the custodial care of the mentally ill. Though in 1806 the city council set aside one relief dollar for the insane for every five relief dollars for the aged, poor, and infirm, by the 1830s that disparity had become even more pronounced. In August 1832 the city council authorized $3,500 for the care of the elderly, the poor, and the disabled and only $500 for the "support and maintenance of lunatics." The amount provided for sane dependents increased by 133 percent between 1806 and 1833, while the increase in the support of the mentally ill was a much more modest 66 percent.[11]

Institutional care for the insane in Washington was complicated by the unique administrative relationship between the city and the federal government. Unlike the states in the union, Washington had neither the political sovereignty nor a sufficient revenue stream to adequately handle its mentally ill population. The substantial debt owed to the federal government for initial capital outlays and continuing operating expenses, combined with the tax-exempt status of federal property, significantly impaired the ability of Washington's taxpayers to maintain a robust social welfare fund. Moreover, the fact that many of the dependents who were served by poor relief were transient placed an even greater burden on local property owners. In order to establish a public insane asylum, municipal officials had to turn to the federal government for assistance. Although there were earlier attempts to solicit Congress's help, the city leaders' campaign started in earnest in the mid-1830s, in response to what was perceived to be an increasing number of insane individuals who were driven to Washington by their delusions of governmental persecution or a deranged self-importance. In January 1835 President Andrew Jackson survived an assassination attempt by an unemployed English housepainter, Richard Lawrence, who was confined to the Washington County jail after officials determined him to be insane. One of Washington's papers, the *Intelligencer*, pointed to Lawrence's deed and the prospects of the nation's capital being "visited by more than its proportion of insane persons" as the primary justifications for the construction of an insane asylum within the city's borders.[12]

Local government officials increased the pressure on Congress in the latter half of the 1830s. In January 1838 Mayor Peter Force, writing on behalf of the Grand Jury of Washington County, petitioned President Martin Van Buren and Congress for the construction of a new penitentiary and insane asylum. "The number of persons now confined in the jail as lunatics, whose release would be dangerous to society," Force wrote, "shows that it is equally necessary that a public asylum should be provided for those unfortunate persons." Force's assessment of the District's ability to reform criminals and care for the insane was confirmed by two District circuit court judges, and the petition was endorsed by Van Buren and forwarded to Congress. The matter was referred to the House of Representatives' Committee for the District of Columbia, and in April the committee reported favorably on the issue of providing "the benefits of some suitable lunatic asylum" for the insane who were currently incarcerated in the county jail, including Jackson's would-be assassin. Apparently Congress lost interest in the issue, and efforts to authorize the establishment of a public asylum languished, prompting city officials to petition once again in 1840 for both a hospital and an asylum.[13]

The following year Congress passed legislation authorizing the transfer of indigent insane District residents to the Maryland Hospital in Baltimore. The federal government had an established relationship with the hospital, contracting with it to receive and treat sick and injured sailors. The institution functioned primarily as a marine hospital from 1802 to 1807, neglecting its principal responsibility of providing care for the indigent and the insane. The federal government stopped sending naval personnel to the hospital in 1807, and within a decade it had become a highly functioning general hospital that served paying patients, the indigent, and the mentally ill. The Maryland Hospital became exclusively a mental institution by an act of the Maryland legislature in 1839.[14] The federal government transferred only those District residents whose insanity and state of impoverishment had been determined to the satisfaction of a grand jury, and the transfer could be done only under the supervision of the US marshal.[15] At $5 per patient per week, plus transportation-related expenses, the costs of confining the District insane in the Maryland Hospital bordered on prohibitive, especially compared to the roughly $2 per week Maryland spent on in-state patients. In 1843 and 1844 Congress was delinquent in paying a bill of approximately $3,900 for fifteen patients at Maryland Hospital.[16]

It may have been the judgment that the per-patient fees charged by the Maryland Hospital were exorbitant that prompted Congress finally to respond to the entreaties of the local board of health and explore the possibility of building an insane asylum within the District. In 1842 Congress appropriated $10,000 to convert the former jail, located at Judiciary Square in Washington City, into an asylum for the indigent insane as well as "sick, disabled and infirm seamen, soldiers or others." This first attempt by Congress to authorize the establishment of a public asylum for the District failed, however. Representatives and senators disagreed about a variety of issues, including the question of federalism and whether care for the insane should be a national, state, or local responsibility; the necessity and efficacy of a professionalized treatment model; and the location and suitability of the proposed facilities. The District would continue to send insane people in need of institutionalization to Maryland Hospital, as well as a private hospital, Mount Hope Institution, which had opened in Baltimore in 1840.[17]

African Americans were among those District residents who were institutionalized in Maryland. Maryland Hospital admitted African American patients from its earliest days. On the other hand, Mount Hope Institution, founded by the Sisters of Charity as an asylum for indigent and well-off insane people of all religious denominations, drew the line at admitting African Americans. Nonetheless, of the forty-three District residents who were confined to these two institutions in 1852, three were black men and two were black women. It is not entirely clear how African American inmates were treated compared to their white counterparts. The administrative staff of Maryland Hospital certainly spent less money on provisions for them, as it charged the federal government only $3 per week for this class of patient, as opposed to $4 per week for whites.[18] Mentally ill African Americans probably also wound up in either the District's jail or the Washington Asylum's workhouse. But most would have been cared for in the households of family members, the predominant site for the care of the insane through the first half of the nineteenth century.[19]

The stability of black families and their ability to provide care for mentally ill members of their households was certainly influenced—though not determined—by the District's demographics, the characteristics of its economy, the biased nature of its poor-relief policies, and its laws regulating slavery. From the founding of the capital to the eve of the Civil War, the District's African American community changed from primarily enslaved people to predominantly free individuals. In 1800 enslaved people of African descent constituted almost a quarter of the total population of the District; there were twenty-four free African Americans for every one hundred bondspeople. By 1860 the absolute number of enslaved African Americans had actually declined by roughly 2 percent, while the total population increased by 432 percent and the number of free African Americans increased by an astronomical 1,321 percent. For every enslaved person of African descent, there were 3.49 free people of color.

In part, the growth of the free African American population was the result of a transformation in the regional economy. As farmers in western Maryland and northwestern Virginia shifted from the cultivation of tobacco to less labor-intensive cereal production, their need for slave labor diminished. This new labor consideration and liberal manumission laws in Maryland and Virginia combined to produce an increase in the numbers of free African Americans relative to the number of enslaved people of African descent. Another contributor to the growth of the free black community was the quite common practice of skilled slaves purchasing their freedom with the accumulated savings they made through "hiring out." Moreover, the development of the free black community made the District an attractive destination for runaway slaves from northern Virginia and southern Maryland.[20]

An enslaved African American population continued to exist within the District during the antebellum era, but the regional economy inhibited stable household formation. The majority of urban slaveholders owned fewer than a half-dozen slaves—fewer than three in the 1850s. There was little economic incentive for urban masters to have a large number of slaves, and selling younger slaves or transferring them by deed was a standard strategy for limiting the size of their slaveholdings. They generally kept enslaved women as household servants and hired out enslaved men and older children to farmers in outlying counties or to urban proprietors in need of both skilled and unskilled laborers. The small size of the average slaveholding and the gender imbalance among the urban enslaved population meant that the enslaved families that did form tended to stretch across households, often at a substantial distance from one another.[21] Additionally, because of the practice of hiring out, conjugal pairs that were owned by the same slaveholder often did not live together for significant stretches of time. This extra-household family formation would have inhibited the ability of enslaved African Americans to care for their mentally ill relatives. While it was possible for a spouse, parent, or child to travel to another household to minister to a loved one with an acute illness, they would not have been able to dedicate the time and energy required to take care of someone with a condition that was perceived as chronic.

As such, the responsibility for providing for the health care needs of the enslaved individual with an unsound mind or the bondsperson who had "epileptic fits" fell principally upon the slaveholders. They may have consulted the domestic medicine manuals of the period or employed a physician to apply some of the heroic treatments aimed at reducing inflammation of the brain or bringing the afflicted slave's bodily humors into balance.[22] Enslaved people who were considered to be dangerous to themselves or to others may have been sequestered in an attic or an outbuilding. Whether slaveholders confined or provided medical care for their mentally ill bondsperson would have been shaped by the economic, and perhaps emotional value they had invested in their human chattel.

In a complex personal relationship based both on the violent logic of property rights in human beings and the recognition of mutual interdependence, power and resistance became important lenses through which urban masters assessed the mental state of their bondspeople. Because feigning illness was a common form of defiance, slaveholders had to determine the veracity of the signs and symptoms of insanity exhibited by enslaved people. Indeed some physicians endorsed the use of harsh medicinal compounds, and even physical punishment, to expose slaves' false claims of sickness. Enslaved African Americans may have used the ruse of epilepsy—thought by nineteenth-century physicians to be a cognate disease of insanity—to avoid work or to discourage a prospective buyer from purchasing them on the auction block, even as some clearly suffered from the disorder.[23] It would have been much more difficult, however, to feign the kinds of mental diseases that would have prompted slaveholders to turn to institutional care or confinement for their bondsperson—disorders such as chronic melancholia, mania, dementia, or idiocy.

In these cases, many slaveholders may have attempted to relieve themselves of their responsibility simply by manumitting their deranged or mentally disabled bondsperson. This was always a concern of colonial and state legislators. As early as 1752, Maryland law, which regulated slavery in Georgetown and the areas that would become Washington City and Washington County, allowed for the manumission of slaves as long as they were younger than fifty and "with a healthy constitution, of sound mind and body and capable of labor to procure sufficient food and raiment." Between 1796 and 1832 the age threshold was lowered to forty-five. In 1824 Virginia passed a law aimed at reducing the number of abandoned slaves by threatening a fine of up to $50 for those slaveholders who failed to provide their bondspeople of "unsound mind, or aged or infirm," the proper support. This law governed slavery in the portion of the District south of the Potomac River until Alexandria was ceded back to Virginia in 1846.[24]

Despite these legal restrictions, the abandonment of mentally ill and disabled bondspeople—through manumission at least—was an option for slaveholders, especially when they were unsuccessful in selling them. Slaveholders were also likely to shed their responsibility by allowing the free relatives of their dependent slaves to purchase their freedom. Getting a few hundred dollars for a slave who consumed resources that were greater in value than the revenue he or she generated was a good economic decision for slaveholders and helped them to avoid possible violation of the District's manumission laws. Even as they welcomed the ability to free their relatives from bondage, this shifted the burden of caretaking onto free African American families and potentially undermined their own economic stability.[25]

As in free African American communities in urban areas throughout the United States, free people of color in the District of Columbia lived fairly precarious lives. Racial discrimination and competition with Irish immigrant laborers impeded occupational mobility and the accumulation of wealth. While there were African American men who were artisans, the overwhelming majority of them—three-quarters in 1850—were employed in the unskilled, semiskilled, and service sectors of the labor force. Similarly, most African American wage-earning women worked either as domestic servants, cooks, or washerwomen. To be sure, some men and women were able to exploit the patronage of elite whites and parlay their positions as servants, stewards, barbers, tailors, and seamstresses into successful businesses. African Americans' entrepreneurial opportunities, however, were diminished in 1836, when the District's city council issued an ordinance prohibiting free African Americans from obtaining licenses to operate restaurants or taverns—presumably to prevent blacks from selling or distributing liquor. Free African Americans were still allowed to hold licenses to drive carts and hackneys, although the ordinance prohibited the issuance of any license to free people of color entering the District after November 9, 1836. The limited occupational mobility available to free African Americans meant that all able-bodied adults in the household had to engage in some form of wage employment in order to make ends meet.[26]

This set of circumstances certainly made taking care of a mentally ill or intellectually disabled family member an enormous challenge for free African American families, as it would have been for any working-class family. Although these families would have activated a network of kinswomen to take care of young children while parents and older children were working, it would have been more difficult to rely on older, non-wage-earning women to look after family members whose disorders may have expressed themselves in erratic and potentially violent behavior.[27] Mutual aid or benevolent societies might have functioned as a resource for free people of color who were dealing with a mentally ill and dependent relative, although there is no evidence that this was common. But associational assistance would have been a critical supplement in light of the racial inequities in the District's poor-relief distribution. Taxes for public relief were collected at the ward level and relief funds were disbursed according to neighborhood. Free African American households were not concentrated in any one enclave within the District, but the assumption that they were a naturally indolent race contributed to a discriminatory process in which overseers of the poor neglected to distribute relief funds to African Americans that were commensurate with the larger free black community's overall economic contribution to the city.[28]

If free African American families could not depend on outside relief that might allow a member to withdraw from the labor market for short stints of caretaking, neither could they rely on the option of placing their insane or intellectually disabled relative in the almshouse. Between 1845 and 1851 African Americans constituted between 8 and 11 percent of the admissions to the District's almshouse, even though they made up 22 percent of the city's population. On the other hand, in the 1850 federal census enumeration of the almshouse, the percentage of African American inmates was roughly equal to their percentage of the total population. One explanation for this is that by the time African Americans were admitted to the almshouse, they were experiencing such economic deprivation that it was impossible for them to benefit from the reformatory mission of the institution, resulting in much longer stays than those of white inmates.[29] Another explanation, however, might be that a significant portion of the almshouse inmates were chronically ill or considered incurably insane. If so, this would suggest that free African American families waited until they could no longer possibly care for a mentally ill family member before they sent him or her to the almshouse. Understanding that public assistance—in the form of either outside relief or custodial care—would most likely be denied to them, free African American families probably delayed removing their mentally ill relatives from the home as long as they were not an undue financial burden on the household.

But some inevitably did become a financial burden or a danger to themselves and those around them. What would have triggered this recognition was different for every family, as was the way they would have sought to resolve the problem. Like slaveholders, free African American families may have sought to treat their mentally ill relative with the domestic remedies of the day. Those without a spare room may have confined them in a garret or a shed. In the case of those whom they simply could no longer sustain economically, families may have allowed them to roam the city streets, occasionally providing them food and hoping that the courts would commit them to the almshouse.

By the early 1850s a more permanent option began to take shape. Writing to Commissioner of Public Buildings William Easby in 1852, the president of the District's Board of Health, Dr. Thomas Miller, complained about the city's inadequate policy with respect to the insane. "It is notorious that a number of Lunatics are every year committed to our County Jail for the want of a more fit place of confinement," he remarked. "Others are strolling about the streets of Washington and Georgetown, merely because they are *inoffensive*, and have no friends to take charge of them." Even though the federal government's policy of removing insane paupers to the Maryland Hospital was a decade old, Miller was convinced that the District needed a more enduring solution. "It is also well known that the number of this unfortunate class of individuals has much increased and as the population of the District multiplies so will they continue to increase," he suggested, "besides, the provision made by Congress has [and] will induce many to turn their Insane loose in our cities, that they may be taken care of under that provision."[30] Miller made only general references to Washington's insane inhabitants, and it is impossible to know how many of those "strolling about the streets" or in the county jail were African American. Within three years of Miller's letter, however, the Government Hospital for the Insane would be open and admitting mentally ill African Americans. The recognition that this would be an inescapable reality meant that ideas about race and racial difference became central to the planning and design of the federal institution.

"An Unnatural Association": Creating a Racial Topography of the Asylum

Four years after Congress opted to forgo the creation of an asylum in the District and to reauthorize the transfer of the city's mentally ill residents to hospitals in Maryland, the reformer Dorothea Lynde Dix submitted a memorial to the legislative body proposing a national scheme to provide care for the indigent insane. Dix had been successful in convincing individual states of the need to build public hospitals for their mentally ill populations, and in 1848 she turned her attention to the problem on a national scale. She proposed that the federal government sell a small portion of the hundreds of millions of acres of public land and turn over the proceeds to states so that they might build more hospitals and improve existing facilities.

Dix's proposal was informed by the medical consensus of the era, in which insanity was considered to be a curable disease as long as there was early and proper intervention. "Under ordinary circumstances, and where there is no organic lesion of the brain, no disease is more manageable or more easily cured than insanity," she optimistically stated, "but to this end, special appliances are necessary, which cannot be had in private families, nor in every town and city; hence the necessity for hospitals, and the multiplication, *not enlargement*, of such institutions." Throughout her memorial, Dix remarked on the current condition of facilities for the mentally ill in all of the states and the District of Columbia. She found the prospects for treating the District's insane to be somewhat improved over previous years, yet she believed that more could be done. Dix wrote that she had "witnessed abuses in some of these [jails and almshouses] in 1838, in 1845, and since, from which every sense recoils. At present," she continued, "most of these evils are mitigated in this immediate vicinity, but by no means relieved to the extent that justice and humanity demand."[31] Although access to Maryland institutions had ameliorated the problem of the mentally ill in the District, Dix implied, an institution needed to be built in the nation's capital.

From Dix's perspective, the imperative to build an institution in the District was driven by the need to avoid the "evils" of confining the insane in jail cells, almshouse basements, and overcrowded hospitals. By the time she submitted her memorial to Congress, Maryland's asylums, and particularly Maryland Hospital, were straining under the weight of the growing numbers of inmates. The probability of curing insanity decreased in these kinds of environments, and incurable lunatics deserved to be spared from the inhumane conditions that accompanied overcrowding. The need to reconsider building an asylum in the nation's capital became particularly acute when the superintendent of Maryland Hospital announced in the summer of 1852 that it would cease accepting District residents and would expect the US marshal to remove all current District inmates by January 1, 1853. Congress considered utilizing insane asylums in Philadelphia and Virginia to house the District's mentally ill, but overcrowding in those institutions made this policy untenable.[32]

In August, Representative Edward Stanly, a Whig from North Carolina, proposed an amendment to an appropriations bill increasing the federal support for insane District residents from $10,000 to $19,000 for that year. Stanly included in his remarks from the floor a letter written several months earlier by Dr. Thomas Miller, stressing the urgency of building a hospital within the nation's capital. "The practice and experience of the medical faculty here," Miller wrote, "have demonstrated to them that a very large proportion of the insane in this District and city are either foreigners or non-residents—those, in short, who come to the seat of Government, some to prosecute claims, and others to procure clerical or other employment. Among so many of this class, a large number must of necessity be disappointed; and coming here with high expectations of success, when poverty, vexatious delays, and 'hope deferred' overtake them, it unfortunately happens that the reason of some becomes more or less deranged, and humanity requires all the relief which can be afforded."[33]

With this anticipated growth in the number of insane in the District and the imminent severing of relations with Maryland Hospital, Stanly declared that "Congress must take care of them, or they will be turned at large upon the community."[34] In fact the numbers had been growing over the previous several years, and Congress was well aware of it. Between 1844 and 1850 the amount spent on committing District residents to Maryland institutions more than doubled. Whereas the federal government had spent less than $4,000 for fifteen residents in 1844, by 1850 it was spending over $8,000 for thirty-one residents: roughly $204 per patient plus an additional $10 to $12 for transportation.[35]

Stanly also proposed an amendment authorizing the executive branch to spend up to $110,000 for the "purchase of a site, and for the erection of a suitable building for the proper accommodation of insane persons." That same month, the Senate took up the bill and Robert Hunter, a Virginia Democrat, modified Stanly's amendment, reducing the appropriation to $100,000 and specifically delineating the responsibilities of the asylum to house and treat residents of the District of Columbia as well as members of the US Army and US Navy. In light of the diminished opportunity to transfer District residents to hospitals in Virginia and Pennsylvania, Hunter pleaded with his fellow senators to recognize the need for an institution in or close to Washington. The Senate agreed to Hunter's amendment, and after reconciliation with the House, the appropriations bill was passed on August 31, giving the executive branch "the proper measures . . . to carry this beneficent purpose to effect."[36]

Shortly after congressional authorization, Secretary of the Interior Alexander Stuart began the search for a superintendent. Dix was instrumental in the search, much to the chagrin of Thomas Miller. In addition to being the president of the District's Board of Health, Miller was a prominent physician in the city. He was particularly interested in the problem of insanity. In his February 1852 letter to William Easby, in which he laid out the most important features of a prospective asylum in the District, Miller demonstrated a familiarity with the standards of care that were being promulgated by the Association of Medical Superintendents of American Institutions for the Insane (AMSAII), the professional organization of asylum superintendents that had formed in 1844.[37] It is not surprising, then, that Miller was upset when he was passed over for the position of superintendent. In fact he enlisted the assistance of President Millard Fillmore, who informed Dix of his disgruntlement. "Dr. Miller has been to see me and protests very strongly against '*importing*' a physician to take charge of the hospital," Fillmore informed Dix. "He claims much merit, and for aught I know, truly, in having procured the passage of the law, and desires the appointment of governing or consulting physician." Fillmore declined to intervene further in the selection process, which had already begun by the time he wrote Dix.[38]

The physician who was "imported" into the nation's capital to run the Government Hospital was Charles H. Nichols. From the very beginning of the process, Fillmore and Stuart had consulted with Dix about an appropriate person to serve as the first superintendent, and Dix pointed them toward Nichols. A Mainer by birth, Nichols was also a Quaker, which situated him firmly in the genealogy of philanthropically minded asylum reformers who were also Quakers, stretching back to Samuel Tuke of England's York Retreat and the founders of the Pennsylvania Hospital. When the superintendency of the Government Hospital became available, Nichols had only recently resigned as resident physician of New York's Bloomingdale Asylum, whose founding in 1821 was the result of Quaker philanthropy.[39] His departure from Bloomingdale was not a particularly amicable one, and there is some evidence that he was embittered by the process. Nonetheless he remained committed to "promote the welfare of that class of my fellow men, a fraction of which, stricken with the most terrible of temporal afflictions, comes up here for the comfort [and] health that home [and] its endearments deny," he confided to the superintendent of the Pennsylvania Hospital, Thomas S. Kirkbride. His time at Bloomingdale had convinced him that the best way to promote such welfare was in the role of superintendent. "I think I am well fitted to manage an Insane Hosp.," Nichols wrote to Dix in February 1852, "[and] hence am inclined to regard that as *my mission*, but I do not wish to go into another Institution unless it is, or is likely to be, well sustained pecuniarily, [and] unless it would be expected that I should virtually have the entire management of it."[40]

Within two weeks of Congress's appropriation, Dix had let both Nichols and Stuart know that she had Nichols in mind as the hospital's superintendent. Nichols was not particularly impressed with the size of the appropriation or the amount of land Congress authorized the secretary to purchase, but he was interested in learning more about the position from Dix. He let her know that he would accept an appointment if "the conditions are liberal" and if there were truly the resources and freedom "to make it what it ought to be, *a model hospital*." In order to increase the likelihood of turning it into an exemplary asylum, he wanted to be appointed before the site was selected so that he could "assist in devising the plan of the Institution [and] *Superintend its construction*."[41] Fillmore, who had a great deal of confidence in Dix's judgment, had no hesitation in offering the position to Nichols. In late October, Nichols assumed the superintendency with an annual salary of $2,500. His formal appointment came two weeks later, in a letter from Stuart that revealed the hopes that he and Fillmore had for the hospital. "It is the desire of the President," the appointment letter stated, "that the proposed hospital shall be a model institution, embracing all the improvements which science, skill, and experience, have introduced into modern establishments."[42]

At least a month before he officially took on the role of superintendent, Nichols began to help Secretary Stuart and Dix select a location for the hospital. AMSAII standards dictated that, for maximum efficacy, asylums should be located at least two miles from urban areas and on a bucolic expanse of land no less than one hundred acres, with proper drainage, accessibility to a fresh water source, and preferably a good view of the surrounding area. Nichols believed that the distance from the city should be greater than two miles, so as to avoid being "annoyed to death by visitors [and] its usefulness greatly impaired."[43] Dix and

Nichols ended up recommending a parcel of land owned by Thomas Blagden, located on the southern side of the Potomac River's Eastern Branch (also known as the Anacostia River), approximately two and a half miles southeast of the center of Washington City. Blagden's estate covered roughly 185 acres, divided equally between farmland and forest. The tract's high elevation afforded stunning views of Washington City, Georgetown, Alexandria, and Uniontown—what is now the Anacostia neighborhood of Southeast Washington, DC. After visiting the site, President Fillmore authorized the purchase of Blagden's property plus an additional eight acres adjacent to it for $27,000.[44]

The overriding concern of everyone who was involved in the site selection was the healthfulness of the environment. The District was known for its many low-lying, marshy areas which made their inhabitants susceptible to fevers and agues. Secretary Stuart solicited testimony from local physicians and residents

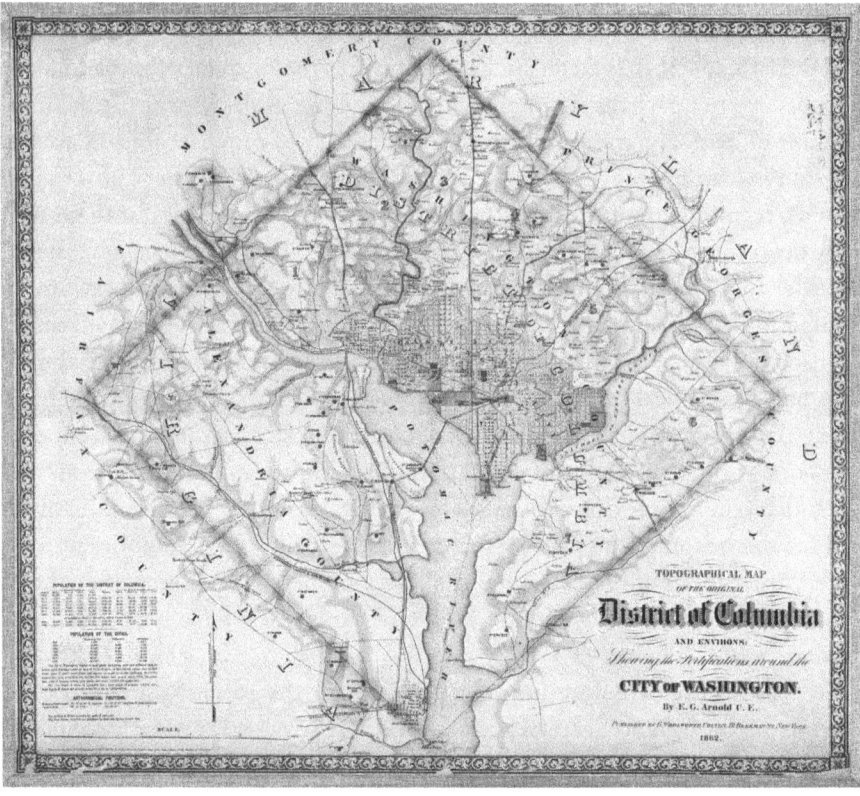

A map of the District of Columbia in 1862, including Washington City, the City of Georgetown, Washington County, and Alexandria County (which was ceded back to Virginia in 1846). Saint Elizabeths is located in the southeastern corner of the District, south of Uniontown and near Fort Snyder, one of the many forts that protected the capital from Confederate forces. *Library of Congress, Geography and Map Division.*

who were familiar with this particular tract of land in order to establish its reputation as a salubrious location. The overall positive assessments by six individuals left the secretary with "no doubt that the locality selected is, in a remarkable degree, exempt from diseases which ordinarily arise from malaria." This assessment was seconded by Nichols in the report that he prepared for Congress in late December. After inspecting the property, he concluded that miasmatic fevers would not pose a problem due to the absence of marshes and stagnant pools of water, the windward location of the hospital in relation to the Eastern Branch, the high elevation, and the presence of a large wooded area, which would serve as a buffer between the hospital grounds and any disease source.[45]

Interestingly, race was a significant factor in the site selection. Nichols felt confident in pronouncing the salubrity of the locale because there was no evidence that whites there succumbed to disease. "Five white families reside at distances from the proposed site of the institution," he indicated in his report, "and I cannot learn that more than one death has occurred within the territory they occupy for four years." Nichols reinforced his point by remarking, "These people generally *look* healthy."[46] To be sure, on the assumption that the majority of inmates would be white, Nichols's concern that the environment be hospitable for people of European descent made sense. He was also most likely less concerned about the impact of the environment on African Americans—not because their health did not matter to him but rather because he assumed that they were relatively impervious to the threat of contagion.

In the mid-nineteenth century, people of African descent were widely believed to be more resistant to fevers associated with malaria, which at the time referred to the miasmatic atmosphere resulting from putrefying organic matter rather than a disease caused by a specific pathogenic organism. While physicians acknowledged that African Americans were susceptible to malaria, they also generally agreed that cases of fever within the black population tended to be less virulent and fatal than for whites. In the District the assumptions about innate African American resistance to malaria were reinforced by the fact that there were black residential enclaves in the low-lying, marshy areas of Tiber Island in the southwestern part of the city—sandwiched between the Mall, the Potomac, and the Washington Canal—and Foggy Bottom, just west of the Mall and north of the Potomac. These were considered to be unhealthy environments and uninhabitable by the city's white middle- and upper-class residents. The fact that the mortality rate for African American Washingtonians was higher than that of the capital's white inhabitants did not dislodge the assumptions about blacks' proverbial physiological protection against miasmatic fevers.[47]

Nineteenth-century Americans were especially cognizant of the environmental advantages and disadvantages of areas they settled, and they took steps to maximize those advantages at the expense of others. This manifested, for instance, in slaveholding families occupying land at higher elevations while their bondspeople lived and toiled in the lower-lying areas, or in the concentration of African American Washingtonians in Tiber Island and Foggy Bottom.[48] But it was more than just assumptions about the demographics of the future inmate population or different races' susceptibility to malaria that led Nichols to specify the race of the current residents as an indication of the healthiness of the local environment. In his conceptualization of the ideal therapeutic environment for the insane, Nichols considered the protection of the *white body* from disease and the shielding of the *white mind* from stimuli that might impede its recovery of reason to be paramount.

In his late December report, the superintendent remarked on the absolute importance of a tranquil, natural landscape in the therapeutic process. The physical features of the grounds, as well as the views the site commanded, Nichols argued,

> are of immense consequence. This is so well understood among practical persons, that there is no establishment in the country that has not, in some one or more of its published documents, attempted to laud the attractive beauty of the landscape about it. The moral treatment of the insane, with reference to their cure, consists mainly in eliciting an exercise of the attention with things rational, agreeable, and foreign to the subject of delusion; and the more constant and absorbing is such exercise, the more rapid and effectual will be the recovery; but many unbroken hours must elapse each day, during which it is on every account impracticable to make any direct active effort to engage and occupy the patients' minds. Now, nothing gratifies the taste, and spontaneously enlists the attention, of so large a class of persons, as combinations of beautiful natural scenery, varied and enriched by the hand of man.[49]

But the landscape consisted of more than just geological formations, the natural elements, and flora and fauna; it also consisted of other human bodies. Just as less than beautiful physical surroundings could foster the development of external stimuli that might compound inmates' mental derangement or interfere with their recovery, people who threatened an inmate's sense of self were also an obstacle to rehabilitation. For many superintendents, and particularly those in the South, insane African Americans were a human part of the landscape that potentially hampered the curative possibilities of the asylum.

This concern with the recovery-retardant potential of proximity between the races extended to the built environment and contributed to the design of the hospital campus. Moral treatment—alternatively referred to as moral management and considered by nineteenth-century physicians to be the most progressive therapeutic regimen—was based on the premise that the insane could regain their full faculties if they were removed from the environment that was the source of their mental distress, given a structured daily routine that consisted of both physical activity and rest, and provided with nutritionally sufficient meals and appropriate medical care. Advocates of moral treatment believed that a mentally ill individual was more likely to recover if he or she was housed and associated with other individuals who suffered from a similar form of insanity or who were at the same stage of the disease. An architecture that accommodated this therapeutic rationale was critical for moral treatment to succeed.[50]

Officially superintendents were more concerned with the separation of asylum inmates on the basis of gender. At its annual meeting in Philadelphia in 1851, the AMSAII adopted a set of standards regarding the construction of asylums, one of which was to have "distinct wards for each sex."[51] Although the AMSAII did not have an explicitly stated policy with respect to race or ethnicity, segregation was a subject of some importance to hospital superintendents. In the first year of its existence, the organization impaneled a committee to study the issue of separate asylums for "colored persons." The head of the committee was John M. Galt, the superintendent of Virginia's Eastern Lunatic Asylum, which had begun segregating free black inmates only three years earlier, when Galt assumed control of the hospital from his father, Alexander D. Galt. Prior to 1841 free black and white inmates occupied the same wards. This was a tolerable situation because of the small number of black patients and the fact that all patients had private rooms, spartan and uncomfortable though they were. When John M. Galt became superintendent, he expanded the hospital in order to accommodate more patients—including free blacks. The increased African American presence, in addition to the fact that Galt subscribed to the principles of moral treatment, led to the implementation of a policy of segregation at Eastern Lunatic Asylum.[52]

Nonetheless Galt approached the issue of racial segregation for the AMSAII without any preconceptions. He surveyed several superintendents in different regions of the country to ascertain their thoughts on the subject, including Samuel B. Woodward, superintendent of Worcester State Hospital in Massachusetts. In a letter to Woodward inquiring about racial attitudes in the Bay State, Galt indicated that many superintendents "refused admission [to mentally ill African Americans] either because of the odium which might consequently attach itself to the institution, or because of the want of some separate compartment." On the other hand, the numbers of insane blacks in many northern and midwestern states were so small that it did not make fiscal sense to superintendents in those areas to create separate hospitals or separate wards for them.[53] The report that Galt completed for the AMSAII reflected this diversity of opinion, blending a pragmatic sense of what might be possible given the local conditions of specific hospitals and a larger belief in the powerful influence of race on the nature of mental illness and the prospects for its treatment.

Although Galt acknowledged that it might be in the best interests of states that had comparable numbers of mentally ill African Americans and whites to create separate hospitals, the reality was that the small numbers of African Americans who required institutionalization meant that they were more likely to be treated in asylums where the majority of the inmate population was white. Galt's commitment to treating the mentally ill led him to declare, with only a bit of equivocation, that "nearly the identical rules of moral and medical treatment are applicable to the colored insane" as to whites. However, he was clear that racial segregation should be a key feature of moral treatment. "In the first place," he wrote, "it is supposed that in the insane, the same feelings exist upon this point as with the sane, and hence from any admixture of races, a train of irritating circumstances would be likely to follow which must materially interfere with the comfort, the management, and the cure, of both the white and colored patients." Galt's concern over the potentially deleterious impact that racial mixing would have on the prospects of recovery extended only to white patients. He suggested that, in situations where superintendents could not avoid integrating wards, they should house African Americans among whites suffering from dementia, on the grounds that individuals with dementia "take less notice, as a general rule, of their situation and companions."[54]

In short, Galt's classification scheme underlying moral treatment ultimately prioritized white mental health. Since harmful external stimuli—including especially people of different races—might disrupt the mind's ability to heal itself, superintendents had to take every precaution to protect their patients from exposure, unless those patients were African American. "Although amongst the colored insane as with others," Galt wrote, "a just classification is preferable, yet we do not consider the principle to assume here that extreme importance which it holds as regards insane whites. For the tendency of a mind approaching rationality to be shocked by witnessing the conduct of the more deranged, seems less intense in patients belonging to the former, than in many of those of the latter class. Hence in looking to the welfare of the colored insane, the less difficulty in assigning them a fit position amongst white patients."[55] In other words, although African Americans were capable of suffering the same mental illnesses as whites, they were less sensitive to their surroundings. Though not explicitly expressed, this understanding of black insanity converged with larger cultural perceptions of African Americans as dull in temperament and less sensitive than whites to pain or tactile sensation.[56] Galt's reasoning also implied that black insanity was inherently more deranged than white insanity. This would become a refrain within psychiatric discourse in the postbellum era and continue into the twentieth century. Written in the early 1850s, Galt's recommendations to the

AMSAII revealed a preoccupation with the recovery of white sufferers of mental disease.

Another solution Galt proposed to superintendents who either did not have enough African American patients to justify segregated wards or the resources to house them separately was to provide space for them in the servants' quarters of the asylum. "The facility of assimilating lunatics of this class with the servants of the institution," he suggested, "will render their isolation from the white patients a very easy matter."[57] His recommendation was shaped by his own practice at Eastern Lunatic Asylum, where free black inmates were not only segregated but made to maintain their own rooms and employed in menial chores to supplement the labor of the hospital staff. Not an uncommon practice in nineteenth-century southern asylums that admitted black patients, it drew on the associations that whites made between African Americans and drudgery and was aimed at shoring up white patients' sense of superiority, even as it was advocated as a form of therapy. Galt and other superintendents believed that successful moral treatment of mentally ill African Americans depended on rehabilitating them as laborers and servants, in effect reproducing the racial hierarchies that existed outside of the asylum.[58]

Nichols firmly believed that it was "the duty of all State, County, [and] City Hospitals for the Insane" to accommodate mentally ill African Americans. Although he thought it was the government's responsibility to provide for the "colored insane," Nichols adamantly argued that African American patients should not reside in the hospital proper; rather they should be located at some distance from the wards containing white patients. There is some indication, however, that he had not always subscribed to this idea but came to the conclusion only in the process of designing the Government Hospital. In a letter to Dix in January 1853, Nichols suggested that he was thinking about it as a feature of the Government Hospital but had not yet made up his mind. He had just returned from a visit to Western Lunatic Asylum in Staunton, Virginia, which, unlike its counterpart in Williamsburg, excluded African American patients altogether. Nichols was seeking the advice of the superintendent, Francis T. Stribling, who, he related to Dix, suggested that he "place the kitchen in the rear of the Centre building by itself [and] ... place separate wards for the Colored insane 300 or 400 feet in the rear of the distant extremities of the [illegible]." Stribling found the racial integration of the Maryland Hospital repugnant and cautioned Nichols to avoid a similar situation at the new federal asylum. Although he did not express unequivocal support for Stribling's recommendation, Nichols told Dix that he thought "his views on these subjects [are] entitled to particular respect."[59]

By the year the Government Hospital opened, Nichols was resolute in his commitment to racial segregation. He was probably influenced on this matter by Thomas Kirkbride—a good friend for whom the standard asylum construction plan was named—as much as by Stribling. Kirkbride's Pennsylvania Hospital apparently excluded African Americans, and he expressed disdain for Galt's earlier practice of integrating the wards at Eastern Lunatic Asylum.[60] Asylums modeled on the Kirkbride, or linear, plan consisted of a central administrative building with wings on both sides. As each successive wing—generally two to three stories—was added on, it was slightly offset from its antecedent wing, creating a stepped or tiered footprint. Rather than confine African American inmates to one particular wing, Nichols planned the construction of a "detached cottage for colored insane." As a proponent of moral treatment, he had come to believe that "placing white and colored insane in the same wards [was] not best calculated to promote the comfort nor the welfare of either party, by such an unnatural association." Nichols's chief concern was to accommodate African American patients in such a way as to avoid offending the sensibilities of white patients and staff members, on the one hand, and to bring them under the necessary surveillance that their illnesses demanded, on the other. This led to a very precise positioning of the lodge on the grounds of the hospital. Nichols argued that it should be between two hundred and four hundred feet from the main building: "Any distance within that range would exceed an objectionable proximity, but not the pale of an easy inspection by the officers."[61] This lodge, and an additional one that would be built in 1860 and sit equidistant between the central building and the stables, in effect reproduced the racial topography of the plantation.

Like segregation and exclusion policies in general, the construction of separate lodges for African American patients set at some distance from the main building used space to reinforce social hierarchies.[62] But it did more than reproduce the racial boundaries that existed outside of the asylum. As in the case of prioritizing white health in the selection of the site for the hospital, the exclusion of African American patients from the main building privileged the white patient while it also worked to construct the white psyche as the norm.

Nichols's policy of accommodating mentally ill African Americans resembled some institutions' solution to dealing with another group of insane that represented a potential obstacle to the recovery of reason for patients not suffering from chronic mental disease: those lunatics whose insanity caused them to be particularly disruptive, degraded, and dangerous. "The disposal of the violent and noisy class has always been a subject of much diversity of opinion, because every practicable mode involves some unavoidable disadvantage," Isaac Ray, superintendent of Butler Hospital for the Insane in Providence, Rhode Island, wrote in his 1854 survey of American asylums. "The course adopted to some extent in Europe, and generally here, is to place them in smaller buildings at a little distance from the main edifice."[63] Although Ray did not specifically allude to race, the association of mentally ill African Americans with the basest forms of insanity would go on to shape psychiatric thought and institutional practice

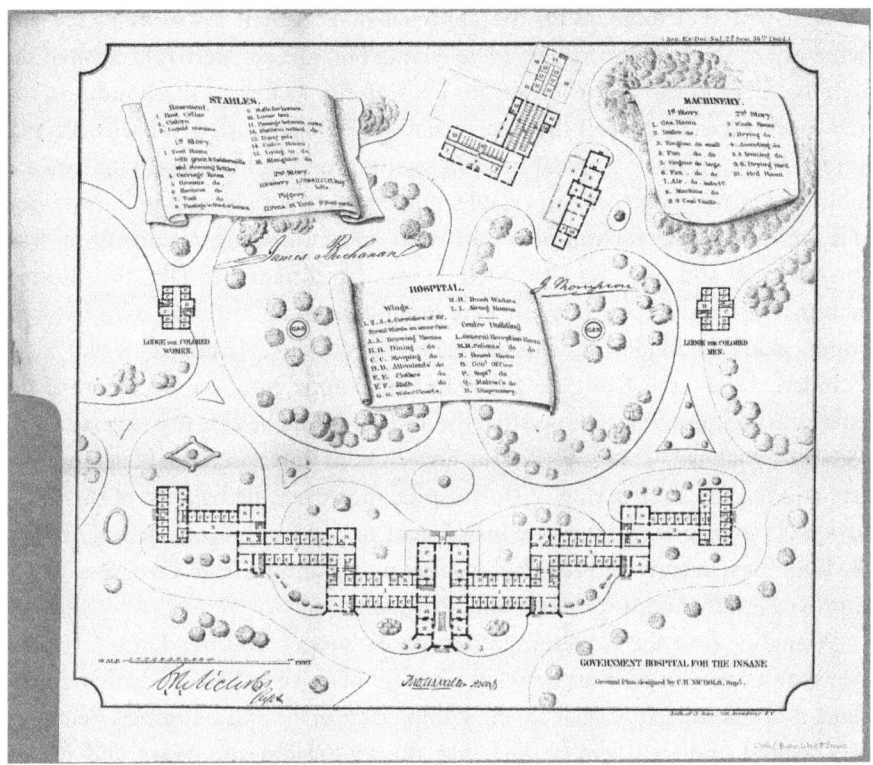

An architectural plan of the Government Hospital for the Insane from the early 1860s, including drawings of its main building, separate lodges for black female and male patients, maintenance facilities, and barns. Although the shortage of space occasionally led to black patients being housed in wards in the main building, the positioning of the colored lodges close to the hospital's livestock quarters and physical plant reflected Superintendent Charles H. Nichols's views about the importance of racially segregating the mentally ill. *Government Hospital for the Insane Ground Plan. Courtesy of American Antiquarian Society.*

in the postbellum period and well into the twentieth century. In Nichols's design of the Government Hospital, the location of the "colored lodges" was shaped less by a fundamentally racist attitude toward African Americans. As a physician with a very paternalistic sense of his duty toward the insane, he felt that he was as responsible for the care of mentally ill African Americans as for the care of anyone else. Rather, the racial segregation embedded in the hospital's initial design was the product of a limited vision of what was possible with respect to psychiatric care and, more important, who should be the main beneficiaries of that care.

Bringing Nichols's architectural vision to fruition was not without its challenges. The superintendent threw himself into the work of planning the hospital with full force. With the approval of President Franklin Pierce and Secretary of the Interior Robert McClelland, Nichols enlisted T. U. Walter, the architect behind the extension of the US Capitol, to design the buildings, but he oversaw every aspect of their construction. He also busied himself with planning for the hospital's operations, including ordering furniture, kitchenware, tools, and farming equipment; establishing contacts with local suppliers of food and fuel; arranging for the hiring of staff; and cultivating relationships with congressmen and local leaders. Nichols was, he confided to Dix, the "busiest man in Washington," so busy that he bought a young enslaved man who, he hoped, would be manumitted in six years "if he conducts [himself] well."[64]

In late 1852, after Congress made its initial appropriation, Secretary of the Interior Alexander Stuart hoped that the asylum would be able to begin receiving patients by January 1, 1854. After the government purchased the Blagden property and began construction of the hospital, however, the balance of the initial $100,000 appropriation became insufficient to pay for the completion of all of the buildings. In early 1854 Nichols sought more funding from Congress, which approved another appropriation bill by the summer.[65]

Wrangling over the Government Hospital's budget continued into 1855, the year that it opened. Nichols drew up a budget of close to $30,000 to cover both general operating expenses and the completion of several buildings. Secretary McClelland endorsed the budget, but the Committee on Ways and Means balked at the amount and pared back Nichols's request. The $8,000 that Nichols requested for the "colored lodge" was met with particular skepticism by members of the committee. Nichols was indignant that the committee would question his medical authority and judgment about what was needed, and he put even more energy into lobbying members of Congress to commit the necessary funds to the hospital. He recounted to Dix:

> In about one fortnight after the opening of the last session, the committee of ways [and] means reported the Civil [and] Diplomatic bill to the House, [and] included in it the $16,800 asked for the support of the institution next year, [and] rejected all the other items. The Com[mittee] stumbled at the 2nd item—"the doctor's nigger house" as they styled it, [and] finally rejected it [and] all the balance. Now imagine the work on my hands. The Com[mittee] had rejected what the Sec'y had recommended, while I felt that I *must* not only have that, but some $20,000 more that no-body had recommended! Suffice it to say that I went to work, determined if possible to accomplish a desperate possibility, [and] I *did* get *all* I had asked [and] all I had contemplated asking, [and] I thank God for it.[66]

Members of the Ways and Means Committee were not convinced that public monies should be used to build accommodations for African American patients, although the language they used suggests that they were not promoters of racially integrated wings of the hospital either.

But despite some members' clear hostility toward the idea that the federal government should provide care for mentally ill African Americans, Nichols managed to get full funding for the rest of his capital and general operational budgets. Alongside the $16,000 for support of patients, Congress appropriated an extra $22,512 for the completion of the main hospital building and $12,020 for additional capital expenses, including "the erection of a lodge for the colored insane."[67] The construction of the colored lodge would be as much, if not more, for the benefit of white patients as for African Americans. While it would allow Nichols to receive mentally ill blacks into the institution and provide them care, the ability to maintain the separation of the races would enhance the institutional experience of insane whites and perhaps improve their chances for recovery.

The colored lodge would not be completed before the hospital opened. But neither would the main building. On January 15, 1855, Nichols received the first patient in the Government Hospital for the Insane, an individual who had been ordered there by the District criminal court. A week later he began the process of removing District residents from Maryland's asylums. The main hospital building was still incomplete in early 1855, which necessitated housing white male and female patients in the same sections but on different floors, a "highly inconvenient" arrangement as far as Nichols was concerned. The fact that the colored lodge was not yet habitable also forced Nichols to quarter African American patients in the "house," his euphemism for the center building.[68]

By late October the main building was complete, and Nichols informed the Department of War and the Department of the Navy that the hospital was ready to receive insane soldiers and sailors. The massive main structure, 711 feet long and in "the collegiate style of Gothic architecture," was vastly superior in construction to the wooden cottage that, by the time of its completion in 1856, was barely large enough to hold twenty African American patients.[69]

Nichols was rightly concerned that the small size of the colored lodge would lead to housing mentally ill African Americans in overcrowded conditions. In his October 1855 report, he intimated that there was a high demand in the District—whether from the community or local officials, he was, unfortunately, not specific—for an institution to confine the "colored insane." "So numerous and urgent have been the appeals for the reception of more of this class," Nichols wrote, referring to the nine black patients already in the hospital, "that only a word would be wanting to bring at once to our doors more than the additional

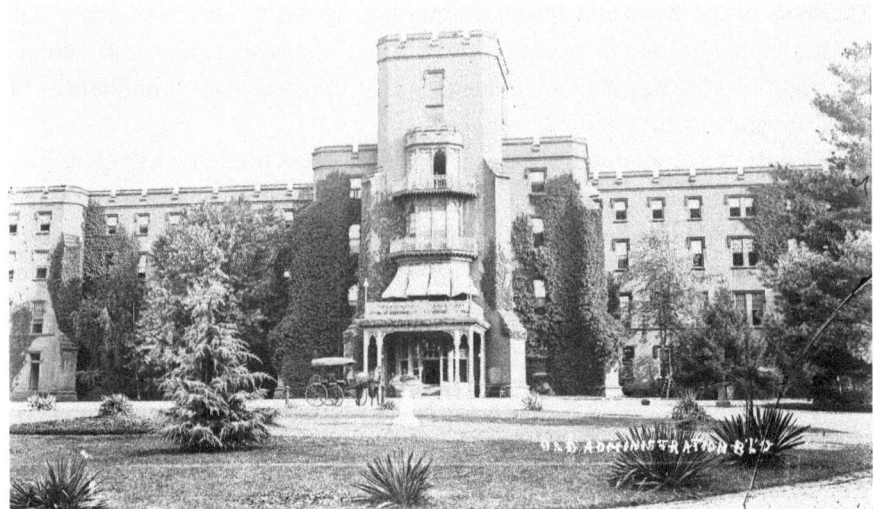

A view of Saint Elizabeths' central administration building around the turn of the twentieth century. Originally opened in the fall of 1855, the imposing red-brick Gothic revival structure was typical of the architectural style of nineteenth-century insane asylums. *National Archives, photo 418-G-9.*

eleven (11) necessary to fill the lodge were it now ready for use."[70] The potential for overcrowding was exacerbated by the combination of Congress's piecemeal funding of the construction and Nichols's desire to accommodate as many indigent insane as could reasonably reside in the hospital with some level of comfort.[71]

Overcrowding would remain a problem at the Government Hospital through the initial years of its operation; in no small way this was due to Nichols's commitment to institutionalizing pauper and civilian insane residents of the District. This became one of the principal pathways for the majority of African American patients at the hospital, although there were certainly some who were members of the military and were committed on the orders of the secretary of war or the secretary of the navy. Regardless of the route they took to the Government Hospital, however, mentally ill African Americans (as well as those African Americans whose unusual behavior may have been interpreted as insanity) found themselves in an institution whose design and operation were based on the premise that their recovery and well-being was secondary to that of their fellow white inmates.

2

The Paradox of Enlightened Care

Saint Elizabeths in the Era of Moral Treatment, 1855–1877

The first inmates actually arrived at the Government Hospital some six weeks before Congress passed legislation establishing how the institution would operate. Nichols was instrumental in the development of the legislation, drafting a version of the bill while he was overseeing the construction of the asylum. A draft bill for the hospital's organization that he submitted in a December 1854 report to the House of Representatives and Secretary of the Interior Robert McClelland became the template for a bill that was reported out of the House's Committee for the District of Columbia in February 1855. The administrative and operational arrangements of the hospital were very much based on the organizational principles espoused by leading insanity experts. At the center was the superintendent model, in which an experienced physician assumed total responsibility for the functioning of the hospital and the care of its inmates. The superintendent had complete control over the institution. He had the power to appoint an assistant physician to help with the diagnosis and treatment of patients, a matron to supervise the care of female inmates, a steward to oversee the provisioning of the hospital, and a support staff consisting of attendants, custodians, farmers, gardeners, cooks, laundresses, and general laborers. The power of the superintendent was checked, to a certain degree, by a nine-person Board of Visitors. Serving in staggered two-year terms, members of the board were primarily responsible for conducting periodic inspections, crafting necessary bylaws for the institution, overseeing the hospital's finances and operations, and submitting annual reports to the secretary of the interior. The active involvement of the board notwithstanding, the expectations were that the superintendent would exercise all necessary control over the institution, its staff, and its inmates.[1]

There were a few differences between the language proposed by Nichols and the language of the bill that was passed by Congress on March 3, 1855, including Nichols's identification of the institution as the National Hospital for the Insane, whereas the official act authorizing the asylum endowed it with the title Government Hospital for the Insane.[2] But neither of these names would remain in vernacular use for very long. As Nichols remembered, shortly after the hospital opened, "both certain patients and their friends were shunning in various ways the use of the organic and legal title of the Institution and groping for some designation of it for familiar use that did not in any manner imply its special character" as an insane asylum. After several different names, including "Anacostia Heights," failed to catch on, the hospital eventually assumed the name of an extant portion of the tract on which it was located: Saint Elizabeths, "the name of the 'Sainted daughter of Hungarian Kings' which suggests nothing but what is 'lovely,'" Nichols proclaimed.[3]

On March 12 Nichols received the first African American patients into Saint Elizabeths. The three men and two women were among the last of a group of fifty-one people who Nichols had begun transferring from Baltimore's Maryland Hospital and Mount Hope Institution in late January.[4] These five individuals—along with hundreds of others whose admissions were the result of the military casualties and larger social dislocations associated with the Civil War and its aftermath—were entering the hospital at a time of great optimism and confidence on the part of physicians regarding the curability of insanity. Superintendents' commitment to a moral treatment model contributed to the location and design of asylums in ways that were intended to maximize the physical and figurative distance between the mentally ill and the sources of their psychic distress. In asylums that had a racially heterogeneous population, such as Saint Elizabeths, this model of care included, and indeed relied upon, racial segregation. But this meant more than just the physical separation of white and black inmates. The imperative of producing an ideal social environment for the mentally ill created a particular therapeutic regime—especially with respect to what physicians considered to be the restorative benefits of leisure and labor—that drew from and reinforced the dogma of racial difference in American society.

The intersection of this dogma and Nichols's commitment to ameliorating the terrible effects of mental disease produced a paradoxical, at times contradictory approach to African American inmates. On the one hand, Nichols's New England ancestry and Quaker faith contributed to a paternalistic sense of duty toward the insane that transcended racial lines. On the other hand, his acceptance of the premise that the white psyche was the norm allowed for the development of a therapeutic paradigm and system of care that privileged white patients at the expense of African Americans. However, African American inmates and their families did not sit by and unmindfully adhere to the expectations laid out for them by Nichols and his staff. In both significant and minor ways, blacks sought to shape their own and their loved ones' experiences in Saint Elizabeths. In the end, African Americans' presence influenced the ways that moral treatment, as both an idea and a practice, evolved in this mid-nineteenth-century asylum.

Prisoners, Paupers, and Slaves: Black Admissions in Saint Elizabeths' Early Years

In addition to the administrative and operational features of the hospital, the March 1855 bill laid out the specific classes of patients who were eligible for admission and the legal procedures by which they would be committed. As indicated in the bill's title, An Act to Organize an Institution for the Insane of the Army and Navy, and of the District of Columbia, in the said District, the hospital's primary concern was the treatment of mentally ill soldiers and sailors, who were to be committed on the orders of the secretaries of the war and naval departments. None of the original five African Americans committed to Saint Elizabeths was in the military.[5] Of the approximately fifty African Americans admitted to the hospital prior to the Civil War, there was only one service member: an ordinary seaman from Massachusetts who was diagnosed with dementia in April 1856 and remained in Saint Elizabeths until his death in December 1864.[6]

A similar category of patient was the federal convict, although the original bill contained no specific references to this class. The hospital had admitted three African American convicts, two men and one woman, by the fall of 1861. One of these was William D., a native Washingtonian who was convicted of larceny and sentenced to the US Penitentiary in the District of Columbia in March 1858. Apparently he was an extremely difficult prisoner. He was punished at least eight times over the course of one year for infractions such as "making noise in cell," "quarrelling and wanting to fight in shop," and "whistling and singing." William's punishments included being placed on a restricted diet of bread and water, being shackled in irons, and being whipped while hoisted in the air by his wrists. One week after being punished for writing a letter to a woman and "cursing depty [sic] warden," William was admitted to Saint Elizabeths with a diagnosis of mania. He remained there for less than three months before he was deemed to be recovered and was released.[7] It is unclear whether penitentiary officials truly believed William was suffering from mental illness or just saw Saint Elizabeths as a practical option for this particularly obstreperous prisoner. By the late 1850s officials were less optimistic about the reformatory potential of the District penitentiary. One chaplain, for instance, pointed out that some prisoners were "suffering great mental depression" because of the conditions of the institution. Given that he made this statement in 1858, it is certainly possible that William was one of the prisoners he had in mind.[8]

Convicts and military personnel who ended up in Saint Elizabeths essentially moved from the custody of one government institution to another. The vast majority of the hospital's early inmates, however, were making the transition from private individuals to wards of the state. Those individuals who were not previously under government custody upon their admission to the hospital were identified as either "civil independent" or "civil indigent." "Civil independent" inmates were also known as "private" or "pay patients." The 1855 law organizing Saint Elizabeths allowed for the admission of private patients, space permitting, whose stay would be paid for by a third party. In order for a pay patient to be admitted, his or her unstable mental condition needed to be certified by "two respectable physicians of the District," and an interested party—"the nearest relation, legal guardian or friend"—had to submit a formal request of admission and prepay for thirteen weeks of room and board.[9] There were a few African American "civil independent" inmates in the hospital's early years, although without more information than their age and diagnosis, it is impossible to know how their stays were financed.[10]

Ironically slaves were one category of "civil independent" patients for whom there is no question about who paid for their hospital stay. Between August 1859 and August 1860 Saint Elizabeths admitted three enslaved African Americans, a number that constituted less than 1 percent of the patients admitted in the first five and a half years of the hospital's operation.[11] That few bondspeople would end up in Saint Elizabeths is not surprising, given the small number of enslaved African Americans in the District of Columbia to begin with and the requirement that slaveholders pay for their slaves' institutionalization. While slaveholders may have tried to sequester a mentally ill bondsperson in an attic or relieve themselves of the burden through manumission or sale, particularly troublesome bondspeople would have presented slaveholders with special challenges. Slave law in Maryland penalized slaveholders who allowed their bondspeople "to depart from their respective habitation or quarter, and remain at large, begging or becoming burthensome to the respective neighbourhoods, or to other persons." On the first such instance, slaveholders were forced to post a $100 security, which was forfeitable in the event that their bondsperson subsequently "depart[ed] and remain[ed] at large." In their posting of the bond and public acknowledgment that they were responsible for a potential nuisance, slaveholders also exposed themselves to civil liability.[12] Given the inchoate nature of tort law when it came to slavery, there was certainly no guarantee that a court would find a slaveholder liable for his insane bondsperson's actions.[13] Still, when dealing with a recalcitrant or completely disconnected enslaved person who was unlikely to respond to punishment (or the threat of it), slaveholders might have made the calculus that $52, the cost of prepayment for Saint Elizabeths' private patients, was a better deal than forfeiting a $100 bond or opening themselves up to a lawsuit.

To be sure, it is possible that, having exhausted all home remedies and the services of a private physician, slaveholders turned to Saint Elizabeths out of genuine concern for the well-being of their mentally ill bondsperson. This may have been so in the case of an enslaved woman, Maria B., who spent four months in the hospital after being diagnosed with acute mania in August 1859. Her master, George Waters, sent for his "woman Maria" on Christmas Eve and promised to pay his account in full as soon as Nichols informed him how much he owed.[14] Why Maria was released at that particular time is impossible to know. Did Waters and his family consider her to be a vital part of their household who they did not want to have to spend Christmas alone in a hospital, or were her services required for the holiday festivities? Was Waters retrieving Maria after Nichols sent word that she had recovered, or did Waters initiate the release? If the latter, the judgment that Maria had recovered from her acute mania would have been influenced by the desires of the individual who had property rights in her body more than the considerable medical expertise of her caregiver. In such a case, Nichols would not necessarily have interpreted Waters's request as a challenge to his medical authority. In the interests of institution-building in the mid-nineteenth century, superintendents did not reflexively disparage vernacular ideas about madness and its treatment or oppose the families and friends of insane people who acted upon those ideas. Rather, acknowledging the common overlap between lay and medical understandings of insanity and reinforcing it through institutional practice was one of the ways in which superintendents integrated asylum medicine into the intellectual and social landscape of local communities.[15] Any deference that Nichols showed to Waters, however, was surely intensified by the legal relationship between the patron of the asylum and the superintendent's patient. The proprietary authority of the slaveholder ultimately trumped the medical authority of the superintendent.

The last class of patient, and the one that predominated among African Americans, was the civil indigent. Whereas the 1855 act and the hospital's bylaws were quite specific about the procedures for admitting members of the military and private patients, initially there was less clarity around who was eligible for admission under the category of "indigent insane" and the procedures through which they would be committed. The act authorized the secretary of the interior to commit to Saint Elizabeths civilian residents of the District who, "after due process of law" were demonstrated "to be insane, and unable to support himself (or herself) and family (or themselves, if they have no family) under the visitation of insanity."[16]

What exactly constituted due process of law, however, was not entirely clear, at least not to Nichols. Three months after the hospital opened, he wrote to Secretary McClelland to request clarification—and to offer advice—on the commitment procedures for the indigent insane. Nichols was convinced that the local law governing commitments, the *writ de lunatico inquirendo*, was too cumbersome. Requiring a proceeding in which an assembled panel of laymen heard testimony from physicians, family members, and neighbors before making a determination of insanity "involves more time, expense [and] publicity than would be necessary in ordinary cases," Nichols contended. He advocated for a more streamlined process, authorized by common law in the District, in which a grand jury of the criminal court or a circuit court judge could issue a finding of insanity upon hearing sufficient testimony. Nichols also supported an enhanced role for community members in the commitment procedure, including the responsibility of covering any expenses associated with the process, especially the transportation of the inmate to Saint Elizabeths. From Nichols's perspective, this would further destigmatize institutionalization, as it would reduce the role of local or federal law enforcement officials in overseeing the transfer of inmates to the hospital and strip commitment "of the odor of criminal detention which is associated with the functions of jailor [and] keeper highly offensive and injurious to a respectable [and] perhaps well educated patient, whose double misfortune of indigence and insanity has rather exalted than depressed his natural moral sensibilities."[17] Nichols was making his argument at a time when superintendents throughout the country were trying to make the commitment process as simple and burden-free as possible. In order both to differentiate the curative function of the asylum from the punitive and custodial nature of the penitentiary and to diminish the popular stigma associated with insanity, asylum physicians sought to minimize the legal impediments in what they considered to be a primarily medical proceeding.[18]

By the winter of 1856–57, Congress had taken up supplementary legislation to its 1855 act that was aimed at establishing clear commitment protocol. Instead of requiring a *lunatico inquirendo* proceeding, the bill authorized the secretary of the interior to commit an individual to Saint Elizabeths once he was presented with documentation from a judge or justice of the peace certifying that the individual was insane and destitute. The judge's determination was to be based on the testimony of "two respectable physicians" and "two respectable householders," all of whom needed to be District residents. Despite some expressed concern that without the "inquisition" process of the *lunatico inquirendo* the commitment procedure invested too much power in the hands of the magistracy, the House followed the Senate's lead in passing the bill, and it became law on February 7, 1857.[19]

Though that year's annual report captured the optimistic humanitarianism with which the Board of Visitors viewed institutionalization—characterizing it as the "protection [and] care of all classes of the insane of the District"—it also clearly articulated the limits of the institution's magnanimity.[20] When it came to admitting mentally ill civilians, their residency had to be established. In their testimony, the two physicians needed to state with certainty that the prospective inmate had become afflicted with insanity *while* a resident of the District. As an institution that "rejects no physical malady if it be complicated with any form of mental alienation," Saint Elizabeths could not afford to provide care for transient lunatics, a particular problem in the nation's capital, in perception if not in reality.[21] Ideally individuals who had come to the District after they had become insane or who were temporarily residing in the District when they became insane would be removed from the capital and committed to the public institutions in their home states. Identifying nonresidents was critical, especially given the increase in the number of inmates in the institution between 1856 and 1860. The number of inmates "in the house" almost tripled in those years, from 60 to 167.[22] The number would continue to increase over the next decade. The chaotic years of the Civil War, moreover, would wreak nearly as much havoc with the admissions policy as it did with the minds of soldiers, sailors, and civilians.

"An Asylum for Free Negroes": The Impact of the Civil War

As was the case with a great many institutions and American society more broadly, the Civil War had both short-term and long-term effects on Saint Elizabeths. Its location made the hospital a valuable resource for the federal government, which was using the District as both a supply depot for the Army of the Potomac and a center for the care of wounded Union soldiers and sailors. In addition to the army-maintained cavalry depot that was adjacent to the hospital, the staff and inmates of Saint Elizabeths had to share the campus with the navy's Ordinance Bureau and a company of US marines. Because of its proximity to the Washington Arsenal and Navy Yard, two of the forty-eight forts in and around the District of Columbia were located on the hospital's grounds. The urgent need for hospital beds led to the recruitment of Saint Elizabeths into the medical service for the army and navy.[23] Despite Nichols's concern that the presence of recuperating soldiers and sailors would impede the recovery of insane inmates, the army established a 250-bed hospital in the east wing. By the summer of 1862 increasing numbers of sick and wounded troops necessitated the erection of tents for the "shelter of convalescents." Two years into the war, R. W. Jewett, a patent holder for an artificial limb, set up a shop on the grounds, and soon military hospitals began transferring amputee soldiers and sailors to the campus's Army General Hospital, where they were fitted for, and learned to use, their prostheses.[24]

The war also affected the hospital personnel. Nichols served as a volunteer surgeon for the Army General Hospital and accompanied regiments into the field as they engaged in battles around Washington, certainly putting more pressure on his assistant physicians to provide medical care for the hospital's insane inmates. There was a significant turnover in the Saint Elizabeths staff, since roughly a quarter of its male employees split their duties between service on the battlefield and in the wards.[25] Nichols found it difficult to fill some of the positions on his staff due to the demands of the military. "The Army has absorbed all doctors, good and bad, who had not remunerative practices," S. Preston Jones, the assistant physician at the Pennsylvania Hospital for the Insane, wrote to Nichols, "and as to recent graduates, they find places in military hospitals, which they decidedly prefer to our kind."[26]

But undoubtedly the war's largest impact on Saint Elizabeths was the increase in admissions of people diagnosed as insane and, if only temporarily, a change in the inmate demographic. In fact the hospital's administration was unprepared for the sheer numbers of Union soldiers and sailors who required commitment to an insane asylum due to the mental stress and trauma resulting from military service. In a three-month span in 1861, the Board of Visitors calculated, the number of admissions had amounted to 80 percent of the number during the entire preceding year. The massive increase of the military, the suspect constitutions of the conscripts, and the nature of modern warfare and military life created a potent combination that laid the etiological groundwork for an epidemic of insanity. "A large proportion of the land forces are men of no little moral and nervous susceptibility, quickly transferred from the quietude, comforts, and sympathies of home to all the hardships and profound excitements of the camp and field," the board claimed. In emphasizing the various factors that contributed to increased mental strain among service members, the board was indicating to the secretary of the interior and Congress the hospital's need for a larger appropriation. The board also signaled its patience given the extraordinary pressure for funds that the war was placing on all federal agencies and institutions; nonetheless it reminded the secretary and Congress of their obligation to provide the best treatment for "citizen soldiers whose reason has given way in the services of their country."[27]

Although they may not have been considered citizens, many of these soldiers were African American. Between August 1863 and July 1865 twenty-three African American soldiers and one sailor were admitted to Saint Elizabeths. All were enlisted personnel, and only one was a noncommissioned officer. The majority of men were from regiments of the US Colored Troops, but a few were from volunteer regiments, including the 54th Massachusetts Volunteers. The increase in the commitments of black soldiers reflected the growing involvement of African Americans in the military. From July 1, 1861, to June 30, 1863, there were no soldiers or sailors among the thirteen African Americans admitted to Saint Elizabeths. The US Colored Troops were established in 1863, and enlistment of African Americans remained robust for the remainder of the war. In fiscal year 1863–64, soldiers made up 40 percent of African Americans admitted (six of fifteen), and during fiscal year 1864–65, 54 percent of those admitted (eighteen of thirty-three). The military-to-civilian commitment ratio was not as high as it was among the overall population of the hospital, which was approximately six to one.[28]

Despite the astronomical increase in the commitments of soldiers and sailors, hospital officials recognized early on that among the war's casualties would be civilians who were mentally incapable of handling the turmoil and uncertainty that accompanied military conflict. In the same meeting in which it discussed the war's psychological effect on soldiers and sailors, the board acknowledged the devastating repercussions that would ripple throughout the noncombatant population. "The profound political agitations and alarms and the domestic dissensions and ruptures which are doubly incident to a national capital and a border region in a time of civil war," the board reported, "must likewise render the number of the indigent insane of the District of Columbia larger than was anticipated at the time of preparing our last annual statement of the condition, prospects and wants of the institution."[29] The capital was indeed a volatile, at times chaotic environment during the war. That was particularly true for African Americans given its location between two slave states (one of which had seceded from the Union and the other precariously perched to do so), the somewhat ambiguous status of fugitive slave law, the confused nature of military policy toward slaves, and the early abolition of slavery within its borders.

The capital's location between Virginia and Maryland posed obvious political and strategic problems for the Union, yet it also created opportunities for enslaved African Americans in the District and the surrounding Maryland and Virginia counties. President Abraham Lincoln had come into office as a moderate on slavery—committed to its nonextension but not to its abolition. The necessity of keeping secessionist sentiment in Maryland to a minimum led to a fairly cautious approach to the bondspeople who had begun fleeing to Union lines once the war started, an approach that was all too often undermined by overly zealous commanders and soldiers in the field. Despite the orders of Lincoln and some of the generals in the field that soldiers were not to facilitate the escape of bondspeople or prevent slaveholders from retrieving their fugitive slaves, they routinely did so, prompting more enslaved African Americans to try to get to Union-occupied territory. The Fugitive Slave Act, passed in 1850, was still officially in effect, however, and it was strictly enforced by the Metropolitan Police and the US marshal for the District of Columbia. Through the early part of 1862, it was not uncommon to see loyal slaveholders from Maryland searching for their escaped bondspeople among the hundreds who were confined in the District jail. This generated a great deal of opposition from free blacks and abolitionist-leaning whites, including Republican members of Congress.

After an investigation of the District jail in which fugitive enslaved people were being held, Congress took up a bill to abolish slavery in the nation's capital, which in turn was opposed by the Maryland legislature and not a few Washingtonians, including a majority on the Washington City Council. Fearing that such an act would turn the District into "an asylum for free negroes" by virtue of its being "between two slaveholding areas," the council, led by Mayor Richard Wallach, passed a resolution against abolition. Pressing forward, Congress passed the District of Columbia Emancipation Act in April 1862, immediately freeing more than 3,100 enslaved people. The act also provided compensation to loyal District slaveholders and set aside $100,000 for the colonization of either Liberia or Haiti by those freed.[30]

In many ways, the Emancipation Act did turn Washington into a safe haven for enslaved African Americans, although they had been entering the city (and also Georgetown) from the very early days of the war. But the act certainly intensified the in-migration of enslaved African Americans from Maryland and Virginia, despite the fact that the Fugitive Slave Act was still in force.[31] Estimates vary, but between twenty thousand and forty thousand African Americans migrated into the capital during the war, substantially augmenting the 10,983 black Washingtonians and 1,935 black Georgetowners who resided in the District in 1860. The Freedmen's Bureau census in March 1866 counted 27,287 African Americans in Washington City, and in 1870 federal census takers recorded 35,455 African Americans, an increase of 223 percent over the city's black population in 1860. By 1870 blacks made up 32.5 percent of Washington's total population and 28.7 percent of Georgetown's.[32]

The majority of enslaved African Americans making their way into the District were placed in contraband camps.[33] The first such facility, Duff Green's Row, located near the Capitol and administered by the District's military governor, James Wadsworth, housed approximately four hundred refugees. Black "contrabands" were registered after it was determined that their masters were disloyal to the Union, given military protection papers, provided clothing and rations, and, if physically capable, either transported to the front lines to help construct fortifications or employed locally in military support services. In the summer of 1862 Duff Green's Row was converted to a military prison, and Wadsworth, with the assistance of the Freedmen's Relief Association, transferred the inhabitants to a larger facility, the former barracks of General George McClellan's troops, located at 12th Street and Vermont Avenue. Camp Barker, as the new contraband camp was called, dwarfed the operation at Duff Green's Row. By October an estimated 4,200 refugees were residing in the camp. The massive influx of African Americans—as many as three hundred in one week—prompted local whites to call for the removal of the contraband camp to the outskirts of the city.[34]

Although freedom was certainly better than enslavement, life in the camps was scarcely an improvement over the plantation for most refugees. The concentration of so many refugees in one place made the camps an easy target for rowdy crowds of white Washingtonians who were resentful of the potential racial equality that emancipation portended. In terms of the environment of the camps themselves—and the four tenement complexes that were established and run by the Freedmen's Bureau in the immediate postwar years—overcrowding was a persistent problem, substandard infrastructure created unsanitary conditions, and the lack of basic supplies and insufficient rations exacerbated the poor health of many inmates. Infectious diseases such as smallpox, dysentery, and tuberculosis ran rampant throughout the camps and tenements. Camp Barker averaged twenty-five deaths a week in the summer of 1863. These conditions elicited the complaints not only of local residents but also of military officials, camp inmates, and the African American community, all of which led to the closure of Camp Barker by that fall.

The refugees were then transferred to the six-hundred-acre Freedmen's Village, located on Robert E. Lee's confiscated estate across the Potomac, in Arlington, Virginia. Established by two members of the abolitionist organization, the American Missionary Association, and later administered by the Freedmen's Bureau, Freedmen's Village operated in a fashion similar to Camp Barker, although refugees worked on a government-run farm, and camp residents were required to pay rent. Even though some of the same conditions obtained at the Village, the mortality rate was not as high as at Camp Barker, with the number of deaths averaging 2.0 a day as opposed to 3.5 per day at the District facility.[35]

Infectious disease and malnutrition were not the only health problems that camp inmates experienced. The mental stress that accompanied dislocation, not knowing the fate of family members, and the overall uncertainty about the future must surely have had a debilitating effect on some individuals' psyches, just as the poor conditions of the camps must have aggravated the incipient mental illnesses of others. Camp officials did occasionally report the existence of insane inmates and sought to have them transferred to Saint Elizabeths. In late June 1863 the medical director for the Department of Washington and a US Army surgeon, R. A. Abbott, requested that Thomas Boston, "now a patient in the Contraband Hospital in this City, and reported by the Surgeon in charge, as insane," be admitted to the asylum.[36] Apparently Boston was not admitted—at least his name does not appear in the register. The Department of the Interior refused to authorize the commitment of individuals when it could not be determined that the onset of their insanity occurred while they were residents of the District. The department rejected, for instance, the request of the acting military governor, Major John P. Sherburn, to admit "sundry persons now in said camp into the Insane Asylum," invoking an 1861 law passed by Congress which required that testimony on the residence of prospective patients come from physicians rather than District householders.[37]

The strict residency requirement, however, was rendered impracticable by the uprooting and movement of people caused by the war. In its 1862–63 annual report, the Board of Visitors addressed the necessity of dealing with the presence of insanity within an increasingly transient population, pointing out that mentally ill refugees "have, in many instances, been a serious charge upon the War Department, which has [been] compelled to take care of them in camps and other unsuitable places for such persons, and consequently at great expense and inconvenience."

Hospital officials exhibited a particular concern that any possibility of recovery for mentally ill refugees would be thwarted by the disordered environment of the camp. In order to maximize the therapeutic potential of the hospital, the board recommended that Congress amend the law to allow the staff to admit transient lunatics—primarily refugees from Maryland and Virginia—until such time that "they can be more properly disposed of."[38] Within a year of the board's report, Congress passed an act removing the residency requirement for admission of the transient insane to Saint Elizabeths. Two physicians still needed to attest to an individual's insanity, and two District householders needed to give testimony that he or she was incapable of self-support before being admitted. Moreover those requesting admission were expected to gather enough information about the prospective inmate's background for officials at the hospital or the Interior Department to track down his or her family and friends. Removing them from the harmful environment of the camps and then transferring them to private or public hospitals or households in their home states became Saint Elizabeths' primary approach to the transient insane.[39]

Debates over jurisdictional authority and interdepartmental wrangling also affected the commitment of freedpeople to Saint Elizabeths. Although Nichols was generally supportive of the 1864 amendment that allowed for mentally ill transients inside the District to be admitted to the hospital and treated free of charge, his sense of charity stopped at the banks of the Potomac. To his mind, Saint Elizabeths had no responsibility to provide uncompensated care to insane refugees residing in Virginia's contraband camps. In June 1864, for instance, the chief quartermaster of the Department of Washington requested that Eliza Matthews, "the crazy contraband woman," be admitted to Saint Elizabeths. Matthews had been tried in February for attempted arson at Freedmen's Village. Considering her to be "crazy and dangerous," camp officials confined her for three months but were eager to have her "turned over to the civil authorities." Nichols was not averse to admitting Matthews, but he suggested to Secretary of the Interior John P. Usher that she be admitted as a private patient, whose care would be paid for by Freedmen's Village.[40]

Nichols took an even harder line one month later in response to a request that Saint Elizabeths admit an "entirely Insane" freedman who had been "confined to the 'Slave pen' for safe treatment" at a contraband camp in Alexandria. Even though the camp surgeon suspected that Phillip might have served in the military, the lack of documentation rendered his situation the same as Eliza Matthews's in Nichols's opinion: the military requesting Saint Elizabeths to admit and provide free treatment to an insane refugee from another state.[41] In short, in order for mentally ill transients to be properly considered eligible for what amounted to free treatment, they had to be physically in the District at the moment it was determined that they needed to be institutionalized. Nichols was clearly perturbed that one arm of the federal government, the US military, would seek to pass its expenses on to another government institution, Saint Elizabeths, especially when the latter was comparatively starved for resources.

Whether to admit a freedperson into Saint Elizabeths was clearly not the issue for Nichols. His firm belief in the efficacy of institutionalization in retarding the advancement of mental illness did not stop at the imagined racial boundary between whites and blacks; he argued only for an equitable distribution of the burden of providing care for the indigent insane. In his letter to the secretary of the interior explaining his rationale for recommending against Matthews's admission as a civil indigent patient, Nichols hoped "that there need be no delay in placing all insane persons for whose care Government officials are in any way responsible, under proper treatment immediately after the existence of insanity is established. Early treatment," he reminded the secretary, "greatly enhances the probability of recovery and self support."[42]

Even as the District became first a way station and, later, the permanent home for thousands of African Americans fleeing slavery and war, however, the federal government was loath to become their permanent warden. This was as true of Saint Elizabeths as it was of the Freedmen's Bureau, which, among many of its duties, served as a labor broker of sorts, facilitating the employment of freedpeople up and down the Atlantic seaboard.[43] The attempt to prevent the permanent settlement of formerly enslaved African Americans in the District largely failed. Even though Mayor Wallach's fear that Congress's 1862 Emancipation Act would make the nation's capital an "asylum for free negroes" did materialize, African Americans continued to constitute a fairly small percentage of the admissions to Saint Elizabeths in the immediate postwar years. This was the case throughout the South, as public asylums resisted efforts by Freedmen's Bureau officials to admit insane freedpeople.[44] Unlike other southern asylums, however, African Americans remained a significant presence within the federal hospital, and their presence would shape the development of a mid-nineteenth-century therapeutic regime.

Race and Moral Treatment at Saint Elizabeths

Of the approximately 280 African Americans admitted to Saint Elizabeths in the first two decades of its existence, perhaps the most enigmatic case is that of Leutitia B. The thirty-nine-year-old native Virginian was admitted to the hospital almost a year to the day after the end of the Civil War. Residence was not typically listed in the hospital's register, so we do not know if Leutitia was a longtime denizen of Washington, if she lived in one of the District's four tenement complexes set up and run by the Freedmen's Bureau, or if she was an inmate of one of the camps located in northern Virginia whose officials may have managed to circumvent Nichols's opposition to accepting Virginia refugees as public wards.[45]

There is very little about Leutitia that is actually remarkable. Like more than two-thirds of African Americans admitted to the hospital in 1866, she was an insane pauper. Her diagnosis of mania was not unusual either. Since the beginning of the hospital's operation, 63 percent of the African Americans admitted were diagnosed with some form of mania—mania, chronic mania, and acute mania being the most common.[46] What makes Leutitia a particularly interesting case is the cause of her insanity. Similar to most of her fellow African American inmates, the diagnosing physician attributed Leutitia's mania mainly to moral, in contrast to physical, causes. As opposed to the small number whose insanity was thought to be brought on directly by an underlying bodily infirmity—such as epilepsy, pulmonary tuberculosis, idiocy, or paralysis—the sanity of the majority of admitted African Americans was disrupted by unnerving events or processes, such as "religious excitement," the death of a close family member, alienation from their social network, "domestic trouble," "fright," or "jealousy." But even with the elastic and amorphous quality of moral causation, it is difficult to make sense of the precipitating factor in Leutitia's descent into madness: the "blackness of her husband."[47]

The opacity of the early register books at Saint Elizabeths makes it impossible to fully understand what the hospital staff meant by this provocative phrase. She was admitted several decades before hospitals began creating and maintaining patient case files, and there are therefore few clues to Leutitia's commitment. Was "the blackness of her husband" the considered opinion of one of the two physicians who had to attest to her insanity, and, if so, was the doctor literally referring to the man's skin color? The medical profession generally accepted the proposition that insanity could occur when an underlying morbid condition was aggravated by "a powerful impression from without producing some great moral shock"; as such, Leutitia's husband's dark complexion might very well have been the catalyst as far as the diagnosing physician was concerned, although presumably Leutitia would have been accustomed to it.[48] Or did the phrase mean something less tangible, such as her ill treatment at her husband's hands, his "black-heartedness," as it were? If so, was this information provided to the physicians by one of the two District householders who had to confirm Leutitia's inability to self-support or by Leutitia herself?[49] The possibilities are many, but all are ultimately nothing more than speculation. Leutitia's presence jumps off the page of the hospital's registry demanding our attention and is, at the same time, frustratingly confined by the limits of the record-keeping process: nothing more than a few words jotted down, perhaps by an uninterested clerk who was merely following institutional procedure. Nonetheless the cryptic reference to blackness is emblematic of how race loomed over clinical encounters between white physicians and African American patients even if the sources are not always precisely clear how it did so.

Although there was no uniformity of thought among mid-nineteenth-century physicians as to the precise nature of mental illness and the best scheme by which to classify it, all asylum superintendents understood insanity to be a disease of the brain that impaired the ability to reason and overpowered individual volition. There was disagreement over whether the derangement of one's moral faculty, or affective life, without an accompanying deterioration of one's intellectual faculty, constituted insanity. This debate over the existence of moral insanity was a central feature of the professional development of psychiatry in the Civil War era, but there do not appear to be many individuals admitted to Saint Elizabeths with this diagnosis during Nichols's administration.[50]

Within the broader category of mental disease affecting an individual's ideation, experts on insanity identified three general forms: melancholia, mania, and dementia, or, as the Austrian psychiatrist Maximilian Leidesdorf summed it up, "states of mental depression, states of mental excitement, states of mental weakness."[51] These forms were differentiated according to the perceived source and stage of disease and the nature of one's delusions and behavior, leading to more specific diagnoses, such as acute suicidal mania, chronic paralytic dementia, acute puerperal mania, chronic melancholia, dipsoic mania (mania brought on by excessive alcohol consumption), senile dementia, and so forth.

Medical professionals acknowledged that the boundaries between these forms of mental illness were hardly rigid, in terms of either symptoms, etiology, or pathology. The British physician Henry Maudsley, for instance, suggested that, in certain cases, the symptoms of acute melancholia and acute mania were so similar that the diagnosis of one or the other was often "a matter of caprice or accident." Even as he recognized that dementia, melancholia, and mania were discrete mental disorders, Maudsley argued for a developmental relationship between dementia and the other forms of insanity. That is, the longer an individual's mania or melancholia remained untreated, the greater likelihood that his or her abnormal mental state would devolve further into dementia.

Nichols articulated a similar set of ideas about the mercurial nature of both insanity and psychiatrists' understanding of it at the 1862 meeting of AMSAII. "I doubt whether we often meet with cases that belong exclusively to one of the cardinal subdivisions of that disease which are generally made in the text books," he remarked to his colleagues, "unless we mention dementia, which, it may be contended, is rather a negative condition, than a form of positive disease."[52]

For the medical profession, wrote Maudsley, mania, melancholia, and dementia were not so much distinctive "pathological entities" as they were "different degrees or kinds of the degeneration of the mental organization." Nonetheless they had different manifestations. As Maudsley argued, melancholia produced a "great oppression of the self-feeling with corresponding gloomy morbid idea," whereas mania resulted in an "excitement or exaltation of the self-feeling, with corresponding lively expression of it in the character of the thoughts or in the conduct of the patient."[53] Mania could also have more dangerous manifestations than melancholia, at least in terms of the possibility that people suffering from it might harm others. It was the rare person, indeed, who was diagnosed as an acute homicidal melancholic. John Charles Bucknill and Daniel H. Tuke, for instance, associated mania with anger, fear, hatred, and, in general, "malevolent" emotions. "All that can be said is, that one or more of the passions is almost always exalted in mania," they pointed out, "and that a furious condition, although not constituting an essential symptom, is very generally present in the acute form."[54]

The racial differential in Saint Elizabeths' diagnosis rates during the first two decades of its existence indicates that melancholia and mania had not yet been racialized during this period. Although proportionately more African Americans than whites were diagnosed with mania, the prevalence of mania among whites and the infrequency of melancholia diagnoses across both racial groups suggest that neither form of insanity had become associated with any particular race. Mid-nineteenth-century diagnostic criteria were relatively murky, and asylum physicians were more likely to evaluate their patients by their behavior for the purposes of assigning them to appropriate wards than they were to approach their mental illness with the goal of understanding its underlying pathology.[55] As such, the initial diagnoses of Saint Elizabeths patients were unlikely to be made through primarily a biologically determinist lens. In the post-Reconstruction period mania would become more attached to African Americans and melancholia to whites, at least in the medical literature; in the decades surrounding the Civil War, however, no such connections were made. If race played little to no role in diagnoses at Saint Elizabeths, however, the same cannot be said about the hospital's therapeutic regime.

Like most asylum superintendents in the mid-nineteenth century, Nichols subscribed to a moral treatment philosophy. Not possessing a great deal of confidence in the curative possibilities of some of the medical remedies meant to treat mental illness by altering the body's physiological processes—such as hashish, chloroform, and electromagnetism—adherents to this form of therapy stressed the importance of immersing the insane in an environment that was conducive to mental wellness. Mentally ill individuals needed to be removed from the surroundings that contained the source of their mental stress and resocialized to be responsibly functioning members of society. Central to this therapeutic philosophy was the idea that the sooner insanity was identified, the greater the chances that its progress would be arrested. "The curability of insanity," the hospital's 1865–66 annual report indicated, "is in inverse ratio to its duration before proper treatment."[56] In addition to an isolated environment, moral management dictated that patients be placed in a hygienic setting. This meant not only a natural environment free of disease but also a commodious built environment and the conditions necessary for the maintenance of physical health. "Comfortable accommodations, liberal diet and warm clothing now constitute established, settled means of treatment in insanity," Virginia physician John M. Galt wrote in 1850. These "comfortable accommodations" were essentially the accouterments of a respectable, bourgeois household: a library full of virtuous literature, sewing rooms, perhaps a piano.[57]

Nichols exhibited quintessentially Victorian values in his approach to therapy, opposing a "liberal diet" in favor of more parsimonious fare and advocating for more routine employment of patients. His assessment of the American asylum demonstrated that he was committed to a reform ethos, grounded in a New England evangelical temperament that conceptualized the asylum as a home and the superintendent-patient relationship as a paternalistic one.[58] Even though Nichols was committed to the principles of moral management, however, the therapeutic model was not equitably applied across racial lines. To be sure, Nichols expressed the desire to palliate, if not cure, all of the lunatics who crossed the hospital's threshold. But there were limits to his medical altruism. These limits were ultimately imposed by the larger cultural context in which he lived and worked, but this observation does little to deny the fact that the therapeutic regime of the hospital was characterized by racial ambivalence and, in many instances, racism.

Documenting racial discrimination within Saint Elizabeths in the mid-nineteenth century is a challenging project. In the absence of detailed case files, there is very little documentary evidence of the day-to-day interactions between the superintendent, his assistant physicians, attendants, and inmates. Outside of the annual reports and correspondence of the superintendent—with other superintendents, members of the hospital's Board of Visitors, and occasionally inmates' family members—the most accessible archival artifact that allows a glimpse inside the institution is the board's inspection report. Conducted monthly, sometimes by the entire board but most often by two or three of its members, the inspection report was intended to "be an efficient practical means of preventing frauds and abuse from creeping into its service, and also, of affording the medical head that support before the public, under difficulties, to which he is entitled."[59] But the inspection reports were more than this. They also functioned as a legitimating ritual, one whose goal was less to objectively assess the assets and deficiencies of the institution than it was to invest the institution with the cultural authority as arbiter for the treatment of the insane.

Inspection reports occasionally pointed out the work that was being done to improve the conditions of the hospital, but more often than not the reports were filled with some slight variation of the following language with such monotony that it bordered on mantra: "The undersigned Committee of the Board of Visitors, have this day made a tour of inspection of all the buildings and grounds, and take pleasure in reporting the condition of this establishment throughout, to be in the highest degree conducive to its humane design. Perfect order in every department, remarkable cleanliness and as much contentment among the patients as could be expected in their unfortunate state of mind." Board members did interact with inmates during their visits, but any evidence that the latter were less than content, such as inmate complaints, did not undermine the former's confidence in the asylum. "A very few patients, as usual, ask to leave the Hospital," two board members reported in 1873, "but with this exception there is evidently all the contentment possible, and these doubtless complain from the disease that is upon them." Attributing inmates' indignation or expressions of unhappiness to their insanity delegitimized any self-protective behavior that they may have engaged in while simultaneously validating the hospital's therapeutic regime.[60] Rather than approach the board's inspection reports as unproblematic representations of life within Saint Elizabeths, then, we should understand them as self-serving representations of the virtues of institutionalization.[61]

There are also few independent accounts of what confinement in Saint Elizabeths was like for African Americans. In his tour of American insane asylums in 1868, the Scottish physician Alexander Robertson visited the hospital and gave a fairly detailed description of its operation. But he expressed regret that he did not get an opportunity to observe the conditions for African American inmates, although he did not explain why he was unable to do so. It is possible that Nichols or his assistant physicians purposely kept Robertson away from the buildings that housed African American inmates. An editorial writer for the *New National Era*, a Washington newspaper that had been edited by Frederick Douglass until 1872, made the following complaint about Saint Elizabeths in 1873: "When inquiry is made for colored patients they are represented as being so mad as not to admit of being seen." Even though the editorialist did not get an opportunity to visit the colored lodges, he nonetheless wrote about the rumor that African Americans were being treated less well than the white inmates. "This suspicion is aroused," the editorialist explained, "because of the fact that the colored patient is isolated from the white patient; that persons visiting the Asylum are never shown the corner set aside for colored patients, while the commodious and well furnished halls for the white patients are to be seen with the patients surrounded by musical instruments, billiard tables, &c." Reflecting the radical republicanism of Douglass, the editorialist informed his readers that the asylum was "supported by the General Government out of the taxes of all its citizens," and as such, just as the "colored man's rights" were respected in certain government institutions, so too must they be "respected in our Government Insane Asylum."[62]

The hospital's policy of segregation itself can be considered a clear indication of racial discrimination, especially in the wake of the Civil War and emancipation, when black Washingtonians were actively engaging in a battle for equal rights. But even during Radical Reconstruction, when Congress was squarely behind the expansion of citizenship rights for African Americans, there was very little integration of public institutions and accommodations. In the considered opinion of Nichols—and the larger psychiatric community—racial segregation was critical to the long-term prospects of recovery for the mentally ill—or at least mentally ill whites. "It is deemed so essential to the welfare of the insane," the hospital's 1865 annual report stated, "that all their innocent domestic and personal comforts while in a hospital should correspond to those to which they have been accustomed in health, that when civil patients of refinement and liberal education—who 'have seen better days'—are sent to us by the department... we, as far as practicable, make the food and clothing and all the personal relations of such patients conform to their previous habits."[63] Successful treatment depended not only on a healthful physical environment but also on the reproduction of the social environment to which an insane individual had become habituated. As the hospital's report indicated, it was primarily the respectable patients who Nichols and the board thought would most benefit from this mode of therapy. Nonetheless the racial segregation policy dissolved the lines of class within the white civilian inmate population, even as it was based upon a presumption that white inmates had no interracial interactions prior to their institutionalization.

In Nichols's case, this ethnocentric model of therapy combined with a paternalistic philosophy to produce a paradoxical, sometimes contradictory posture toward African American inmates. From the earliest years of Saint Elizabeths' operation, Nichols found himself constantly requesting funds in order to construct more buildings to accommodate African American inmates because he felt the need "to take care of them just as we take care of the other insane."[64] Within three years of the completion of the colored lodge in 1856, he asked for

$10,000 to build another lodge so that African American men and women could be housed separately. This was completely in line with the moral treatment principle of gender segregation. Nichols acknowledged the importance of paying attention to gender difference in the prognosis of black mental illness, calling the situation of African American men and women occupying the same lodge "obviously objectionable." In the spring of 1860 he began overseeing the construction of a lodge for colored females; within a year he expressed confidence that "the interior . . . will be finished" and that this would accomplish "the very desirable separation, in different buildings, of the colored men and women." This separation was short-lived, however. Beginning in the summer of 1861, the colored male lodge, along with the gardener's house, was converted into a naval hospital and the African American male inmates were moved to the colored female lodge. Wounded and sick sailors occupied the male lodge until October 1865, when they were moved to a newly built hospital in the District. Nichols and the board were pleased with the vacating of the male lodge, as the annual report stated, "As soon as some needful repairs can be effected the colored men will be transferred to it from the first story of the lodge for colored women, and the welfare of both sexes will be promoted by their entire separation, and the additional room and freedom each will enjoy."[65]

Nichols was clearly attentive to the housing conditions of African American inmates. But ultimately the resources expended on the buildings for them were a fraction of the overall capital budget of the hospital. In 1875, for instance, he proposed the construction of another building for white female patients that would be at least a third of a mile from the center building and completely closed to white male patients. To be sure, there were fewer African Americans who needed to be housed, so comparing a $10,000 budget for a colored lodge and a $375,000 budget for a building with a capacity of up to 250 white female patients is not prima facie evidence of racial discrimination.[66] But if per-patient cost is considered, then the racial disparities in the hospital's expenditures become clear. The original colored lodge was expected to hold up to twenty individuals. At $12,020, the cost per patient ended up being $600. It is unclear what the expected capacity of the colored male lodge and the renovated colored female lodge was, but by 1876 each housed approximately forty people. Assuming that the hospital kept close to its original budget of $10,000, at worst the cost per patient was $250 and at best $500, but with massive overcrowding. Either way, the cost per patient paled in comparison to the $1,500 per-patient cost associated with the planned separate building for white female patients.

The cost differential is clearly apparent in the use of wood, as opposed to brick, to construct the lodges for African American inmates. Also, the colored lodges did not have a forced-air ventilation system, a standard feature considered "indispensable to give purity to the air of a hospital for the insane" but somewhat expensive to install. Nichols himself admitted the race-based prioritization of the hospital's spending early on, reporting in 1859 that the colored male lodge could "be erected and fitted up at less cost, and with less disturbance of the patients and detriment to the general interests of the hospital, as such, than at any future time."[67] He may very well have been asking for the minimum he thought he would be able to get from Congress and framing his request in language that would have made it more palatable to the kind of members who expressed skepticism of the "doctor's nigger house" a few years earlier. This does little to diminish the larger reality, however, that race played a vitally important role in how the therapeutic regime within the hospital emerged.[68]

The quality of hospital staff and the proper interaction between staff and inmates were other critical components of moral management, and here, as in the case of housing, Nichols inhabited a paradoxical position with regard to his African American charges. The person who was most responsible for the care of the inmates was the superintendent himself. Subordinate to the superintendent were his assistant physicians, the steward, the matron, attendants, and even, according to Isaac Ray, superintendent of Rhode Island's Butler Hospital for the Insane, the superintendent's wife, who, "with her whole heart and strength she sympathizeth with her husband, appreciating the worth of his labors, and upholding his hands."[69] The individuals with whom inmates had the greatest contact were the attendants and, for female patients, the matron.

There were some basic requirements for being employed at Saint Elizabeths as an attendant. Male attendants needed to be strong enough to handle excitable patients yet sufficiently patient and sympathetic to do so with "kindness and good-will." All attendants—indeed all employees—were expected to possess the utmost virtue, including comporting themselves respectably, not interacting with patients of the other sex except under direction of the medical staff, and refraining from the use of alcohol and tobacco. Racial and ethnic background was also an important factor in employing attendants. Andrew McFarland, an Illinois superintendent and AMSAII president in 1860, thought it was less important that hospitals hire attendants who shared the ethnicity of their inmates than it was that attendants be able to identify with the ethnicity, and hence the worldview, of the superintendent. "I cannot say from experience that any nationality more than another—colored races of course being left out—can be relied on to supply us with recruits for this service," he suggested to his colleagues. "Good attendants may unquestionably be made from Teuton, Scandinavian and Celt." While there was some disagreement among superintendents over the wisdom of hiring Irish attendants, there was a general consensus against employing African Americans—except in the South, where, for instance, the superintendent of Tennessee's Hospital for the Insane found that the enslaved women owned by the hospital made "the most excellent attendants on his female department."[70]

The use of bondswomen as attendants, while by no means widespread throughout the South, did not violate the therapeutic principles of the day because it essentially replicated the racial hierarchies that existed outside of the asylum. However, no superintendent, including Nichols, contemplated hiring African American attendants, especially males, who would have exercised some authority over white patients.[71] The preservation of "personal relations," as Nichols wrote in an annual report, mandated that the only interracial encounters in the hospital be between white staff and black inmates. Still, in keeping with his liberal sensibility, Nichols did not countenance overtly racist treatment of patients. Prior to the Civil War, for instance, he extended an offer of employment to a white woman but stressed to her that she should approach her job as attendant with the utmost impartiality. "You better not come if you have any religious, social or sectional prejudices," he wrote to her, "which would interfere with your usefulness and contentment in a community and among patients composed of persons of all colors, religions and nativities."[72]

One reason in particular that dissuaded Nichols and other superintendents from employing African Americans as attendants, particularly in the male wards, was the prospect of their using force to subdue "excitable" patients. The use of mechanical restraint as a form of inmate management was a controversial issue in asylums in the mid-nineteenth century. By the 1840s a movement among British physicians to abolish the use of straitjackets, muffs and mittens (devices used to immobilize a patient's hands), and bed straps had emerged, leading to British criticism of their continued employment by American asylum superintendents. The Americans recognized that mechanical restraint was a less than ideal form of inmate management, but given the large populations of some asylums and the extremely destructive behavior of some patients, they pointed to its utility in extraordinary circumstances. Still, the British position influenced some American physicians who believed that the use of mechanical restraint gave asylums "too much the air of prisons."[73]

For his part, Nichols had concerns about mechanical restraint and used it sparingly.[74] These qualms notwithstanding, he began to employ this particular form of inmate management more regularly as the hospital's population grew. The British physician John Charles Bucknill disapprovingly observed during his tour of American asylums that at Saint Elizabeths there "were eight out of seven hundred and fifty patients under mechanical restraint at the same time." Bucknill did not remark on the racial or gender breakdown of this group, and there is no evidence to suggest that African American patients were subjected to this type of coercive control more than white patients. Nor is there any evidence to suggest that black inmates were placed in isolation with any greater frequency than white inmates. On his visit to Saint Elizabeths in 1868, Alexander Robertson remarked on the extensive use of seclusion rooms to manage acute cases. Apparently he observed only one patient being mechanically restrained, whom he described in the following way: "A man of colour was walking about quietly in the hall adjoining the strong rooms, with his arms firmly secured in stout leather muffs. He was stated to have been violent and excited for six months, and it was considered that it would be dangerous to attempt to dispense with the use of mechanical restraint in his case. They seemed tight about the wrists; but on remarking that, I was assured that they did not chafe the skin."[75]

Again, this anecdotal evidence is too thin to draw any conclusions about whether mechanical restraint was inequitably applied along the lines of race. What is interesting in this case is that the lines of racial segregation broke down among the "excitable" inmate population. The only patients of color who resided in the main building, the only facility that Robertson observed on his visit, were those whose acute conditions warranted their placement alongside other patients considered to be dangerous.[76] The decision to purposefully integrate this particular ward, however, was not just rationalized by the lack of space to achieve racial separation of the most violent inmates, although it was certainly a factor. It was also made more palatable by the larger logic that condoned racial integration among the most degenerate, demented, and dangerous populations. In this sense, the decision was an early manifestation of a broader tendency in the psychiatric profession in the late nineteenth century—within the United States and beyond—to tolerate the blurring of racial boundaries in ways that conflated blackness with depravity and criminality.[77]

In addition to creating a comfortable environment for patients and ensuring that they were attended to by responsible and virtuous staff members, the moral treatment model dictated that the insane be appropriately employed at some useful task. Idle hands left the mind susceptible to morbid and disturbing thoughts, thwarting any possibility of recovery. Yet Nichols was also somewhat circumspect about inmate labor. He cautioned that "compulsory labor" could be just as damaging as it was curative, depending on the state of the inmate's disease. Moreover, Nichols, like most superintendents, saw in labor a dual purpose. On the one hand, "industrial exercise" served as an important therapy, particularly for those individuals who were in the early stages of their insanity. On the other hand, the employment of inmates reduced the labor costs of the hospital. In the latter case, it was primarily the chronic insane whose labor would function as a cost-saving device. But Nichols's belief in the therapeutic value of labor was grounded as much in his bourgeois paternalism as in any medical theory. "If such a sense of the importance of labor as a sanity measure in treating the insane, especially of the working classes, prevailed here as appears to prevail abroad," he claimed, "the *systematic* employment of our patients would probably become a constant feature in the administration of our hospitals, with an improvement in the health, contentment, quietude, cheerfulness, and happiness of their inmates."[78] His singling out of working-class lunatics as being the most in need of the type of labor that predominated in the asylum illustrates the importance of resocialization that lay at the center of this therapeutic model.

There are few records that provide a clear picture of which patients engaged in what kind of work at Saint Elizabeths. Much of the evidence is anecdotal and yields no conclusive information. Like other hospitals, there was a clear gendered division of labor, with male patients working at the hospital's farm, stables, tailor and shoemaker shops, bakery, kitchen, boiler room, and wharf. Women engaged in more domestic chores, such as sewing and laundering. According to Alexander Robertson, employment on the hospital farm was the more coveted form of labor. He estimated that between a quarter and a third of the male inmates worked on the farm.[79] However, there do not appear to be any racial patterns in inmate labor at the hospital. Despite Nichols's mention in an 1858 letter that he had "several black women who can wash very well—can rub all the wrist-bands [and] collars, [etc., and] iron plain garments," there is no definitive evidence that African American female patients were overrepresented in the hospital's laundry during his administration.[80]

Whether racial discrimination existed in other areas of treatment is also a question that requires some speculation. Appropriate forms of leisure were deemed to be critical to therapy, leading asylum staffs to provide opportunities for inmates to engage in various types of recreation. As John Galt suggested, "for several reasons there is a disposition in the insane to have their attention withdrawn to their own mental operations, rather than to enter into any intimate fellowship with each other; amusements tend to break down this wall of separation, and, by arousing social feelings, they wean the morbid spirit from so hurtful an introspection."[81]

Inmates at Saint Elizabeths could expect to be educated and entertained by weekly lectures, musical and dramatic performances, and dances every now and then. Pliny Earle, who occasionally served as one of Nichols's assistant physicians during the Civil War, gave lectures to Saint Elizabeths' inmates on such topics as astronomy, England, Malta, electricity, and "the laws of the beautiful." Some of the lectures were accompanied by a musical performance by the hospital band, which consisted of both patients and staff members, and others were paired with stereopticon presentations, as when patients were treated to a lecture about Pompeii replete with magic-lantern slides. In addition to in-house musical performances, Nichols brought in local groups to entertain the patients. In November 1875, for instance, the Joe Jefferson Dramatic Club, a group affiliated with the legendary comedic actor, performed for the patients and the Board of Visitors.[82] Robertson noted that there were "occasional dances in the winter, but this form of amusement is not held in much estimation." Robertson did not give details as to who held the dances in low esteem, but it was most likely the

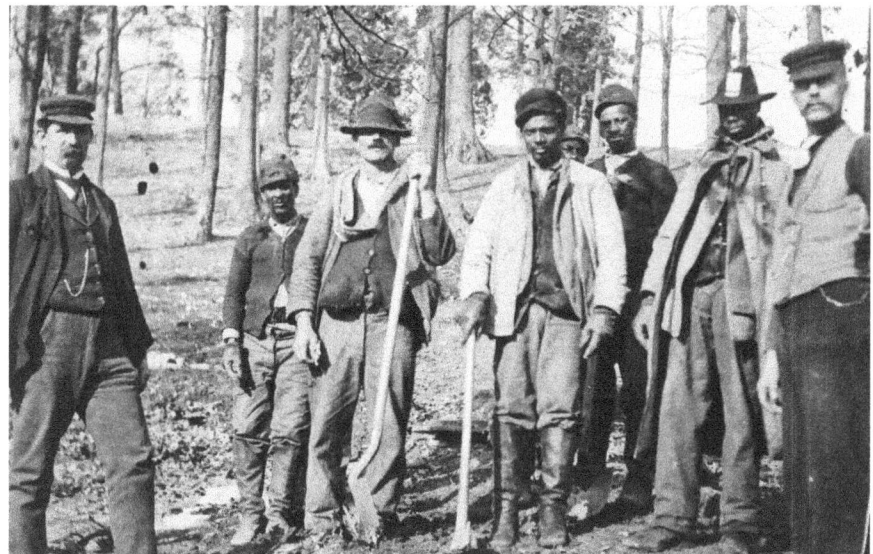

An interracial group of male patients, flanked by two attendants, takes a break from working to pose for a photograph. Whether clearing surrounding forest land for the hospital farm or digging a trench for a water pipe, the labor they engaged in was thought to have a therapeutic benefit. *National Archives, photo 418-L.*

inmates themselves. Most superintendents agreed with Galt's caution against allowing dancing between male and female patients because it had a tendency to "awaken sexual feelings." This kind of Puritanism cloaked in a therapeutic rationale led to the strict supervision of social interaction that would have annoyed adult patients who were self-aware enough to attend a dance in the first place.[83]

Although there is no direct evidence, it is likely that African American inmates were subjected to at least segregation within, if not full exclusion from, the institution's recreational spaces. Galt, one of the foremost promoters of moral management, emphasized the need to separate the races in their living quarters—an aspect of patient life that Nichols strove to achieve; it is difficult to imagine the Saint Elizabeths superintendent not adhering to this principle in the realm of leisure. And there is documentary evidence that forms of recreation in the early to mid-twentieth century—excursions, patient-staged shows, dances—were segregated, and it is unlikely that the racial environment during Nichols's tenure would have been more liberal.[84] At a minimum, hospital staff would have taken measures to separate African Americans from whites in the hospital's chapel or auditorium, just as they separated men and women. But it is entirely possible that African Americans were left in their lodges altogether when Earle gave a lecture on St. Peter's Cathedral or when there was a New Year's Day minstrel show in the hospital chapel.[85] If they had attended the minstrel show, we can only imagine how African American patients would have felt about this racist form of popular culture. For many, it would have likely reinforced for them their doubly marginalized positions as institutionalized people of color.[86]

Even though Saint Elizabeths' therapeutic regime prioritized the mental well-being of white patients, neither African American inmates nor those who were concerned about them placed their welfare solely in the hands of Nichols and his staff. Rather, they engaged moral treatment in a variety of ways. Some family members sought to shape the treatment of their loved ones while others deferred to the medical authority of the superintendent and his assistant physicians. Some patients accepted their new identity as a sufferer of mental illness while others resisted their institutionalization.

Although there were certainly some mentally ill blacks whose institutionalization went unnoticed by anyone but themselves and the hospital staff, there were many whose relatives actively and anxiously monitored their custody. Samuel F. wrote to Nichols at least six times between August 1873 and February 1874 inquiring about his wife, Rosa, who was admitted to Saint Elizabeths in January 1873 suffering from periodic mania. "Will you please to Oblies me by sending me word how my wife . . . is at present[?] Tell her all are well hopeing when These few lines reaches her they may Find her the same as we can say of our selfs."[87] Julius Nelson sent at least fifty-two letters to the hospital staff over a nearly twenty-year period, requesting information about his nephew, Robert F. "Will please let me hear how Robert . . . is for the Day I was there he was in a very poor state of mind," Nelson wrote to the superintendent. Like many of the inmates' relatives, Nelson took a keen interest in his nephew's well-being, sending him clothing and other items that might make his stay more comfortable and asking Nichols to let him "know if you have got them."[88]

Most of the family members of African American inmates who wrote to Nichols did not challenge his medical authority. Archibald Lester was eager to have his mother paroled for a visit after he was "informed that she is now in possession of her usual health and mental faculties." Five days later, in response to a letter from Nichols expressing his desire to keep her in the hospital, Lester accepted the superintendent's assessment. "I shall conform to your judgement and have her remain in the Hospital," he wrote. "If any influence is [brought?] to have her removed while in her present condition you can say it is my wish she should remain."[89] As this letter suggests, Nichols actively kept the families of his patients apprised of their condition and progress. "I received a letter from you once at Willards Hotel stating the condition of my wife," Jacob Foster wrote to Nichols, most likely referring to his place of employment. "And since then I have heard from her through her sisters that were over there last week. And I would be very glad if you would let me know how she is getting along. . . . I have not the time to come over myself and I am very anxious to hear from her."[90]

Some individuals sought to shape the treatment of their institutionalized family members, if only through epistolary requests. Lucinda Callaway, most likely an employee at the House of Representatives, wrote to Nichols to inquire as to whether her grandmother Jane W.'s spiritual needs were being met: "How is Jane ... geting a long now my grand mother is her mine geting better dose the preast to viset her or dose she wish to see a preast she is cathlic." In another letter, Callaway sought to serve as an intermediary between her grandmother and the hospital staff, particularly in the case of her diet. "How is my Grandmother ... is she well in helth how is her mind dose she talk just as much as she uster what is her talk," Callaway inquired. "Will you please see she is kept warm has she a good supplie of cloes to keep her warm Dr please see she gets a plenty to eat she said when I was there she did not get a nuf to eat will come and see her next week if possible would have been to see her but have been sick please [answer] this letter as soon as recived please."[91]

Lucinda's letters are significant on a number of levels. They illustrate a woman who was keenly interested in the mental health of her grandmother. But rather than requesting a general assessment from Nichols, she was eager to hear specifics about the form and content of Jane's communication so that she might judge for herself if her grandmother was improving or getting worse. Lucinda also wanted assurance that the hospital was properly ministering to Jane, reminding Nichols that her grandmother was Catholic and informing him that she suspected Jane was not being sufficiently fed. The letter in which she suggested this was written on the letterhead of the US House of Representatives. It is entirely possible that Lucinda felt that a letter with the imprimatur of the federal government would both secure a prompt response and lead to first-rate treatment of her grandmother. At the very least, she made it clear to Nichols that she would continue to be involved in Jane's care as long as she remained in the custody of the hospital.

Others were even more assertive with the hospital staff. The wife of Joseph D. Harris, admitted to Saint Elizabeths with a diagnosis of chronic epileptic mania, sought to manage her husband's custody and, in doing so, challenged the staff's medical authority. Joseph Harris was an African American physician who had served as the superintendent of two Freedmen's Bureau hospitals in Virginia, an assistant physician at the South Carolina Lunatic Asylum, and a ward physician at Freedmen's Hospital in Washington, DC, before experiencing a seizure in July 1876.[92] Because of some questionable financial decisions he had made, Elizabeth Harris was particularly concerned that he not be allowed to leave the hospital or conduct any business while institutionalized. She was careful to remind the hospital staff that her husband was mentally ill and that any instances of lucidity should not be taken as evidence of his improvement. "Ever since Dr. Harris has been subject to spasms and fits he has been unsafe at home and unfit to transact business," she wrote to assistant physician A. H. Witmer. "He sometimes writes beautiful letters and he talks very well, but he is easily excited and he *is not responsible* for anything he says or does. I hope that you will take every precaution that Dr. H. hold no conversation with anyone from outside, and that no letters from him relating to business or asking to see any one, be allowed to leave your office." Elizabeth Harris persuaded staff members to share with her any letters her husband had written before mailing them off. In one communication she sent to Nichols's successor, W. W. Godding, she expressed gratitude that she was able to see his letters. "Such expressions give one no idea of his condition, and result in no good," she stated. "Indeed, his letters abroad are generally *so well written* as to *mislead* his friends *as to the state of his health*."[93] She was invested in keeping her husband confined to Saint Elizabeths so that he would not squander any more of her family fortune. In order to ensure his continued institutionalization, she interposed herself between her husband the sufferer and the trained personnel who had the medical knowledge to treat him.

Perhaps it was necessary for her to do so. Joseph Harris was what many superintendents and asylum physicians would probably have considered a difficult patient—not because he was particularly violent or dangerous but because he constantly challenged the terms of his institutionalization. In November 1876, for instance, he wrote to Nichols requesting an eleven-day parole, which was permitted under a hospital policy that ranged from granting patients short-term visiting privileges with families to allowing patients to wander the hospital grounds without being accompanied by an attendant. Harris wanted time away from the hospital in order to spend Thanksgiving at home as well as to attend a session of Congress. In his letter, he positioned himself both as a respectable citizen and as an inheritor of the radical self-assertiveness of black abolitionists. "Frederick Douglass said he prayed two years for freedom but never received it until he prayed with his *legs* also," Harris remarked. "And so, also, while I have prayed for your and my divine guidance in this matter I concluded to pray again with my *pen*." He displayed in this letter and others a sense of entitlement, undoubtedly encouraged by his status as a pay patient but perhaps also by his sense of belonging to a confraternity of doctors. The fact that he was a civil independent patient whose board was most likely paid by his wife explains the influence she had on the hospital's treatment of him. But his status also merited a more flexible parole policy, even though it did not entirely satisfy him. On one occasion, the doctor had obtained permission to go into Washington City in order to tend to some business but was prevented from bringing the matter to a close because of the hospital's curfew. This prompted a letter to Nichols that barely obscured Harris's indignation behind his complaisant language: "*Next day* I asked permission to return to the city, *without inconvenience to the Hospital*, but as yet have received no answer. Now, if there be rules preventing my going to the City as occasion requires, I most respectfully beg leave to inquire what is necessary to obtain my discharge?"[94]

In other communications with Nichols, Harris's identity as a physician came to the fore. In one letter he felt the need to revisit a conversation he had had with Nichols in order to establish his own medical authority. "When you unexpectedly called yesterday I had just been exhausted by too much exercise in walking over the grounds [and] up the stairs," he explained to the superintendent. "I beg you will forget my last [parting?] note. The cause of it has been removed. *Petit mal* is, of course, my present disease. I meant to say the cause of my coming here was something more called 'sun-stroke.'" In the same letter Harris requested a meeting with the surgeon general the next time he should visit Saint Elizabeths. It is not clear whether Harris knew John Woodworth, but it is not improbable, given his experience at various federal medical facilities during Reconstruction. As such, it is difficult to say whether Harris's request was motivated by the desire to see an old acquaintance or something else, such as to lodge a complaint about his confinement. If the latter, it would have done him no good, given that the US Marine Hospital Service had no jurisdiction over Saint Elizabeths. Nonetheless his appeal for an audience with the nation's highest-ranking medical officer and his nonchalant comment that cast his relationship with Nichols as one between peers rather than doctor and patient, are both telling. Ultimately his wife succeeded in making sure that he never got out of Saint Elizabeths, but Harris would continue to assert his citizenship status and professional identity in order to take back some of the control the institution and his wife had over him.[95]

Other inmates sought their release from the hospital through even more confrontational means. One of these was Emily S., a thirty-seven-year-old woman from Virginia who was admitted to the hospital in September 1869 with a diagnosis of chronic melancholia. She was released approximately six months later as "improved." In the late 1880s she ended up in Freedmen's Hospital, and an investigation into a staff physician's abuse of patients provides some clue as to why she was released from Saint Elizabeths twenty years earlier. Dr. Charles B. Purvis was charged with hitting Emily in the face and throwing her to the floor. It is not clear whether Emily herself accused Purvis, but the investigative board sought specific information about her time at Saint Elizabeths in order to help it adjudicate the charge. Godding, who was an assistant physician at the time, provided to the board a transcript of a portion of Emily's medical record. According to the record, she had been a patient at Freedmen's Hospital before winding up at Saint Elizabeths and had exhibited a particular pattern of interacting with the staff and her fellow patients. "This girl appeared to be a bright, intelligent girl of the best class of house servants," the record indicated. "Complained that she had been maltreated by the nurses at the Freedman's Hospital. Soon began to complain in the same way of the help here. Fussy and particular about everything. Worked some at the laundry but thought she was abused by everybody; would weep and lament about herself and her hard lot." Emily had expressed a desire to leave the hospital and live with her brother in Texas. When it became apparent that her brother would not be in a position to support her, Emily turned to her sister, a resident of the District. Nichols and his assistant physicians reported that Emily was "improved somewhat and . . . harmless" and agreed to release her into her sister's custody.[96]

We do not know exactly what happened between Emily and the nurses and physicians at either Freedmen's Hospital or Saint Elizabeths. Nor do we know, if the accusations were false, whether they were manifestations of Emily's mental illness or a conscious attempt to register her discontent with being institutionalized. Perhaps it was a combination of the two, her depressive state shaping the way she perceived her interactions with the staff and her belief that any slight that went unchallenged gave the institution more power over her. It is actually not clear who had more power in this situation. Certainly Nichols had the prerogative power of the state on his side, in that he could deploy the instruments of local and federal government—the law, the bureaucracy, and the police—to confine Emily as long as he considered it necessary. On the other hand, it is entirely possible that Emily's nettlesome behavior forced Nichols's hand and caused him to prematurely release her as "improved somewhat" rather than "recovered." What Emily's case does suggest is that patients and physicians engaged in a struggle in which neither had exclusive possession of the upper hand.[97]

The End of the Nichols Era

In the last eight years of his administration, Nichols was the target of two investigations. He survived a Board of Visitors investigation that was triggered by an exposé in the *Saturday Evening Visitor* in 1869 that purportedly uncovered his mismanagement of the hospital.[98] Renewed troubles for Nichols began in the summer of 1875, when the *New York Times* reported that Saint Elizabeths had abandoned three of the hospital's patients in Maryland. The "three demented creatures" who were driven to Maryland by two officers of the Metropolitan Police Department were only a few of the many who had been unceremoniously turned out of the hospital, according to the newspaper. "It is said that patients have been frequently given in charge of the Police," the *Times* alleged, "taken in the cars to the larger cities North, and abandoned upon their arrival at the depot, their custodians sneaking away and leaving their victims without even the means to obtain a meal or a night's shelter." To the newspaper, Saint Elizabeths was emblematic of the corruption associated with the Republican administration of Ulysses S. Grant. It acknowledged that some of the abandoned patients were most likely not residents of the District and the hospital was merely returning them to their home state. Yet the newspaper could not help but wonder why the $150,000 congressional appropriation to provide for the indigent insane was not enough to take care of the few "who may be discovered here [Washington, DC] without known residences and sent there for treatment by competent authority."[99]

The charges prompted an inspection of the hospital by the House Committee on the Army and Navy. After the committee failed to turn up any evidence of maltreatment of patients or of institutional mismanagement, the House Committee on Expenditures in the Department of the Interior began an investigation. Several months of fact-finding and witness testimony produced a harrowing image of life inside Saint Elizabeths. Inmates were allegedly manhandled by sadistic attendants; served spoiled meat and rotten produce; kept in overcrowded, cold, and vermin-infested rooms; and not given sufficient clothing. Witnesses also claimed that Nichols spent more time away from the hospital than he did tending to his patients. One former female attendant alleged that during her employment there was a stretch of three months in which he did not visit the wards where she worked. To make matters worse, several witnesses suggested that Nichols and his staff duped the Board of Visitors into thinking that the hospital was well-run by sprucing it and the patients up right before the monthly inspections.[100]

Nichols and his supporters mounted a defense in both the congressional hearings and in the court of public opinion. They challenged the credibility of the accusers, the witnesses, the congressmen supporting the investigation, and the press.[101] His supporters pointed out that many of the problems in the hospital stemmed from overcrowding, over which Nichols had little control. When more than 700 people were crammed into a space with a capacity of 550, patients were bound to be underserved and management techniques were destined to occasionally become crude. Nichols's defenders deflected the charges of mistreatment of patients back on the government and suggested that it was federal policy—in both admissions and resource management—that was ultimately the cause of the hospital's problems. As long as Saint Elizabeths was required to admit insane paupers who were not residents of the District—a policy that Nichols had supported during the Civil War—then officials and the press should not be surprised when the hospital discharged and returned patients to their home states once their residency was determined. In the meantime it was the federal government's responsibility to provide sufficient funding to accommodate the large number of patients in Saint Elizabeths, a perennial reminder delivered in the hospital's annual reports. In the end, the evidence provided by Nichols's defense swayed the committee, and it issued a finding that exonerated Nichols of corruption, mismanagement, and mistreatment of patients.[102]

But exoneration did not make life easier for Nichols. Congress continued to ignore his pleas for funds to construct a building for female patients—which would have addressed the "evils of great overcrowding." In fact an 1877 appropriations bill recommended cuts of more than $9,000 to the proposed budget for patient care (from $154,583 to $145,000) and $20,000 to the proposed budget for general upkeep and repairs (from $25,000 to $5,000). In a letter to the chairman of the appropriations committee, the Board of Visitors cautioned, "The very closest economy will be necessary in order to make the inmates of this Institution here justly provided for by law, simply comfortable and give them such medical and moral treatment as their welfare requires."[103] But Nichols was no longer interested in employing "the very closest economy." After spending twenty-five years planning the hospital, overseeing its construction, and serving as its superintendent, he had no desire to continue to try to make Saint Elizabeths a beacon of psychiatric care with such anemic support. Approximately a year after the conclusion of the investigation, he resigned his position and returned to head the hospital in which his career began: Bloomingdale Asylum. Taking his place was William Whitney Godding, one of his former assistant physicians, who had left the hospital in 1870 to become superintendent of the Massachusetts Hospital for the Insane in Taunton.[104] Godding would oversee the growth of the hospital—both its inmate population and the campus itself—and his superintendency would coincide with the emergence of a particularly racialized concept of black insanity, which would also shape the ways that African American inmates at Saint Elizabeths were managed.

3

"From Slave to Citizen"

Race, Insanity, and Institutionalization in Post-Reconstruction Washington, DC, 1877–1900

In the late 1880s the Australian physician George A. Tucker published *Lunacy in Many Lands*, an encyclopedic volume containing information on scores of asylums that he had visited in the first half of the decade. In addition to his personal observations, excerpts from annual reports, and texts of lunacy legislation, Tucker included the responses that superintendents gave to a survey he had distributed. Saint Elizabeths was one of the asylums that Tucker toured. Perhaps it was the hospital's location in the upper South or the sizable African American population in the District in the 1880s that prompted Tucker to inquire whether Saint Elizabeths' superintendent had observed an increase in the prevalence of insanity among the "coloured," but his response was very telling. "Very marked," W. W. Godding claimed, "I think largely growing out of their emancipation. Washington was a city of refuge to which contrabands flocked during the war, and the entire change in their modes of life, the added cares, the new ambitions awakened, the struggle for existence under circumstances by no means the most favourable, all the trials of the transition period from slave to citizen without the advantage that in time may be expected to accrue from the latter; all of these have had their effect in greater mental strain and consequent increase of insanity."[1] Godding was so certain that emancipation had contributed to the mental distress of African Americans that he answered in the affirmative Tucker's question as to whether there was an increase in insanity in the District "beyond the increase in population." Although he suspected that this was the case with whites as well—it was difficult to state so definitively because of the District's high rate of transiency—he was without a doubt when it came to the city's black residents.[2]

Godding's response to Tucker's survey reflected a prominent strain within the national debate over the "Negro problem" in the postemancipation era.

A population that had overwhelmingly been enslaved, African Americans were not deemed equal by whites of any political persuasion, despite their nominal citizenship after 1868. The general consensus among whites—northern and southern, Republican and Democrat—was that freedpeople were incapable of adapting to their new civil status without the assistance of their more civilized counterparts. That assistance could range, depending on where one fell on the ideological spectrum, from advocacy of industrial education to compulsory labor. Alongside this "new paternalism" existed a more malevolent attitude toward African Americans, one that considered them to be completely incapable of surviving and flourishing outside of the relationships of dependency that slavery had engendered. Without the security of bondage, this line of thinking went, freedpeople would revert to their savage ancestral past and eventually become extinct, potentially rending the social fabric of the nation in the process. The child-like negro would prefer engaging in criminal activity to honest labor, would easily allow his vote to be manipulated by corrupt political parties, and would mistake his political power for a license to sexually assault white women. Along with segregation, which also ultimately became a cornerstone of the new paternalism, disfranchisement and extralegal violence purportedly functioned as safeguards against the regressing African American.[3]

Proponents of this particular postemancipation narrative pointed to increased rates of crime and disease among African Americans as evidence of their inability to adjust to their new lives as free people.[4] An alleged epidemic of rapes and attempted rapes of white women in the late nineteenth century was taken to indicate the utter lack of self-control of the negro, a problem that was best solved by lynching and more community-engulfing violence, such as the race riots in Wilmington, North Carolina in 1898 and New Orleans in 1900. From a disease standpoint, according to this narrative, the higher incidence of tuberculosis and syphilis within black communities revealed the inherently weaker constitutions of African Americans and, not coincidentally, reinforced the southern apologist argument that slavery had been a benevolent and salutary institution.

In addition to growing rates of certain somatic diseases, as Godding's answer to Tucker reveals, the medical community suggested that increased diagnoses of insanity were further telltale signs that freedom ultimately had a deleterious effect on African American health. Freedpeople, the argument went, were ill equipped to handle the stresses and strains that were natural to an existence in the competitive, modern world. Within this logic, insanity was still largely defined as a disease of civilization, a refrain that would continue into the early twentieth century. As asylum physicians continued to conceptualize mental illness as an affliction of the most cerebrally advanced races, its growing presence within a race that was supposedly in the process of becoming more primitive presented a theoretical problem concerning the etiology of insanity. One of the ways they sought to resolve this contradiction was to deploy an evolutionary argument that emphasized racial degeneracy and the lack of civilizational advancement of people of African descent. Degeneration, rather than evolution, became the principal explanatory model for increasing rates of black insanity.

The emergence and growing influence of neurology underpinned this argument. By the 1870s advances in understanding brain anatomy and the central nervous system had contributed to the development of a medical field that challenged the hegemony of the physician-superintendents associated with the birth of the antebellum asylum. Neurologists did not depart from the materialist understanding of mental illness that had shaped antebellum psychiatry; rather, they attributed the physiological origins of mental illness to damage to the nervous system. Influenced by a European model of scientific and clinic-based medicine and gaining experience from their work with wounded Civil War soldiers, neurologists claimed greater medical expertise in the study and treatment of insanity. While there was a fairly caustic public split between prominent neurologists and asylum physicians in the 1870s and 1880s, most of the recriminations were motivated by differing opinions on the relative importance of asylum management and scientific research rather than the causes of mental disease. Insanity continued to be understood as having its roots in the physical nature of the brain and nervous system.[5]

The reduction of mental disease to a physical foundation fit well with the late nineteenth-century Darwinian and hereditarian focus on the biological essence of race and ethnicity. Ideas about evolution, group competition, and the hereditary nature of disease crept into asylum physicians' and neurologists' explanations of insanity, and particularly its various racial dimensions. Moreover, as these theories increasingly became frameworks for explaining poverty, mental defectiveness, criminality, abnormal sexuality, and other types of social deviance, the medical profession easily framed insanity among African Americans within these contexts.[6] To be sure, African Americans were not alone in this analysis; the Irish were a group in whom asylum physicians and neurologists were especially interested when they explored the relationship between race and mental illness. In the case of African Americans, insanity was racialized in a way that reproduced prevailing cultural notions of blacks as an ignorant, primitive, criminally prone people who were incapable of adjusting to, much less thriving in, modern America.

This racialization of insanity shaped the experiences of African American patients at Saint Elizabeths. The medical profession developed a new preoccupation with black insanity in the 1880s and 1890s, departing significantly from the antebellum consensus that people of African descent were immune to mental disease. From the late 1860s to the turn of the century, insane asylums throughout the South began admitting more blacks into segregated wards, and several states began constructing mental hospitals exclusively for African Americans.[7] By the 1880s the number of African American patients in Saint Elizabeths began to approach their percentage in the District's total population. The increased presence of blacks on the hospital's wards coincided with a growing tendency within the medical profession to characterize the typical mentally ill African American as more depraved and dangerous than the average insane white. This had always been the case, but the assertion was increasingly expressed in clinical language that associated black insanity with mania. This characterization of black insanity ultimately influenced how African American patients were housed and treated in the hospital.

Even though the attribution of increasing rates of insanity among African Americans to freedom and racial degeneration came to reflect the medical profession's approach to the "Negro problem," actual institutionalization was the result of a host of interactions between, and complex calculations made by, local authorities, hospital staff, and family and community members. When African Americans decided to institutionalize their loved ones, sought the hospital superintendent's advice about the propriety of bringing relatives home for a short visit, or requested that they be retrieved and returned to the hospital, they were not only acknowledging the superintendent's medical authority. In turning to Saint Elizabeths to assist them in managing, protecting, and providing for their relatives, African Americans were also employing the state as an important resource.[8] Many black Washingtonians relied on the institution to address problems that were internal to their families and their communities, even as their own particular social locations—including the circumstances under which their family members were admitted to the hospital, their class position, their understanding of insanity, and so forth—led to different engagements with the hospital. Though they did not employ a language of civic equality, African Americans who interacted with Saint Elizabeths demonstrated a "rights consciousness" in a new era of black citizenship.[9]

A "Natural Access of Insanity": Explaining Black Mental Illness

Although the idea that general emancipation might serve as a catalyst for insanity began to appear in medical literature with some frequency in the 1870s, reaching a crescendo by the mid-1880s, perhaps its first serious articulation was delivered about eighteen months into the Civil War. In the October 1862 issue of the *American Journal of Insanity*, A. O. Kellogg, the assistant physician at New York's Utica State Lunatic Asylum, published an article exploring the themes of insanity and "mental imbecility" in William Shakespeare's *The Tempest*. At the center of Kellogg's analysis was the character of Caliban, the monstrous figure who was intelligent enough to learn language from Prospero but whose naturally libidinous instinct led him to attempt to defile Prospero's daughter, Miranda. Kellogg drew parallels between the relationship between Caliban and Prospero and the relationship between enslaved people and slaveholders in the American South. In a somewhat tortured interpretation of the play, he created two different images of the beastly character that conveniently resembled the contrasting representations of enslaved people that would come to dominate the mythology of the Lost Cause. Some of the "modern Calibans" were the bondspeople who, recognizing the superiority of their masters, demonstrated their fealty through their "readiness to fight for them." The other modern Caliban, which conformed more closely to Shakespeare's character, was the rebellious bondsperson, the contraband who disregarded his natural state of bondage and threw his lot in with the Union troops. "The savage and uncultivated nature of both" Caliban and the rebellious enslaved African American, Kellogg claimed, "made desperate by the years of degrading and abusive servitude, shows itself in the outrages they are ready to commit, when suffered to act unrestrained by the superior intelligences, that have enslaved them and made them beasts of burden."

Even though Kellogg displayed some paternalistic sympathy for enslaved African Americans, ultimately he implied that their release from bondage would have an adverse impact on both themselves and the South at large. While he did not delve deeply into insanity as a specific disease entity, he suggested that emancipation had profound implications for the mental health of blacks, concluding his article with the assertion that the "further consideration of this parallelism between the savage of the poet's imagination and the real Calibans of the actual and the present, would open an interesting chapter in comparative psychology."[10] Whether he was referring to the utility of comparing the psychology of blacks and whites or real people and fictional characters Kellogg did not say.

The presence of insanity among the general American population in the last quarter of the nineteenth century was a matter of some concern for the medical profession and interested observers. The 1880 census of the "dependent, defective, and delinquent classes" documented a marked increase in the number of insane over the previous decade, a much greater increase than in any other decade since the government had begun enumerating this population in 1840. The number of insane Americans had increased a remarkable 145 percent between 1870 and 1880, as opposed to an average of 54.5 percent during the two preceding decades. Although the census's compiler, Frederick Wines, thought the data were misleading due to undercounting in 1850 and 1860, the figures were nonetheless cited by some psychiatrists to illustrate the relationship that many drew between mental illness and modernity.[11]

Judson Andrews, the superintendent of the State Asylum for the Insane in Buffalo, New York, for instance, pointed to the census data in a speech before the Ninth International Medical Congress in which he averred that "the general principle is established that the amount of insanity bears a close relation to the duration of the social and governmental life of the people." Wines himself invoked modernity in his attempt to explain the relationship among insanity, criminality, poverty, and mental defect, and Saint Elizabeths' Board of Visitors resignedly expressed a similar sentiment as it coped with what it perceived to be a disproportionate increase in insanity, a perception no doubt enhanced by the growing number of admissions to the hospital. "It still remains a fact that insanity has come into our civilization to stay and to be provided for," the hospital's 1894 annual report declared. "This is a penalty that we pay for modern intellectual development with its intenser activities of brain and nerve, its high-pressure modes of business with artificial ways of life, and its fierce struggle for existence with the stern law of the survival of the fittest controlling the issue."[12]

The prevailing antebellum belief that whites were more susceptible to mental disease than nonwhites continued to dominate psychiatric thought and was confirmed by the raw data of the 1880 census.[13] Nonetheless, as more and more African Americans required institutionalization—leading, for instance, to the construction of colored asylums in Tennessee in 1865, Virginia in 1869, and North Carolina in 1880—physicians began to speculate about the causes behind this veritable epidemic of insanity. For many, this speculation amounted to little more than a retrospective defense of the benevolence of slavery. A proliferation of articles with titles such as "The Effects of Emancipation upon the Mental and Physical Health of the Negro of the South," "The Increase of Insanity and Tuberculosis in the Southern Negro Since 1860, and Its Alliance, and Some of the Supposed Causes," and "The Effect of Freedom upon the Physical and Psychological Development of the Negro," left little doubt where their authors stood on the question of whether slavery had been beneficial for African Americans, their typical claim that they were reconstructed southerners notwithstanding.[14]

But this particular narrative had wider purchase within the medical profession. The esteemed neurologist William A. Hammond, a Pennsylvanian who served as the surgeon general of the Union army during the Civil War, drew a causal relationship between freedom and rising rates of insanity among African Americans.[15] As such, the narrative reinforced the psychiatric theory that mental illness was a product of civilization more than it undermined earlier ideas that races had particular constitutional predispositions toward insanity or mental health. Indeed culture and biology would awkwardly coexist in both asylum physicians' and neurologists' attempts to explain the presence of insanity in the African American population.

Regardless of what role asylum physicians and neurologists assigned to culture and biology, they generally attributed the increased rates of mental illness among African Americans to their inability to successfully compete with whites. As freedpeople became responsible for providing for themselves and protecting their own citizenship rights and political interests, the nervous strain accompanying their day-to-day struggle accumulated to the point that many were driven insane. In addressing "the undeniable increase of crime, pauperism, and insanity among negroes *since* the war," the superintendent of a Chicago insane asylum and a prolific author on race and mental illness argued that group competition was mainly responsible. "The negro is expected to combat with the white in the struggle for existence much more in Chicago than in New York," James G. Kiernan wrote in 1885. "He has imbibed the speculative spirit of the former city, to the lack of which his race owed its relative immunity from paretic dementia" prior to the war.[16] Whereas a Darwinian conception of group development underpinned the growing consensus about black insanity, medical professionals moved between culture and biology as the phenomenon's principal underlying cause. What unified these two disparate agents for physicians was the idea that neither had substantially evolved in the case of African Americans.

When asylum physicians pointed to the role of culture in producing insanity, they understood it to be connected to, but to also operate independently of, biology and race. They equated culture with the level of social, economic, and political development of any particular group, which accounted for different propensities toward mental illness *within* races. This allowed Judson Andrews, for instance, to explain the lower rates of insanity among whites in the southern and western regions of the United States. The 1880 census figures, he noted, "emphasize the statement that the pioneers of our newer settlements are the more hardy and vigorous citizens, and that the feeble and dependent are left in their former homes, to enjoy the comforts of the hospitals and asylums, which are the special growth of the older civilization."[17] In a great many physicians' estimation, civilization was the sum total of cultural development and it posed the greatest threat to mental health where cultural development was most accelerated and condensed: the city.

In this sense, emancipation and the increasing movement of former bondspeople from plantations and rural areas provided a logical explanation for why there was a pronounced increase of insanity among African Americans. This theory was propounded by the editor of the *American Journal of Insanity* in a précis of an article by the Mississippi physician J. M. Buchanan that originally appeared in the *New York Medical Journal*. Emphasizing the postemancipation movement of blacks even more than Buchanan, the editor posited that "there is [a] great tendency among them to huddle together in cities and towns, and to neglect all provident care and labor for future necessities in favor of present amusements and dissipation." In addition to the emotionalism of their religious worship, the editor continued, the new environment that encouraged decadence "would tend to produce in the southern negroes the natural access of insanity which the statistics go to prove."[18]

Henry Hurd, superintendent of the Eastern Michigan Asylum near Detroit, made a similar point in his discussion of general paresis, a disorder, alternately called paretic dementia and general paralysis of the insane, which was variously characterized by depression, euphoria, loss of muscle coordination, delusions, and progressive dementia. "Prior to the emancipation of the colored race, cases of general paresis among them were unknown," Hurd declared. "After the war when the colored people crowded into cities, took up new conditions of living and began the struggle for existence in competition with a more highly cultured race, the disease developed and is rapidly increasing."[19]

When physicians expounded this line of thinking, they generally pointed to the failure of people of African descent to evolve culturally as the main factor contributing to their mental deterioration once they moved to more civilized environments. As such, the close proximity of African Americans to Africans in evolutionary time figured prominently in their discussion of black insanity in the postemancipation period. J. F. Miller, the superintendent of North Carolina's asylum for the colored insane, invoked this as more or less a remote cause, an underlying condition that increased the likelihood that African Americans would succumb to the inciting causes of mental illness: "A native of Africa and a savage a few generations ago, then a slave for several generations afterwards; this is the man and the race upon whom the high responsibilities of freedom were thrust; a nation literally born in a day." The failure to completely evolve past a state of savagery, despite more than two centuries of enslavement in the West, made African Americans more susceptible to the stresses of modern life.[20]

One of the assistant physicians at Saint Elizabeths, A. H. Witmer, expressed the same sentiment, albeit in a more subtle way. Addressing the topic before the International Medical Congress in Berlin in 1891, Witmer explained the surge in insanity diagnoses among African Americans as having its origins in an undeveloped culture. "Untutored in a knowledge of the world, and without a sound philosophy or a religion deeper seated than the emotions to sustain them in adversity," Witmer asserted, "many minds have failed under the constant strain of their advancing civilization." While Witmer's reference to civilization was a bit ambiguous in this passage, he ended his speech in a way that left no doubt as to whose civilization he meant. "Behold the West to-day!" he exulted. "The empire of intellect as exemplified in the nineteenth century, in its march has held its true course, until the civilization of the occident encroaches upon the barbaric customs and traditions of the orient, pushing them to the wall and dragging them from the temples."[21] To primitive peoples, civilization could be insanity-inducing and quite deadly. Indeed existing alongside the postemancipation narrative about African American insanity was a similar one about mental illness in Africa, in which European civilization was credited with producing insanity among native Africans.[22]

Miller's reference to African Americans as a "nation" in his *North Carolina Medical Journal* article revealed that he was thinking of them as a culture as much as, if not more than, a biologically determined racial group. Admittedly this is a fine distinction to draw in analyzing racial thought in the late nineteenth century, but it was a distinction that some medical experts made. The neurologist Hammond, for instance, acknowledged the difference between the two when he took up the issue of race in his 1883 textbook. Even as he advanced the idea that freedom increased African Americans' "liability to insanity," he held on to the truism that blacks were largely immune to mental illness. Hammond forthrightly confessed that medical professionals were unsure about how much their "immunity is the result of the racial factor, and how much is due to the differences in the mode of life, the degree of activity of the mind, etc." He went on to throw his considerable intellectual opinion behind the cultural argument. "It is certainly true that barbarous nations do not exhibit so strong a tendency to mental alienation as do those that are civilized," Hammond wrote, "but this simply [is] because they are barbarous, and not because they belong to different races." But even with his nod to the primacy of culture, Hammond could not completely disregard the role of race, as a biologically grounded essence, in shaping African Americans' so-called immunity. Despite the fact that the enslaved negro had "been subjected to humanizing and civilizing influences [and] his animal wants . . . supplied," he contended, "except in cases of a mixing of the blood, he presents the same aspects as his progenitors, whose representatives are figured on the mountains of ancient Egypt erected three thousand years ago." To even more succinctly express his belief in the substantiality of race, Hammond concluded, "Certainly within the historic period there has been no change in the characteristics of the white, yellow, brown, and black races of mankind."[23]

Given his background in neurology, it is not at all surprising that Hammond came back to biology—and a framework of Darwinian evolution—as a way of understanding the incidence of insanity among African Americans. As physicians who were influenced by the clinic- and science-based medicine associated with the French and German medical professions, respectively, neurologists reduced mental illness to the abnormal development of or damage to the brain and the nervous system. Where asylum superintendents grouped inmates according to their behaviors rather than their diseases and employed problematic classification schemes, neurologists argued that successful intervention in the progression of mental illness required an intimate knowledge of brain anatomy and the physiological functions of the nervous system. The abnormal behavior that individuals suffering from both psychoses and neuroses exhibited was merely a manifestation of an underlying brain or neural pathology. One of the most renowned American neurologists, Edward C. Spitzka, clearly expressed this idea in the 1880s. "It is inaccurate to state that insanity is itself a disease," he wrote. "It is, strictly speaking, merely a symptom which may be due to many different morbid conditions, having this one feature in common: that they involve the organ of the mind."[24]

While asylum physicians recognized that heredity played a role in predisposing individuals to insanity, neurologists were more willing to contemplate the possibility that insanity-inducing brain lesions themselves could be inheritable. In the etiological paradigms of the mid-nineteenth-century asylum physicians, the mental illness of someone's forebears might serve as a remote cause that set the preconditions for their descent into madness, a descent that still needed to be triggered by an inciting cause such as religious excitement or excessive study. For late nineteenth-century neurologists, it was possible for someone to be born insane, just as social scientists were beginning to identify the innate criminal or the congenital prostitute. Heredity itself was capable of producing the pathological structure of the brain or the abnormal functioning of the nerves. As such, neurologists believed, evolution played a critical role in the increasing incidence of insanity in the United States and other Western nations. In foregrounding the role of heredity and evolution, they subscribed to the concept of degeneration, the theory that hereditary neurological deterioration was responsible for much of the insanity, mental defectiveness, and deviancy that existed in society.[25]

For medical professionals, academics, government officials, and cultural commentators, degeneration posed an existential threat to the nation. The decadence, moral laxity, and torpidity engendered by modern civilization had the potential to strip the dominant races of their intellectual, spiritual, and physical strength. Concerns about losing their superiority to the lower classes were expressed by elites in European, North American, and Latin American countries. Degeneration undermined national strength at a time when Western nations were vying with one another to extend their international power through the acquisition of territory and overseas markets. While biology and culture interacted in interesting ways—in the sense that an ancestor's culturally deviant behavior could indelibly imprint his or her distant descendant with the physical stigmata of degeneracy—national elites generally understood degeneration to be a biological phenomenon with terrible implications for national culture and racial integrity.[26]

By the 1880s and 1890s another concept of degeneration circulated within medical and intellectual circles, positing that African Americans were on the verge of extinction due to their inability to physically adjust to modern society. Heredity figured prominently in some degeneracy theorists' explanations. The "savage" behavior of their ancestors, once kept in check by the "benevolent" institution of slavery, was reappearing in the newly emancipated negro with greater frequency. Atavism, or reversion to type, these theorists argued, increasingly characterized the African American population.[27]

The myth of black immunity to insanity persisted in the thought of some neurologists and asylum physicians, even as they embraced a biological and hereditarian framework for understanding the causes of mental disease. R. M. Bucke, a Canadian physician and superintendent of London, Ontario's insane asylum, for example, employed evolutionary logic to explain what he perceived to be a racial differential in the susceptibility to insanity. Reminiscent of faculty psychology,[28] he claimed that the human mind comprised mental powers that were segregated into bundles: an intellectual bundle that governed self-consciousness, cognition, creativity, and memory; a moral nature bundle that regulated the human capacity to love, hate, fear, and venerate; and a sensory bundle that controlled visual, aural, olfactory, gustatory, and tactile perception. These bundles, moreover, did not evolve at the same pace either within or across races. Bucke collapsed Australian aborigines and people of African descent (including "Bushmen" and American negroes) into a primitive typology against which to measure the predisposition of the civilized Aryan race toward insanity.

Utilizing recapitulation theory, the idea that the evolution of the individual human organism repeated the evolutionary patterns of the race, Bucke asserted that the intellectual faculties of the Aryan had evolved more rapidly than other races. While Bushmen and aborigines had attained self-consciousness, for instance, the other elements of the intellectual bundle, such as genius, were evolving more quickly among Aryans. But this rapid evolution posed a problem. As Aryans experienced a more accelerated evolution of the higher faculties, they were the "most subject to breakdowns." This thought was consistent with neurologists' analogizing of the minds of more civilized races to complex forms of machinery, which were susceptible to complete malfunction in the event that any one component failed. To support his point, Bucke reminded his readers of the truism of insanity and blacks in the United States. "I suppose very few would claim that the negro mind is advancing at anything like the same rate" as people of northern European descent, he wrote. "As a consequence of these different rates of progression we have in the Aryan people of America a much higher percentage [of mental illness] than is found in the negro race."[29]

Spitzka, too, invoked evolutionary theory to explain the relative absence of mental illness among African Americans, although, to a greater extent than Bucke, he acknowledged the interaction between biology and environment as an important etiological factor. The noted neurologist broached the subject of race in his discussion of paretic dementia. He identified it as a neurological disease that could be directly traced back to "diffuse lesion[s]" on the brain or other parts of the central nervous system. Spitzka believed paretic dementia was brought on by the intellectual overtaxing that was necessitated by an advancing Western culture, and as such, it was the races that possessed a sufficiently sophisticated cerebral capacity that were the most susceptible. Drawing his conclusions from the paretic patients at a New York pauper asylum, Spitzka indicated that the Anglo-Saxon race was the most vulnerable to the disease, followed by Celts, Germans, Hebrews, and negroes.

In a period in which there was a great deal of hypothesizing that paretic dementia was a condition that emerged in the tertiary stage of a syphilis infection, Spitzka conceded that syphilis was a "potent" causative factor in the disease, but he also held firm that paretic dementia was different from syphilitic dementia. He resisted earlier hypotheses that susceptibility to paretic dementia was attributable to a race's libidinous character. If that was true, he surmised, African Americans would be represented in greater numbers among the paretic population. But the low incidence of the disease within the black population confirmed his postulate about the correlation among paretic dementia, evolutional development, and brain structure. "When it is borne in mind, too," he wrote, "that where the negro lives under conditions natural to him, and where he is not compelled to enter into competition with a higher race, paretic dementia is almost unknown, the conclusion will seem reasonable that paretic dementia is more frequent with races of a high than of a low cerebral organization, because their higher civilization induces a restless mental activity with its attendant emotional strains, and that the disease is hence attributable to the excessive wear and tear of the brain induced by such civilization."[30]

Even though Spitzka was advancing an increasingly outdated notion about black immunity to insanity, his emphasis on biology was consistent with neurological understandings of mental illness. Further, in locating the origins of mental disease in brain anatomy and neurological physiology, Spitzka participated in the construction of insanity in ways that facilitated the racialization of its specific forms. Nonetheless he acknowledged that the environments in which African Americans lived and the alien cultures to which they were exposed played significant roles in the prevalence of mental illness in the black population.

Another neurologist who considered the interplay between biology and culture in the onset of insanity among African Americans was Kiernan, the medical superintendent for Chicago's Cook County Hospital for the Insane. Like Spitzka, he observed that paretic dementia was more prevalent among the Aryan races than among either Jews or African Americans; however, he was also sufficiently appreciative of its presence among African Americans to speculate on its causes and symptoms. Acknowledging paretic dementia's neurological origins, Kiernan argued that it had psychical symptoms. It was here that African American culture had its most important influence. Among the black patients with paretic dementia that Kiernan observed in the Cook County hospital, "Voudoo superstitions" and "attacks of sexual furor" were the most prominent manifestations of their disease. These were, according to Kiernan, "psychical peculiarities dormant in the race" that emerged when African Americans became "subject to the strain of commercial life."[31] Although paretic dementia had a physiological basis, in other words, the chances that African Americans would become afflicted with it and the particular symptoms that they would exhibit were deeply influenced by a culture that was considered primitive at best, savage at worst.

When Spitzka, Kiernan, and others offered theories about the relationship between biology and culture in the onset of mental illness among African Americans, they were exhibiting the same reluctance to make sharp divisions between the two that characterized social scientific thought more broadly. For example, even at a time when physical anthropologists and cultural anthropologists (the descendants of ethnologists) were beginning to define their fields by rigidly differentiating between, respectively, the role of the physiological and anatomical and the role of the social in the development of human populations, they discovered themselves drawing on each other's intellectual foundations to support their hypotheses. In other words, social scientists who were grappling with questions of the progression of racial groups and the relationships between them tended to refuse a hard distinction between biological and social evolution.[32] Asylum physicians and neurologists, too, blurred the lines between biology and culture when they considered the changing prospects of African Americans becoming mentally ill against the larger backdrop of human and societal evolution.

Where asylum physicians and neurologists felt more confident in declaring the primacy of biology was in their explanations about the specific forms of mental illness to which African Americans were presumably predisposed. Blacks' underdeveloped nervous systems, many of them surmised, contributed to the particular mental pathology that afflicted them. In this sense, African Americans were firmly situated within a racial taxonomy that presupposed a correlation between the "lower mind" of primitive peoples and their tendency to be "more easily excited to terror or anger."[33] The presumed inability of African Americans to evolve at the same pace as people of European ancestry contributed to more violent manifestations of insanity once they did in fact become mentally ill. This particular idea was translated into praxis when mentally ill African Americans were disproportionately diagnosed as suffering from mania as opposed to melancholia.

The tendency to conflate African Americans' mental illness with mania had not always existed within the medical profession. While the mid-nineteenth-century medical experts who subscribed to the basic mania-melancholia-dementia classification scheme regularly associated mania with the crude behavior and visceral emotions that were attached to primitive or savage races, there was little, if any, explicit racialization of either mania or melancholia. By the 1880s and 1890s, however, physicians were constructing a particular racial typology of black insanity. J. W. Babcock, superintendent of the South Carolina Lunatic Asylum, distilled this racial typology into a diagnostic profile when he spoke of the "comparative rarity of melancholia and the prevalence of mania" among African Americans. Even though French psychiatrists had been theorizing as early as the 1850s that mania and melancholia were but two stages of the same disease, the two continued to be seen as separate disease entities even in the late nineteenth century. As distinctive forms of insanity, it was believed they resulted from the deterioration of different regions of the brain, regions that had disparately evolved across different races. Babcock, for instance, quoted the superintendent of South Africa's Grahamstown Asylum, T. Duncan Greenlees, to explain the preponderance of mania among people of African descent: "If we consider the theories of those who maintain that, while mania represents a loss of the lower developed strata of the mental organism, melancholia indicates an absence of the higher and latest developed strata, then this prevalence of mania among natives of low developed brain functions goes far to prove this theory."[34] Given the association between these particular forms of insanity and levels of cognitive development, the observation of disproportionate cases of mania among African Americans confirmed preconceptions about the intellectual hierarchy among the races.

In addition to correlating with African Americans' purported lower level of intelligence, the prevalence of mania reflected the violent emotions of fear, anger, and uncontrollable excitement that formed the center of their psychic lives. Brain anatomy played a significant role in this regard as well. The assistant physician at the East Mississippi Insane Asylum, J. M. Buchanan, suggested as much when he invoked the smaller cerebral capacity of the negro—due to the "premature closing of the cranial sutures"—as a contributing factor to growing rates of insanity in the post-Reconstruction period. The smaller "brain-pan," Buchanan claimed, was "an hereditary physical condition, and any sudden attempt to transform the negro by a system of enlightenment and culture so much at variance with his nature must not only prove futile, but is a source of actual harm to him, viewed from any standpoint." African Americans, according to Buchanan, were particularly irrational and gullible; easily misled by political demagogues as well as religious charlatans, they were prone to "sudden outburst[s] of frenzy and despair" when promises went unfulfilled. "The insane negro," Buchanan wrote, "is combative and homicidal, but suicidal tendencies rarely exist. Dementia and melancholia are common, but the most frequent forms met with can best be characterized as moral or emotional, fraught with hallucinations and delusions. The superstition and credulity of the negro render his untutored mind ripe for ideas and impressions calculated to dethrone his reason, and he falls an easy victim to fear, fright, rage, jealousy, ambition, religious fanaticism, political commotions, and all phases of undue excitement coincident with his surroundings."[35]

J. D. Roberts, a physician in North Carolina, characterized the African American who was susceptible to mania in a similar vein. "He is essentially an emotional character," Roberts declared, "not of the higher order of emotions it is true; feelings easily aroused: superstitious: fearful of hidden dangers; fond of the marvelous, and religious to an extent approaching fanaticism." Roberts went on to disparage mental illness among African Americans as being of a "debasing nature" and exhibiting "animal propensities." Roberts was careful to avoid overgeneralizations. "I do not mean to say here that all insane of the white race are of a mild type and not addicted to a lower order of conduct," he wrote, "or that all colored insane are of a violent, profane and vulgar type, for such is not the case. The comparison is only between the striking characteristics of the two races."[36] Roberts may have been referring to the extreme manifestations of black insanity. His construction of this continuum on which one could locate types of insane behavior that were explicitly racialized, however, not only presupposed racial difference. It standardized a range of abnormal behavior that allowed those who did not conform—for instance, the melancholic or suicidal black or the violently manic white—to be judged anomalies. Roberts was not alone in his characterization of mental illness among African Americans. The medical consensus that people of African descent manifested their mental alienation in extroverted and violent ways dovetailed well with the emergent fiction of innate black criminality around the turn of the century.[37]

Interestingly enough, diagnoses of African American patients at Saint Elizabeths in the late nineteenth century did not conform to this medical consensus. In the first half of the 1880s, African Americans were still much more likely to be diagnosed with some form of mania than with either dementia or melancholia. In both 1880 and 1885, 64 percent of African American patients were diagnosed with mania, while those diagnosed with either dementia or melancholia amounted to 31 percent and 23 percent of admissions in each of those years. By the last decade of the century, however, there was a rough diagnostic parity among mania, melancholia, and dementia, with each falling somewhere between a quarter and a third of diagnoses of admissions.[38] Still, the general idea that mental illness among African Americans approximated the most depraved and violent forms of insanity among whites would go on to shape the ways that many African American inmates at Saint Elizabeths were managed in the late nineteenth century.

Where the postemancipation narrative of black insanity did more closely align with reality was in the increased admissions of African Americans to Saint

Elizabeths. The number of blacks admitted to the hospital remained below their proportion in the total population until the last decade of the century. While the proportion of African Americans in the total population of the District had increased from 19 to 33 percent between 1860 and 1870, African Americans constituted only 17.5 percent of civil admissions to the hospital in 1870. The number of black civilian admissions increased to 23 percent in 1880, even as their percentage of the total population remained at 33. It was not until 1890 that the proportion of civilian African Americans admitted to the hospital exceeded their proportion in the total population, at 40 percent and 33 percent, respectively.[39] This significant increase over the 1880s was occurring as the medical profession was constructing the mentally ill African American as one who was driven to insanity by freedom and the responsibilities of citizenship. But there were a number of dynamics that contributed to the growing presence of African Americans at Saint Elizabeths, not the least of which was black families' efforts to utilize the state on their behalf.

"Across the Branch": Pathways into Saint Elizabeths

Despite the rapid influx of African Americans into the District during the war and an emergent consensus about emancipation's deleterious impact upon the psyche of freedpeople, there was not massive confinement of African Americans in Saint Elizabeths during the 1870s. In fact, in the immediate postemancipation period, the District's police were just as likely to return mentally disturbed people to their families as to seek their institutionalization. On its face, the admission process does not seem to have been a particularly burdensome one, yet one gets the sense from reading the District's arrest records from the 1870s that the police avoided initiating a commitment procedure if they could. For instance, they tended to deal with epileptic seizures as a medical event as opposed to a cause for confinement, enlisting the aid of a physician and returning the epileptic to his or her home after the seizure subsided.[40]

Even individuals whom the police identified as insane were often returned to family members or institutions other than Saint Elizabeths. In April 1870, for instance, an officer on the morning detail arrested John D., "an insane colored man . . . who had escaped from the freedmans hospital," and immediately returned him. In February 1877 police detained an elderly man "in an unsound state of mind, [found] wandering about the streets, without shoes or pants [and] coat on. He was brought to the station and turned over to his son." That same month, the police took control of an "insane col'd woman," Jane C., who had been brought to the precinct by two African American men. Rather than sending her to Saint Elizabeths, they returned her to her husband in a neighboring Maryland county, undoubtedly to the hospital superintendent's relief.[41]

Occasionally law enforcement officials discovered that relying on family members to care for mentally ill individuals was not enough. In such cases, they initiated commitment procedures to relocate them "across the branch."[42] On the afternoon of August 7, 1871, Officer L. B. Anderson brought in a young man in his early thirties who "had been seen wandering about in the woods by [a man?] for several days in the county." Anderson thought the man was insane, and according to the precinct report, he turned him over to the department's sanitary officer. It is not clear what the sanitary officer's determination was, but the thirty-two year old man, Henry M., was not admitted to Saint Elizabeths that summer. Several months later, in early January 1872, the police arrested Henry again and transferred him to the sanitary department. That same day a Private Burns transported Henry to Saint Elizabeths, where he was admitted with the diagnosis of epileptic mania. Given the sparseness of details in the written record, it is impossible to say with any certainty what transpired that January day. It is not clear, for instance, whether Henry was arrested while wandering through the District—as he had been in August of the previous year—or if the police had been summoned to his residence in one of the ubiquitous alleys that honeycombed the poor sections of the city. The latter scenario is quite likely, given that the complainant listed in the arrest book, on both occasions, was Henry's father.[43]

The Metropolitan Police sought to commit mentally ill African Americans whom they considered to be threats to themselves or the safety of the public. Although many of the insane paupers' admissions to Saint Elizabeths began with an arrest in public space, many began with a call to the police by a relative, friend, or neighbor. Contrary to some arguments that African Americans were inclined to avoid institutionalizing mentally ill relatives, for many black Washingtonians in the postemancipation era, Saint Elizabeths was a potential asset as they dealt with the presence of insanity within their homes and neighborhoods.[44] As such, the increasing number of black admissions by the 1880s reflects attempts by African Americans to engage the state in pursuit of their own interests.[45] These efforts were complicated by a host of issues, including the stigma associated with insanity, the tension between medical authority and popular understandings of illness, and the varying degrees of trust and mistrust of the medical establishment within the African American community.

To be sure, some black Washingtonians may have avoided utilizing Saint Elizabeths, or turning their mentally ill family members over to the Metropolitan Police, because of the fear of being tainted with the stigma of insanity. Confronted with the rhetoric of racial degeneracy and race suicide emanating from mainstream culture and the black elite, African Americans of all class backgrounds may have been reluctant to publicly acknowledge the existence of mental illness within their families. Insanity, along with intemperance, venereal disease, high infant mortality, and overall ill health were symptomatic of the inability of African Americans to adjust to modern, urban life and threatened the vitality of the race, which had the potential to lead to extinction. Lest they confirm most whites' assumptions about the innate depravity and debility of their race, some African Americans undoubtedly wove a shroud of respectability that hid from view their mentally ill relatives. This was the case even with some who had relatives in Saint Elizabeths. Seeking information about her sister who was an inmate, for instance, one woman took pains to ensure that her sister's institutionalization did not become common knowledge. "Please find stamp enclosed [and] very kindly use plain envelope when writing me," she requested of the staff physician, "as it would be very embarrassing to me to be the recipient of a missive enclosed in an envelope publicly known to be direct from an *Insane* asylum."[46]

In addition to the stigma associated with insanity—which surely influenced some whites' relationship to Saint Elizabeths as well—mistrust of the medical profession had the potential to shape black Washingtonians' decisions about using the institution. Yet letters written to Godding by the family members of African American patients do not indicate a sense of mistrust of the hospital's intentions among the black community. This is all the more interesting given the suspicion with which blacks viewed professional medicine—a suspicion fueled by a history of medical experimentation on enslaved people and the unauthorized dissections and autopsies of black bodies by medical schools in the second half of the nineteenth century. In fact, the presence of Freedmen's Hospital in the District provided fertile ground for the myth of the "night doctor," the white-robed and hooded physician who, wearing rubber-soled shoes, snuck up on his prey, subdued them with chloroform, and took them back to his lair to drain them of their blood. Freedmen's Hospital's surgeon-in-chief Daniel Hale Williams's remark that the "general public was slow to appreciate and take advantage of the facilities offered here for the proper treatment of the sick" probably reflected this fear, along with the general skepticism that Americans had of hospitals as places of effective acute care.[47]

Of course, letters between the family and friends of patients and the hospital staff are not necessarily the best sources for uncovering community mistrust, given that the correspondence often represented the endpoint of a process in which family members and friends came to accept the medical judgment that their loved one required treatment and care. Still, Saint Elizabeths was apparently not one of the three local hospitals that black Washingtonians suspected of being the greatest beneficiaries of black bodies procured for use as cadavers—bodies that many African Americans believed were abducted by "night doctors" but that were more likely unidentified corpses that were headed for burial in the city's potter's field.[48] Many African Americans who interacted with Saint Elizabeths evinced not mistrust or fear but a high degree of comfort—at times bordering on a sense of entitlement—in their dealings with the institution.

Some black Washingtonians probably felt they had no choice but to seek commitment of their family members. The family of Martin S. had him committed in August 1882. The admitting doctor diagnosed the twenty-year-old man as chronically manic as a result of sunstroke. Apparently Martin was cognizant that he was losing his grip on reality prior to his commitment. According to an interview with his sister some thirty years after his commitment, Martin "told his mother that if he lost his mind not to let him kill himself, then went off into a dead faint, and from that time on has been demented." That summer Martin began to do "queer things": "He would get leaves and make aprons out of them. He would remove his clothes, could not be kept dressed, but would tie his clothes around him. He would go up on top of the house quite often, then he would run his sister out of the house, and she went to police headquarters. It took eight policeman to handle him, he being such a powerful man."[49]

Margaret W.'s family sought to have her committed before she was released from the District of Columbia Jail, where she was serving a sentence after having been convicted of petty larceny. A few days prior to the expiration of her sentence, Samuel Le Count Cook wrote to Godding, "It is the desire of her family that she be adjudged insane or otherwise before her release is obtained." A physician and member of one of the District's elite black families, Cook requested that the superintendent meet with Margaret to determine her state of mind. The thirty-six-year-old seamstress and former slave was admitted approximately a month after Cook's letter, with a diagnosis of acute mania.[50]

Shortly before being discharged as "improved" eleven months later, Margaret sought assistance from her former mistress to obtain her release. Mrs. E. C. W. Chubb wrote to Godding on behalf of Margaret, who, along with her mother, had been "a most faithful family servant." According to Chubb, Margaret "represent[ed] that the Drs[.] in charge think her well enough to leave but her husband will not permit her to do so and [she] has appealed to me." Chubb asked Godding for his assessment and, if he considered her "still out of [her] mind," whether it was possible that "she be retained as a servant in the Asylum at some wages which she seems desirous to be."[51] Although it is unclear how much influence Chubb's inquiry had, it is safe to say that Margaret did not return to Saint Elizabeths, as there is no further record of her in either the hospital register or the case files. Her family members, however, were not the only ones concerned about her presence in the community. Several months after she was released, a neighbor wrote to the hospital informing the staff that Margaret was "wandering around and has got no home and no work to do." She requested that the "Doctor . . . send for her and bring her back" to Saint Elizabeths.[52] In the cases of Martin S. and Margaret W., family and community members expected the hospital and law enforcement to collaborate in managing individuals who were, at best, public nuisances and, at worst, a danger to themselves and others.

In some instances, black Washingtonians perceived the medical authority of Saint Elizabeths' superintendent as a potential counterweight to the coercive power of the District's police force. For both longtime African American residents and more recent arrivals, the Metropolitan Police did not inspire a great deal of confidence or trust. During slavery, the police routinely enforced the city's black codes—including requiring black residents to produce their freedom certificates and fining those who broke curfew—and, prior to abolition in 1862, they also cooperated in hunting down fugitive bondspeople. Even after the Metropolitan Police hired two African American patrolmen in 1869, the black community hardly considered the department to have its best interests at heart. Although the police records do not indicate disproportionate arrests of African American residents during Reconstruction, by the mid-1880s black Washingtonians were complaining of overzealous policing and brutality. Much of this was attributable to the post-Reconstruction tendency to criminalize African Americans, including the *Washington Post*'s December 1877 characterization of black crime as a "reign of terror."[53]

There is evidence that some African American residents of the District sought to use the federal government to address violations committed against their loved ones by local law enforcement. The wife of George F., for instance, complained to the superintendent about bruises on her husband's head. She suspected that the police may have used excessive force in apprehending George, who was admitted to the hospital in May 1884 with a diagnosis of acute mania. Godding was responsive to George's wife, making an inquiry to the Metropolitan Police, who attributed the bruises to George hitting his head on the cell door as he attempted to escape.[54]

The family of Mary H. also availed themselves of the institutional power of Saint Elizabeths. Mary was admitted to the hospital in May 1882 suffering from chronic mania, and although her husband wrote to Godding to register his "disappointment" at having returned home from work to find that she had been "taken away unbeknowing to me," he did not question the superintendent's medical authority. Mary was released approximately three years later as "improved." Having corresponded with Godding over the three years during which her daughter was committed, Mary's mother felt that she had established enough of a relationship with the superintendent that she wrote to him to ask for his assistance eight months after Mary's discharge. Mary had disappeared after going for a walk and was subsequently arrested by the police. Apparently she had been wounded on her forehead during the encounter and her mother wished for someone on the hospital's staff to inspect it. "Dear Sir," her letter began,

> I write you a few lines to inform you how my daughter . . . got lost from home[.] We generally lets her take a walk out and she has been coming back so straight but on Sunday Dec[.] 20th she went out and never returned[.] We taken the best of care of her and she never suffered for a thing to eat or drink[.] We had to telephone just as soon as she was mis[sing] and the authorities arrested her and locked her up[.] We found out where she has a lick on her head above the skull bone and that what set her crazy[.] Please look and see it.[55]

Mary's mother sought to enlist Godding's help to ascertain the physical trauma that she believed was the immediate cause of her insanity. Whether Godding obliged her request is unclear. But the fact that she attempted to use a medical interventionist arm of the federal government to address her daughter's encounter with municipal authorities, as in the case of George F.'s wife, is suggestive of an assertion of citizenship that was attentive to the multiple levels of state power.[56]

The incident that prompted Mary's mother's letter to Godding, and her explanation of it, is evidence that Mary's family for some time had understood that her mental instability was such that she was incapable of living an independent and fully productive life, but that this did not necessarily rise to the level of insanity. Whether or not her mother understood the clinical difference between acute and chronic or between remote and inciting causes, she clearly believed that Mary's mental illness was episodic and the result of physical trauma. The fact that her family treated Mary's chronic mania, as defined by physicians, as a manageable problem reflected a calculus that had to be made by many working-class and poor families in the nineteenth century. At what point did a family member's intractability, likelihood of harming self or others, or inability to care for himself or herself outweigh what he or she might contribute to the household—in terms of either material or emotional value?[57]

In most cases this had to have been a wrenching decision born of economic necessity. While there was certainly a burgeoning black middle class, most black households in post-Reconstruction Washington, DC, relied on multiple wage earners who labored in unskilled and semiskilled jobs. Employment opportunities, especially for those black families who resided in the city's alley housing, were severely limited. African American men were likely to be general laborers, junk peddlers, or rag dealers, with much smaller percentages being employed as skilled laborers and professionals. Among African American women who engaged in wage labor, most worked as domestic servants or washerwomen. Even as civil service employment became more available in the 1880s and 1890s, the majority of black men and women who worked in federal offices did so in the unskilled jobs of messenger, janitor, and cleaning lady.[58] For families that could not spare an employable member to stay home to care for a mentally ill relative, institutionalization may have given them a respite. The alternatives—outside of withdrawing wage-earners from the labor force for short stints so that they could share in caregiving duties—would have been leaving them home alone, putting themselves and perhaps the house at risk, or allowing them to roam the streets of the neighborhood. Either of these could have prompted the intervention of the police or a meddlesome neighbor, as was the case with Margaret W.'s family. This could, in turn, create tension within the community.

The brother of Sarah H. had taken care of her for two decades when, in 1888, out of apparent desperation, he initiated a *lunatico inquirendo* process. Thomas and Sarah owned a piece of property that had been bequeathed to them by their father in 1869. According to Thomas's petition, for most of these twenty years, Sarah had been "an almost helpless invalid." More recently, however, her mental condition had "been decaying with the condition of her body until she is now, as your petitioner believes, completely and hopelessly insane." Thomas was seeking to institutionalize his sister because he thought she might get better care in Saint Elizabeths, but he also needed to do so in order to sell their property, the taxes on which he could no longer afford. Caring for his sister and his family and paying the taxes on his property had become too much for him, as reflected in the following poignant statement: "Your petitioner has labored long and most diligently to support his large family, to take care of said lunatic and to free the property from its incumbrance, but in vain,—he finds it impossible to carry all these burdens." The District's Supreme Court ruled in Thomas's favor and Sarah was committed to Saint Elizabeths in September 1888 with a diagnosis of chronic dementia. She remained in the hospital for some twenty months before she died.[59] Sarah's age at the time of her commitment was listed as twenty-five, which means that Thomas had taken care of her for most of her life. For him and the rest of his family, Saint Elizabeths was a welcome, if heartrending option.

Whereas some families grappled with the question of whether to commit a mentally ill relative, some people who ended up in Saint Elizabeths initiated the process of admission themselves. In September 1883 John L., a private in the 9th US Cavalry, was transferred to Saint Elizabeths from a military prison. While stationed in Pittsburgh, John had gotten into a fight with a superior officer, was court-martialed, and received a two-year sentence. In an effort to reduce his time, he feigned mental illness. In a letter to his friend Elijah in October, he wrote, "[I] was sent to pri[s]on and I play cra[z]y and got here." In retrospect, John felt that he had made a mistake. He opened his letter to Elijah, a letter intended to explain why he had not visited him, with this assessment: "[I] am in a Bad place i am in insane saylum." John L. remained in Saint Elizabeths for approximately six months before being discharged as not insane. It is unclear what happened to him after that. He did not, however, return to prison. In his case file there is a special order from the Adjutant General's Office, which indicates that the remainder of his sentence was commuted and that he received his "liberty upon his discharge from the Government Hospital for the Insane."[60] John's ruse successfully pitted one arm of the federal government against another, and in doing so, he managed to skirt a tougher punishment.

Theresa J., admitted to Saint Elizabeths twice in the mid-1880s after being diagnosed with acute mania, also took the initiative on one of her commitments, albeit in a more straightforward way. Sometime after she was released as "improved," she wrote to the hospital's assistant physician, A. H. Whitmer, with a request that she be readmitted. She was finding it difficult to "wark at home," she explained: "[My] head truble me and dont seam rite." After her final release in 1889, she continued to write to the superintendent, not asking to be readmitted but rather inquiring about the possibility of taking in wash or sewing work from the hospital.[61]

Nineteen-year-old William M., admitted to the hospital in June 1886 with a diagnosis of acute mania as the result of scrofula, or lymphatic tuberculosis, was released as "recovered" a year later. However, shortly after his release, he wrote to one of the hospital's physicians requesting to return. "I would like to return to the asylum again as my leg is no better, since I came home, it has given me considerable pain," William alerted the staff, "so I think it better to come back if I will be received. Please let me know as soon as you can, so I can make my arrangements." William was not readmitted, but it may have been more than a case of hospital staff deciding that he was not insane. He was now a resident of a county in northwestern Virginia, and he had originally been admitted only because of his transient status in the District.[62]

Just as John L. sought to avoid imprisonment by feigning mental illness, others may have sought to enter Saint Elizabeths for refuge from something they deemed to be far worse, such as poverty or an abusive domestic situation.[63] Theresa J.'s request to return to the hospital, for instance, may have been prompted by an inability to secure gainful employment. William M. may have been similarly motivated. His request on the grounds that his leg, not his head, was bothering him illustrates that at a minimum he viewed Saint Elizabeths as a facility that would tend to his overall health needs at no cost. What these cases, as well as the family-initiated commitments, suggest is that, far from being solely the objects of discipline by the state, African Americans sought to conform one of the medical interventionist arms of the federal government to their own individual needs. In this sense, ordinary Washingtonians played as much a part in mapping out Saint Elizabeths' role in their communities as the government officials and medical professionals who were responsible for its operation.[64]

How Saint Elizabeths' staff registered this willingness of African Americans to proactively engage the institution remains an open question. When Godding responded to George Tucker's survey in the 1880s, he was illustrating his adherence to the "freedom equals racial degeneration" narrative that had been circulating for at least a dozen years and that the medical profession would continue to advance for another two decades.[65] For Godding, the apparent increase in mental illness among African Americans was not a result of insane blacks who would have ordinarily remained on plantations or in households under the care of slaveholders or their families now coming within the purview of the state. Rather, the soaring rates of insanity could best be explained by the incomplete transition that African Americans were undergoing from the status of slave to the now burdensome role of citizen. Although he was hardly an apologist for slavery, Godding, like so many other asylum physicians and neurologists, unquestioningly accepted this particular narrative of emancipation and repeated it until it became common sense, an irrefutable argument that both explained African Americans' lack of progress and justified their continued discriminatory treatment.

Black Washingtonians, however, did not subscribe to this particular narrative of emancipation. Although their new status was not without its challenges, they considered citizenship itself neither physically nor mentally damaging. Rather, it was the social, economic, and political inequality that continued to shape their lives that most worried, saddened, frustrated, and enraged African Americans. But even as their economic marginalization and political disfranchisement persisted—and worsened after all District residents lost the right of self-government in 1878—black Washingtonians continued to interact with Saint Elizabeths in ways that reaffirmed their identity as citizens. Indeed their increased number of admissions surely reflected a more assertive use of the hospital by African Americans themselves than it did an actual proliferation of insanity brought on by freedom. But these attempts to make claims on the state did not stop at the red-brick threshold of Saint Elizabeths. They extended into the wards, as African Americans sought to manage the therapeutic experience of their loved ones.

4

Care and the Color Line

Race, Rights, and the Therapeutic Experience, 1877–1900

When African Americans interacted with the staff of Saint Elizabeths, they did so in their legal and moral status of citizens. But what did it mean to be a citizen in post-Reconstruction Washington, DC? By the late 1870s the District was under the direct rule of Congress, meaning both black and white residents were legally disenfranchised. Over the course of that decade, the District government went through a number of political reorganizations, beginning with the consolidation of the separate jurisdictions of Washington City, Georgetown, and Washington County into a territorial government in 1871. Prior to consolidation, Washington City and Georgetown each had some variation of a popularly elected mayor-council form of government, and Washington County was administered by a levy court—although all three, by virtue of falling within the District of Columbia, were still subject to congressional legislative and fiscal oversight and executive enforcement.

The conclusion of the Civil War led to increasingly broad support among elite Washingtonians for a reorganization of the District government, support that was motivated by different priorities and objectives. For many Republicans, consolidation was needed to usher in an era of more efficient management, a pressing concern for those who felt that the city was neither prepared to accommodate an expanding federal government nor sufficiently ordered—either administratively or aesthetically—to represent a reunified and powerful nation on an international stage. For many conservative Democrats, political reorganization would potentially blunt the growing political power of black men, who had acquired suffrage in 1867. Although they placed different emphases on its role, both Democrats and Republicans who supported consolidation attributed some responsibility for the financial and governmental mismanagement of the District to an "ignorant" black electorate. Those Republicans, including African Americans, who were most committed to the Reconstruction principles of universal manhood suffrage and civil equality were more circumspect about, if not overtly hostile to, the consolidation movement.[1]

In February 1871 Congress passed legislation creating a territorial government in the District. The law allowed for eligible District residents to vote for the lower chamber of its legislature and for a nonvoting delegate to Congress. The upper chamber, governor, and five-member Board of Public Works were to be appointed by the president. The law also allowed federal property to be assessed for determining the amount of congressional appropriations to be made for internal improvements, but the District government could not tax federal property directly. The disconnect between the expectations that the District should embark upon a major infrastructure modernization project and the meager resources that Congress provided to the territorial government led the Board of Public Works, headed by a local entrepreneur and former alderman named Alexander Shepherd, to run up a massive amount of debt within three years of the legislation's passage.

Conservatives who were opposed to the territorial government—largely because it invested a considerable amount of power in the board, continued to allow eligible black residents to vote, and included too many black appointees for their comfort—seized upon the excesses of the board. They recast Shepherd as a corrupt urban boss whose base of support comprised the illiterate, impressionable black masses who were unqualified to make informed political decisions. Congress began a series of investigations into financial mismanagement in the District, the result of which was the abandonment of the territorial experiment in 1874 and another political reorganization of the municipal government. That year, Congress passed legislation provisionally creating a three-person commission that would be appointed by the president. The support of local property owners for what amounted to direct rule and loss of self-government was enticed by a congressional commitment, embedded in the 1878 law making the commission permanent, to directly finance half of the District's expenses.[2]

Even though they traded suffrage for federally funded infrastructure, white Washingtonians continued to have significant input into policymaking in the District. Prominent whites wielded influence through the Washington Board of Trade, established in 1889 to boost economic growth and manage residential development. The board's power extended to its ability to shape the president's appointments of commissioners. Although initially upper-class black Washingtonians held seats on the board, by the first decade of the twentieth century most had resigned because of growing support for segregation among the District's white population. White Washingtonians of more modest backgrounds could participate in the political process through their neighborhood-based citizens' associations, which had access to the District commissioners to discuss policies regarding education, housing, social services, public parks, and so forth.

Citizens' associations excluded African Americans, reflecting not only the racist culture of post-Reconstruction Washington but also the ways that justification for segregation and racial discrimination were based on the conflation of whites with taxpayers and citizens.[3]

But African Americans in the District certainly understood that direct rule did not annul their citizenship any more than it did their fellow white residents. A city with a substantial black elite, an established black press, a soon-to-be-flagship institution of black higher education, and a robust black public sphere, Washington witnessed its fair share of legal and political challenges to segregation and racial discrimination in the 1880s and 1890s. Individuals and civic and professional groups filed suits against establishments engaging in discriminatory behavior and submitted petitions urging Congress to pass antidiscrimination legislation.[4]

Racial discrimination extended into the city's charitable institutions, most of which either segregated African Americans or excluded them altogether. Charles B. Purvis, the first black surgeon-in-chief of Freedmen's Hospital, castigated the federal government for its failure to ensure equal treatment of black Washingtonians. "Citizens are citizens," he wrote in a letter to the *Washington Evening Star* in 1889. "Charity must know no color and when the government is called upon to contribute to its support it must see that there is no discrimination made."[5] When it came to government involvement in providing social services—especially medical care—to Washingtonians, it was incumbent upon that government to ensure equal treatment. Yet there certainly was unequal treatment of white and black patients at Saint Elizabeths in the post-Reconstruction period. This unequal treatment was not merely reflected in the segregationist policy that was expected by Congress and the executive branch officials who oversaw the operation of the hospital. It was also reflective of the very therapeutic logic of Saint Elizabeths' staff. Shaped by a postemancipation medical consensus that associated black insanity with depravity and criminality and assumptions about the normative nature of the white psyche, W. W. Godding and his staff subjected African American patients to racially discriminatory treatment even as they represented it as therapeutically valuable.

The racial inequities existing in Saint Elizabeths were not addressed, by and large, by black civic organizations in the late nineteenth century. In fact organized protest against unequal treatment would not come until the World War I era. However, the friends and family members of African Americans committed to the hospital exercised their citizenship rights by drawing on Saint Elizabeths as a resource in the first place and collaborating with the staff to manage—and in some instances endeavoring to control—the therapeutic experience of their loved ones. Black Washingtonians' "rights consciousness" would be expressed in both brash and more subtle, quotidian ways.

Racial Segregation and Its Elusive Reality on Saint Elizabeths' Wards

When Godding was appointed superintendent after Charles H. Nichols's resignation in 1877, he inherited a hospital with 765 patients, 227 employees, and six buildings. By 1880 Saint Elizabeths was one of the largest insane asylums in the country. According to its annual report of that year, the hospital had treated a total of 1,044 patients. There were, of course, admissions, discharges, and deaths during the year, but the number of inmates in the institution on any given day exceeded 800.[6]

Godding was not cut from the same cloth of asylum medicine as his predecessor. He was sympathetic to the neurological community, which included such physicians as Edward Spitzka and James Kiernan, who believed in the deterministic role of heredity. This shared belief led Godding to support Charles Guiteau's lawyers' defense that his insanity absolved him of his responsibility for assassinating President James Garfield in 1881. Godding's receptiveness to neurology also prompted him to appoint a pathologist to the hospital's staff in 1884. Isaac W. Blackburn would spend close to three decades examining deceased inmates "for the purpose of trying to discover the causes of insanity as shown by lesions of the tissues of the brain and spinal cord."[7]

Godding outlined his philosophy in a series of articles for the *American Psychological Journal*, the publication of the National Association for the Protection of the Insane and the Prevention of Insanity, a reformist organization established in 1880 to promote medical research, facilitate cooperation between physicians and lay reformers, and advocate for more progressive public policy regarding the institutionalization and treatment of the mentally ill.[8] Godding believed there should be full transparency surrounding commitment, and he criticized the use of duplicity by family members and friends to get the insane individual to the hospital in the first place. He also deplored the practice, associated with the original asylums, of allowing public visit days, in which anyone could come to the asylum to observe—and routinely make fun of—the inmates. To be sure, the rights he believed the insane naturally possessed did not obviate the paternalistic posture that had characterized an earlier generation of asylum physicians. Godding unapologetically advocated for the inspection and, if necessary, censorship of patients' correspondence. A residue of paternalism also surfaced in his placement of moral treatment on an equal plane with the medical approach that was typically championed by neurologists. "If it be said that the primary object of a hospital is to bring about a cure, not to make a home," he declared, "I admit it; but I deny that the two are incompatible with each other; indeed, the content which the home feeling gives is most favorable to recovery;

the moral treatment, so called, is in a majority of cases more efficacious than medicine."[9]

The effectiveness of moral management was constantly undermined, however, by the conditions of mental institutions. Even though he agreed that asylums were an advancement over almshouses and prisons, Godding excoriated the practice of warehousing the mentally ill in large state institutions modeled on the Kirkbride linear plan. This resulted in overcrowded facilities which made it impossible to effectively house together inmates with similar diseases, necessitated the more frequent use of mechanical restraints, and inhibited the development of the tranquil environment that was required for successful therapy. The current status violated the cardinal principle of therapy, as far as Godding was concerned. The insane had the right, he declared, to "not have their lives endangered, or their chances of recovery lessened," by overcrowded institutions.[10]

By these standards, Saint Elizabeths was abysmally failing to meet the needs of its inmates. Shortly after he left his position as superintendent, Nichols reported on the overcrowded conditions of the hospital's main building. "The floors of many of the corridors are literally covered with beds at night," Nichols observed, "and the night attendants, as they patrol the wards, are compelled to pick their way with care, lest they should step upon the sleeping patients."[11] The tight quarters created an environment inimical to the recuperation of the inmates' mental health and posed a threat to their, and the staff's, physical health. The chairman of the Board of Visitors played up this danger in a request for more funding. Pointing out to the chairman of the House Appropriations Committee that the inmate population exceeded the hospital's capacity by 234, J. K. Barnes raised the alarm about potential epidemics: "Thus far no disease of local origin has appeared, but every additional patient adds to the danger of an outbreak much as [illegible] invariably follows overcrowding, whether of hospitals, ships, or prisons." Godding and the board were able to persuade Congress to appropriate $65,000 between 1878 and 1880 for the construction of two facilities separate from the main building.[12]

However useful the construction of additional buildings would be, erecting separate buildings rather than adding additional wings to the main building ran against the AMSAII's fundamental principles of asylum construction. Godding's advocacy for the cottage plan (detached buildings) isolated him from some of the orthodox asylum physicians. Defenders of the Kirkbride plan argued that expanding hospitals along the lines of the cottage system would make it more difficult for superintendents to monitor their patients; moreover detached buildings would beget more detached buildings, leading to massive institutions. Supporters of the cottage system responded that this problem could be avoided if superintendents increased the number of assistant physicians on their staff. Additionally they pointed out that Kirkbride proponents misunderstood the causal relationship between asylum construction and the size of patient populations. The Kirkbride plan, which operated on the premise that in order to be effective a hospital should not house more than 250 patients, was already obsolete. In fact the population at Thomas Kirkbride's institution, the Pennsylvania Hospital for the Insane, had itself surpassed the 250 mark in the 1860s.[13]

The pressures of providing space for more than 250 inmates had ushered in, according to Godding, a second era of asylum construction in the 1860s. For nearly two decades, state governments invested a tremendous amount of resources to build massive institutions to care for their mentally ill. This phase of asylum construction, which produced what Godding called "cathedrals of lunacy," was necessarily coming to a close. As asylums were increasingly becoming domiciles for the chronically insane, superintendents would do well to expand them by constructing smaller buildings spread out across a bucolic campus rather than adding wings to the original structure. Godding pointed to several state hospitals that were trailblazing what he considered to be the "third step in the progress in provision for the insane," including Willard Asylum in upstate New York (purposely created for the chronic insane) and the Illinois Eastern Hospital for the Insane in Kankakee.[14]

Interestingly Godding also referenced the history of his own institution during the first phase of asylum construction. It was during this period, he reminded his peers, that Nichols pioneered the cottage system by constructing two separate lodges for African Americans: "More than thirty years ago this departure in the direction of distinct provision, for different classes, had here its origin in the far-sighted wisdom of the then superintendent who built his heart into his work and so built nothing unworthily, and made here the first distinct, detached building for the colored insane in America, thereby placing his hospital provision outside of the [AMSAII] propositions by placing it twenty-five years ahead of his time and abreast of the requirements of to-day."[15]

In effect, Godding elevated a planning decision that was rooted in mid-nineteenth-century racist medical thought and political culture into an example of therapeutic trailblazing. John P. Gray, editor of the *American Journal of Insanity* and defender of the Kirkbride plan, published a fierce rebuttal, which he concluded with a critique of racial segregation at Saint Elizabeths. "At this day," he declaimed, "from the Government Hospital this separation of the soldiers and sailors of the Army and Navy of the United States on account of color, would seem a strange proceeding to glory in, when colored men sit in the Legislatures of the States, in the Congress of the United States and in the United States Senate, and when recently a colored man was a most respected Marshal of the District of Columbia under appointment of the President of the United States." Godding responded to Gray's criticism by characterizing it, along with Gray's apparent concern for "down-trodden Africa," as an insincere attempt to defend an outdated model of asylum construction.[16]

The back and forth between Gray and Godding was a skirmish in the larger debate between physician-superintendents and neurologists, in which the latter criticized the former for neglecting the virtues of the medical treatment of insanity through their complacent settling for the institutional care of the insane. The treatment of African Americans was a collateral issue that both Gray and Godding disingenuously sought to use to their benefit. Gray had the luxury of reprimanding Godding on the issue of segregation given that the number of black patients at his hospital in Utica, New York, was so small that accommodating them while ensuring their separation from white patients was not particularly challenging. And while both men used race as a rhetorical ploy, the presence of actual black patients at Saint Elizabeths undermined Godding's critique of Gray and his old-guard peers.[17]

In fact what Godding failed to mention was that the colored lodges themselves were beginning to resemble the center building in terms of their overcrowded conditions. Five years before he even delivered his tribute, each lodge housed more than twice the number of inmates they were originally designed for. Without any new construction between 1879 and 1884, the conditions were surely worse by the time he was vigorously advocating for the cottage system. By 1885 Godding and the president of the Board of Visitors, Joseph M. Toner, felt compelled to request more funding from Congress for the expansion of the lodges. "The number of the colored insane has so increased as to render the buildings originally designed for their use entirely inadequate," read their sober assessment, "and it now becomes necessary to make some further provision for them."[18]

One of the lodges was overcrowded, in part, because Godding had begun housing so-called idiots and imbeciles there. In the absence of a federal policy for removing the feebleminded to the Washington Asylum, the board had begun to explore alternatives, including the construction of a separate building on Saint Elizabeths' grounds. In the spring of 1883 Godding proposed taking the "lower ward and enclosed yard on the East Lodge for that class." When the esteemed British physician Daniel Hack Tuke visited Saint Elizabeths in 1885, he noted that the East Lodge contained "nine feeble children, black, and white," and fifteen "women of colour."[19] Tuke's numbers are not consistent with other evidence that suggests the East Lodge was constantly crowded, so it is possible that Godding, in an effort to put the best face on the cottage system, provided Tuke with false figures.

Equally interesting is the rationale for housing so-called idiots and African American women in the East Lodge. On the one hand, Godding may have concurred with what Tuke characterized as the psychiatric consensus that "idiocy

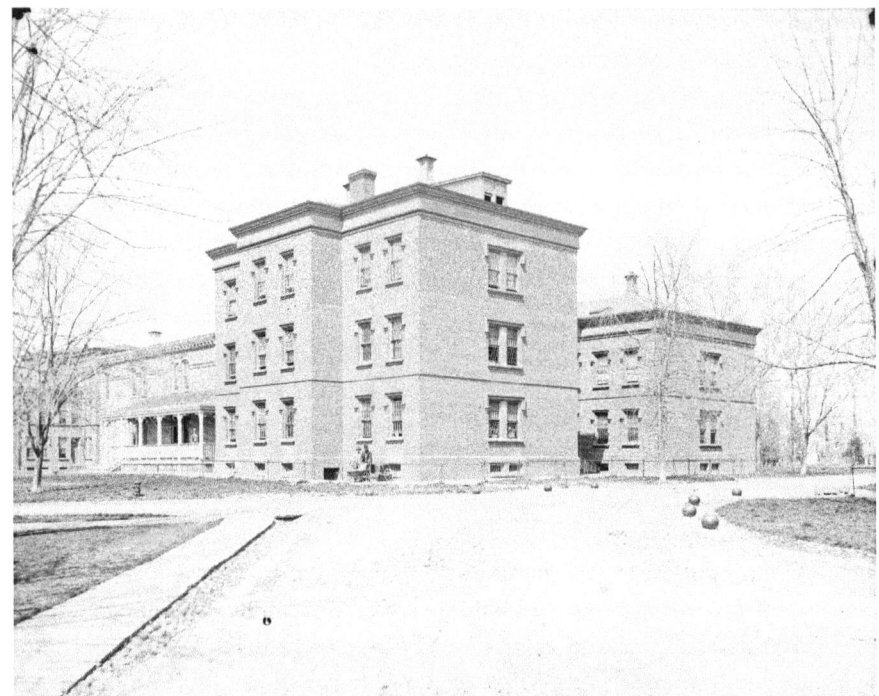

In the foreground sits the three-story East Lodge, the separate domicile for black female patients. The building housed both black men and women during the Civil War, while the West Lodge—initially built for colored men—served as a naval hospital, reflecting the willingness of medical staff to compromise the therapeutic principle of gender segregation when it came to African American patients. *National Archives, photo 418-G-113.*

rather than insanity prevails among the negroes," although the superintendent did not explicitly say so. In his description of the lodge, on the other hand, Tuke indicated that Godding believed that "negroes are less excitable than whites."[20] Of course, these ideas were not incompatible, and the notion that blacks were slow to respond to external stimuli fit perfectly with cultural stereotypes of the dull, idle, and phlegmatic negro. This assumption about black temperament informed John Galt's mid-nineteenth-century prescriptions for placing African Americans in the same wards as whites suffering from dementia in the event that integration could not be avoided. In other words, since African Americans were less aware of or sensitive to their environment, they would be less likely to object to being classified alongside so-called idiots even if they themselves were not. From this perspective the belief that blacks were less excitable would have created a more tranquil environment for a class of patients who were, by and large, considered incurable. Yet this particular characterization of mentally ill African Americans was inconsistent with the emergent medical consensus that insane blacks were inclined to be manic. These multiple, conflicting characterizations—blacks as less excitable, blacks as predisposed to mania—illustrate how ideas about racial difference were malleable enough to allow physicians to justify decisions that otherwise would have been anathema to the profession. At a minimum, the decision to house so-called idiots in the lodge for African American women point to the ease with which hospital administrators compromised the integrity of segregated wards when space was scarce.

The sheer number of admissions in the post-Reconstruction period necessitated violation of the principle of segregation. In his description of the East Lodge, for instance, Tuke also pointed out that eighty African American women were in the center building. Godding informed Secretary of the Interior Lucius Lamar of this intolerable situation in his 1886 annual report. There were close to two hundred African American patients at Saint Elizabeths, and yet the two lodges for "colored insane" had a capacity for only ninety people. "Consequently," he leveled with Lamar, "fully one-half of the whole number under treatment are quartered in rooms designed for other classes, wherever in our crowded wards lodgings can be found. This is not pleasant to the white patients any more than it is to the colored."[21]

The racial integration of wards could certainly create conflict between patients. In 1880, for instance, Dr. Joseph D. Harris wrote to Godding requesting he be moved from Sycamore to Poplar ward. His roommate was a former Confederate colonel from Virginia who kept Harris up at night by calling out the names of places in the state where he had been. There was a racist tone to the colonel's disruptive behavior. Harris reported to Godding, "He sometimes startles me by yelling as he does; it may be in my ears: 'You bald headed negro scoundrel,' etc. etc." While Harris opined that the colonel "probably intends no personal insult," revealing that he occasionally cleared his dishes after meals, the fact that Harris was a black Republican who had run for lieutenant governor of Virginia shortly after the war ended surely played no small part in the colonel's behavior.[22] The racial tensions provoked by occasionally integrated wards were most likely not rare and probably prompted both white and black inmates to request relocation or the removal of others to different wards. Still, when Godding defined African Americans as a "distinct race from the whites, with peculiarities and ways of their own," and suggested that "they are more at home in quarters by themselves and happier in their associations than scattered through the buildings," he was doing nothing more than attempting to justify the racially discriminatory policy of segregation.[23]

And yet Godding framed his efforts to maintain racial segregation in the altruistic language of treatment. In 1887 he had requested funds from Congress in order to expand both the East and West lodges to a hundred beds each. By 1889 the extensions of both lodges were completed, with particularly positive results for the African American female patients, according to Godding. "Crowded into insufficient quarters they had grown careless, noisy, and destructive in habits," he reported, "requiring more or less seclusion and restraint, until both attendants and physicians had accepted the situation as the inevitable, and the best that could be done. Now, changed to new quarters, with their light common dining hall, their fresh and trim associate dormitories and rooms, with everything quiet and orderly about them, they have gone to work, have forgotten to be noisy and destructive, the change in their quarters having wrought in them a notable change for the better, an improvement in those chronic, turbulent cases beyond what we had dared to hope."[24]

Godding and the board further characterized the expansion of the lodges as a fulfillment of the superintendent's vision of the role of the asylum in preserving the fundamental rights of the mentally ill. The minutes of an 1890 Board of Visitors meeting recorded, "The very satisfactory results from providing additional quarters for the colored female patients as shown in their more

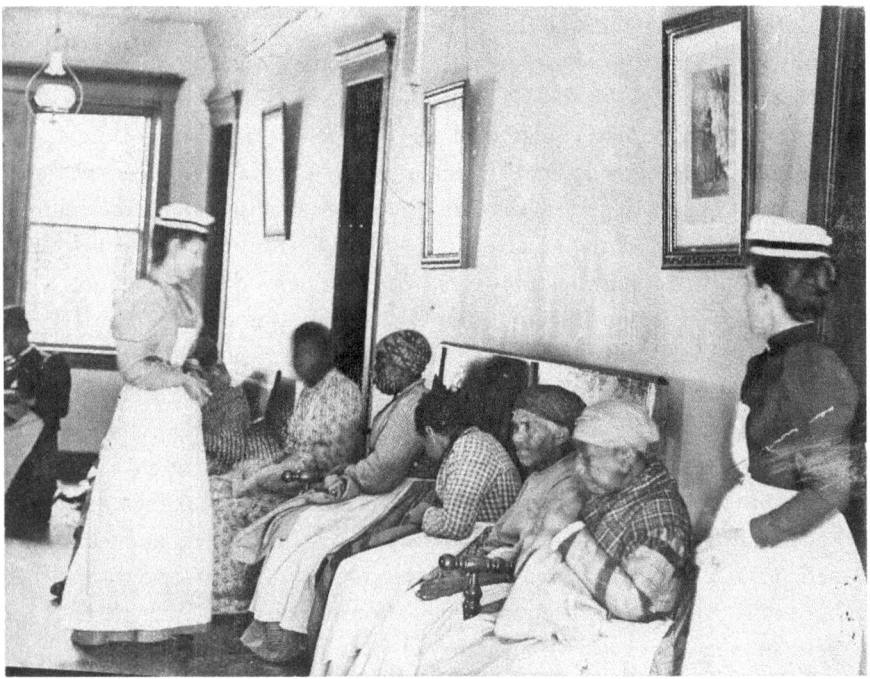

Two white female attendants watch over African American female patients in the East Lodge sitting room in 1898. Although hospital administrators attributed the easier management of the lodge's residents to its expansion (and subsequent alleviation of overcrowding) some ten years earlier, many black female patients continued to resist the power and authority that the institution attempted to wield over them. *National Archives, photo 418-P- box 6A, fol. Miscellaneous Views #3.*

comfortable mental condition, increased amount of work done, and general happiness was pointed out as illustrating the injustice done to the insane by having to keep them in overcrowded wards and the necessity for more hospital accommodations."[25] As these accolades for the East Lodge expansion suggest, it was not just the freedom from cramped conditions that proved to be necessary for an ideal therapeutic environment; patient labor also occupied a privileged place in the psychiatrist's armamentarium.

Despite the optimism expressed by Godding and the board, problems of overcrowding persisted. In 1892, for instance, Saint Elizabeths had three hundred more patients than beds. Godding attributed the expanding inmate population to the fact that the hospital was increasingly becoming a custodial institution for the chronically insane and disabled.[26] The number of indigent insane was also skyrocketing, a concern that the superintendent expressed in 1897. That year there were 332 African American inmates, almost 60 percent of whom were men. Godding was particularly alarmed because the number of African American men had increased by 14 percent over the previous year, compared to an increase of 3 percent for the overall male patient population over the previous year. He suggested that the volatile economic climate was responsible in large part for the growing number of African American men who "come pouring in upon us."

Of the 192 African American male inmates, 107 resided in the 100-bed West Lodge and 55 were "stowed away in narrow quarters that would be full with half the number."[27] The remaining 30, considered by Godding and his staff to be of the "violent and dangerous type," were housed in Howard Hall. Built in 1887 and named after the British prison reformer John Howard, the two-story structure was a remedy for what Godding, and Nichols before him, thought was a potentially cancerous development: the housing of insane convicts, the criminal insane, and homicidal lunatics amid the general population at Saint Elizabeths. Beginning as early as the mid-1870s, the federal government sought to transfer to Saint Elizabeths inmates of federal penitentiaries who had become mentally ill, men found not guilty of federal crimes by reason of insanity, and military prisoners diagnosed as insane. Both Nichols and Godding demurred at accepting convicts from state penitentiaries, pleading overcrowding of the hospital and the lack of accommodations to keep the nonviolent patients secure.[28]

The prospects of housing insane convicts and the criminally insane among the noncriminal and nonviolent mentally ill was considered to be noxious by almost everyone in the medical profession. Opposition to the practice was one thing on which the asylum physicians and neurological iconoclasts could achieve consensus. Whether or not one believed that insanity could exculpate someone from a crime, as many neurologists did, few individuals associated with mental hospitals thought that insane convicts and the criminally insane should come

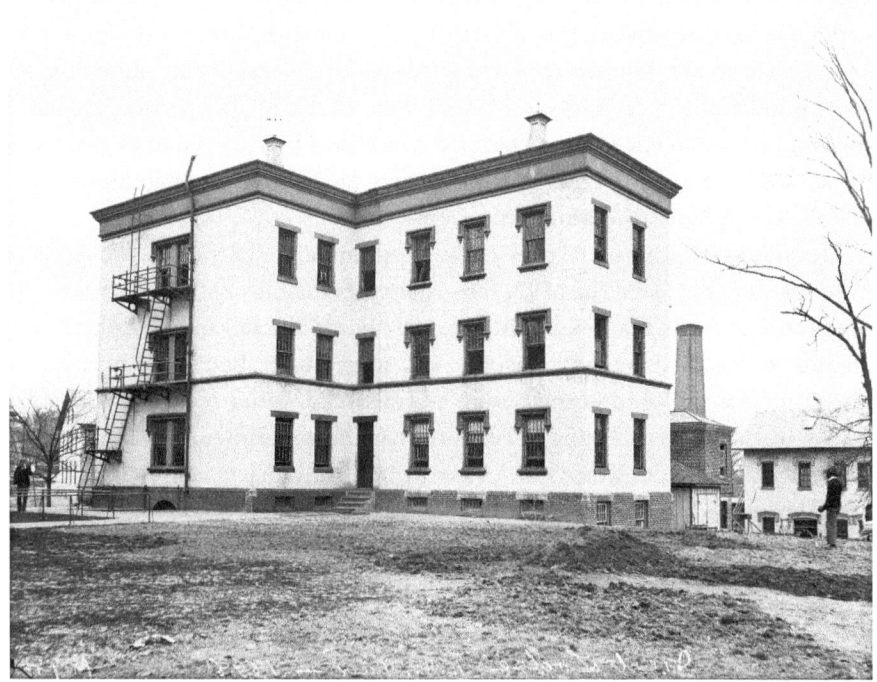

An exterior view of the recently renovated three-story West Lodge for black male patients, 1898. Superintendent W. W. Godding pressed for the expansion of the building in the midst of the economic depression of the 1890s. "The widespread stagnation of business, and the consequent lack of fields for labor has no doubt resulted in the drift of a considerable number of the unemployed colored people of Maryland and Virginia toward Washington, and the ones thus easily dislodged from their homes are apt to belong to the light ballasted, decadent class, who readily round up in hospitals and almshouses," he wrote in 1897. *National Archives, photo 418-G-331.*

under their charge. Physician-superintendents were concerned that the proximity of lunatics with criminal tendencies and the quiet, "reputable" insane would potentially result in the latter being influenced by the former's depravity. In order to prevent this, insane convicts and the criminally insane needed to be housed in buildings that were as secure as prisons; however, doing so would conjure up earlier impressions of the asylum as a more punitive and custodial institution than a curative hospital. Nonetheless it was imperative that the criminally insane be sequestered from the general population. With twenty-eight patients of the "convict class," including military prisoners from Fort Leavenworth, under his care in 1884, Godding recognized this and proceeded with the construction of a separate facility. "The community is to be protected from irresponsible, homicidal cranks at all hazards," he wrote in 1885. "The philanthropist has no call to loosen the necessary restraint on this class; make the glove of silk, but the hand of steel."[29]

Originally conceived as a four-story center building with two wings, by the time it was opened for use Howard Hall consisted of a three-story center building with two two-story wings connected at right angles. Because its population needed to be separated from the rest of the hospital's patients, the building had its own dining room, workshops, rooms for amusement and smoking, and outdoor courtyard so that inmates could exercise. Howard Hall contained the architectural elements of both the prison and the hospital. The wings were laid out so as to block the inmates' access to the rest of the hospital grounds; there was a room in the Hall for the warden; and iron guards were attached to all of the inmates' windows. On the other hand, the inmates' rooms were on the exterior of the wings rather than the interior, giving inmates access to fresh air and sunlight. Howard Hall initially consisted of sixty single rooms (fifteen on each floor of the two wings); within four years, however, the building needed to be doubled in size to accommodate the growing number of dangerous inmates.[30]

Within two decades of its opening, Howard Hall counted among its occupants not only insane convicts and the criminally insane but African American men regardless of their diagnostic classification or their civil status. This was a decision necessitated by the chronic overcrowding of the hospital. Yet it was also a decision that was shaped by and reflected certain assumptions about blackness. A medical consensus that African Americans were more likely to manifest their mental illness in various forms of mania, for instance, could easily shade into racist thinking that presupposed blacks' innate criminality. Physicians Hunter McGuire and G. Frank Lydston, for instance, claimed that there was no "difference from a physical standpoint between the sexual furor of the negro and that which prevails among the lower animals in certain instances and at certain periods... namely, the *furor sexualis* in the negro resembles similar sexual attacks in the bull and elephant, and the running amuck of the Malay race." Referencing the transitory mania presumed to be unique to the Amok peoples of the Malay peninsula, McGuire and Lydston attempted to give scientific and medical credence to the myth of the black beast rapist, a myth that was fueling lynching, mob violence, and attempts to disenfranchise and segregate African Americans in the South in the late nineteenth and early twentieth centuries.[31]

Presumptions about the inherent criminality of African Americans circulated within the field of neurology. Charles K. Mills, a Philadelphia neurologist and president of the American Neurological Association in the mid-1880s, delivered a presidential address in 1886 in which he presented evidence of the links between deviant behavior, mental underdevelopment, and brain morphology. Using earlier comparative studies of primate brain anatomy as a backdrop against which to examine the brains of criminals and mental defectives, Mills claimed that the "low or aberrant type of human brain" was characterized by "simplicity of structure," hemispherical asymmetry, and underdeveloped gyres, or cerebral convolutions. Five of the brains that constituted Mills's sample came from white and black criminals and one "feeble-minded youth." The fact that both the white and black specimens came from criminals suggests that Mills was not mounting an argument that African Americans were particularly prone to criminal behavior. However, one of the claims toward the end of his address suggests otherwise. "Striking differences can be detected between these brains and what is commonly regarded as the average normal human brain, and the brain of high development," Mills contended. "The specimens taken from individuals of the white race exhibit negro, simian, and foetal similarities, resemblances, and reversions in an unusual degree."[32] Mills's conclusion that white abnormality approximated blacks' normal state of being betrays the extent to which ideas about racial difference underpinned medical thought during this period. Similar assumptions, as the early history of Howard Hall suggests, profoundly shaped the logic of classification and management in the asylum.

To be sure, other public hospitals had to compromise their classification systems when the lack of resources led to overcrowding.[33] What makes Saint

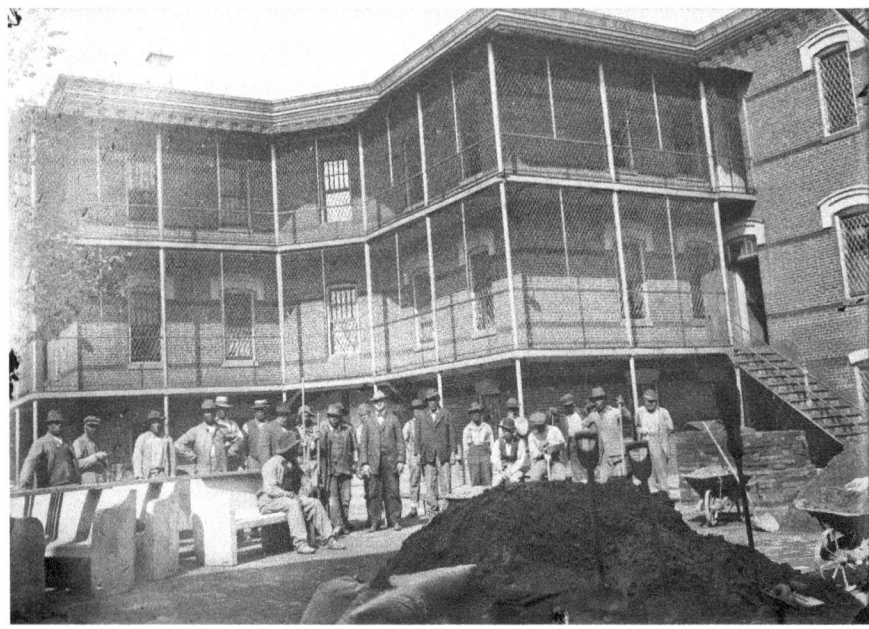

A group of black male inmates either preparing for work or taking a break, in front of Howard Hall, the building for the "criminally insane" and mentally ill convicts, in 1897. The completely fenced-in verandas—along with the mounds of dirt and tools—suggest the association that hospital administrators made between African Americans, their innate criminality, and their natural predisposition toward labor. *National Archives, photo 418-G-342.*

Elizabeths unique is the extent to which race shaped the nature of the compromise. Immersed in a society that constantly framed the "Negro problem" in terms of crime and hypersexuality and embedded in a profession in which his peers were comfortable associating blackness with depravity, Godding addressed problems of overcrowding by housing African American male inmates with insane convicts and the criminally insane. This is where Godding's commitment to preserving the fundamental rights of the insane and to providing a curative environment broke down. In 1894 he reinforced the moral treatment mantra about the importance of one's surroundings in the prospects for recovery. "The successful care, not to say cure, of the insane depends very much on their environments," he wrote in that year's annual report. "In the active stage of his disease if the insane man can be made contented with his surroundings, a great stride has been made toward recovery, if a cure in his case is possible."[34] The fact that he placed African American males where he did does not necessarily mean that he was willing to completely sacrifice their chances of recovering from their mental illness in order to alleviate overcrowding elsewhere in the hospital. With the meager resources provided by the federal government, African American patients would have found themselves in less than ideal conditions regardless of where they were. Nonetheless care was clearly more important to Godding than cure when it came to African Americans at Saint Elizabeths.

Rights Consciousness and Managing the Therapeutic Experience

Although much of Godding's thought aligned him with neurologists—who were intensely critical of the nonscientific basis of moral treatment—most of what went on inside Saint Elizabeths resembled the therapeutic model associated with the earlier generation of asylum physicians. Pharmacotherapy did play an important role in the hospital's therapeutic regime. Godding and his staff routinely employed ethyl carbamate as a hypnotic for insomnia, hyoscine hydrobromide as a calmative for patients with "acute excitement," as well as quinine, strychnine, cod-liver oil, chloral hydrate, and opium. But while it may have been necessary, pharmacotherapy was not a sufficient treatment modality. "The most skillful employment of drugs for the control of morbid processes in the nervous system, and especially in the brain," Godding wrote in 1897, "in the present state of knowledge, leaves much to be desired." As such, he promoted other forms of somatic treatment, medical interventions that worked directly on the physical body. He was especially sanguine about hydrotherapy—the prolonged application of water through the use of wet sheets and blankets, showers, baths, and so forth—which he suggested resulted in "distinct physical and mental improvement" in some patients suffering from general paresis.[35] Saint Elizabeths was one of the first mental hospitals to employ hydrotherapy, which it did in the 1890s. It was joined by relatively few others, however—including Danvers State Hospital and McLean Hospital, both in Massachusetts—largely because of the significant start-up costs associated with installing state-of-the-art facilities.[36]

As much as he touted the use of somatic therapies, Godding recognized that, for the most part, their value resided more in managing patient behavior than in curing mental illness. Consequently he continued to give a full-throated endorsement of moral treatment and its emphasis on providing patients a healthy environment, proper nutrition, and an appropriate balance between labor and leisure. "The modern treatment of the insane depends less on drugs than on moral adjuncts," he stated in the 1885 annual report. "Whatever occupies, interests, and diverts the mind from its morbid broodings is sought out."[37] He and Joseph M. Toner, the board's president, made this statement in connection with a funding request for construction of a greenhouse. The request was part of a larger project to make Saint Elizabeths virtually self-sufficient in terms of the production and consumption of food, and included the acquisition of farmland. But the employment of patient labor was not meant merely as a cost-saving measure or a revenue-generating mechanism. It was also consistent with the therapeutic philosophy of keeping the mentally ill productively engaged. As he pointed out in the 1889 annual report, "Idle men, sane or insane, are seldom happy; those who have steady occupation are generally content."[38]

Godding thought that farm labor was best suited for the "chronic class" as a form of therapy, but these inmates were not the only ones who worked on the grounds. Inmates from other classes, including those deemed to be especially violent, were employed at various tasks, including "mending roads, excavating for building, raking the lawns, and digging in the vineyard."[39] But hospital officials could not compel inmates to work. Instead they utilized a system of incentives, such as "the liberty of the grounds, the excursions to the city, the trips down the river, the visits to the Zoo and the circus, articles of special clothing, and more varied diet," to coax labor out of the patients. The hospital also gave patients some of the profits from the sales of items manufactured at the hospital. This was not enough to induce some patients, however. Because the military provided some extras to officers, and veterans received monthly pension payments, many were less inclined to work for pin money.[40]

Inmates who refused to work could prove frustrating for hospital staff, as the case of John M. demonstrates. The twenty-nine-year-old African American private in the 25th Infantry was admitted in March 1891 with a diagnosis of chronic dementia as a result of a head injury. That summer, Howard Watt, a former soldier and an agent for a Washington lawyer, became John's advocate. He had initially attempted to gain access to Saint Elizabeths in his capacity as a pension agent but was rebuffed by Godding. Apparently Watt managed to visit the hospital as a member of the general public, and on one such visit he met and befriended John. From the little evidence we have, it is not clear if John was already receiving a pension. In 1890 Congress had passed legislation authorizing the distribution of pensions to disabled veterans, regardless of how they became disabled, as long as their disability was not the result of immoral or negligent behavior. Watt most likely met John as he was searching for veterans for whom he could prosecute pension claims. Regardless of the actual status of John's claim—if, in fact, there was one—Watt took it upon himself to defend John from compulsory labor and the racist response when he refused to comply. John, Watt informed Godding, "believes the doctor in charge of the department where he lodges is down on him because he won[']t work, and to use his own words 'has no use for a nigger.'"[41] We have no way of knowing for sure if John's recounting of his exchange with the doctor is reflective of what really happened or if Watt's translation of it is accurate. At a minimum, however, it suggests that John interpreted his institutionalization through his awareness of his racially subordinate position in society. Staff often expected African American patients to work and responded harshly, sometimes violently, if they refused to do so.

While in many ways labor as a form of therapy was thought to have universal value, in other ways it was deeply racialized. This was particularly the case with female patients. Godding thought that mentally ill women were just as likely as mentally ill men to deteriorate if left idle, so he implemented specific practices to keep them steadily occupied. Female patients engaged in sewing and fancy work; some also attended a primary school on the hospital grounds. It is unclear whether these activities were limited to white female patients. However, it is unlikely that integrated groups would have participated in them. On the other hand, Godding used black women exclusively for carrying out laundering duties. The 1886 annual report stated, "In the female department an attendant has been assigned to take a party of the colored women each day to the laundry, working with them there. The result has been so satisfactory that the number of these working gangs will be increased."[42] In the late nineteenth century and into the twentieth, African American women were employed in forms of labor—laundering as well as cooking—that were considered consistent with their station, just as white women were given work that would have been carried out by middle-class homemakers. Godding was not the only superintendent to impose certain forms of labor on certain groups of patients. In the wake of increasing black admissions after the 1880s, the superintendent of the South Carolina Lunatic Asylum began employing black women in the hospital's kitchen and laundry and black men on the grounds. In this sense, forms of therapy within the hospital worked to reproduce the presumed social positions that patients occupied outside of the hospital.[43]

As much as Godding and his staff aspired to hold a therapeutic monopoly—in terms of both moral and medical treatment—patients and their families made their own interventions in the clinical relationship. Some family members sought to insert themselves into the therapeutic experience right away by offering their thoughts on the causes of their loved one's mental illness. Families often framed these illnesses and the medical establishment's prescriptive approaches to them according to their own worldviews. Francis Harding wrote to Godding four years after his sister Mary W. was admitted with a diagnosis of acute mania. He speculated that anxiety was the cause of Mary's insanity. According to Francis, she had converted from Methodism to Catholicism in order to get married, and this, in addition to feeling "poor & helpless pried on her mind untill it gave away." Francis felt obligated to inform Godding so that he "may, by proper remedis in this direction, cur[e] her as ther has been no former [illegible] or any possible reas[on] I could think off, to destroy her mind."[44] Mary J.'s brother, Horace Timmons, interpreted her acute mania within a black vernacular paradigm of

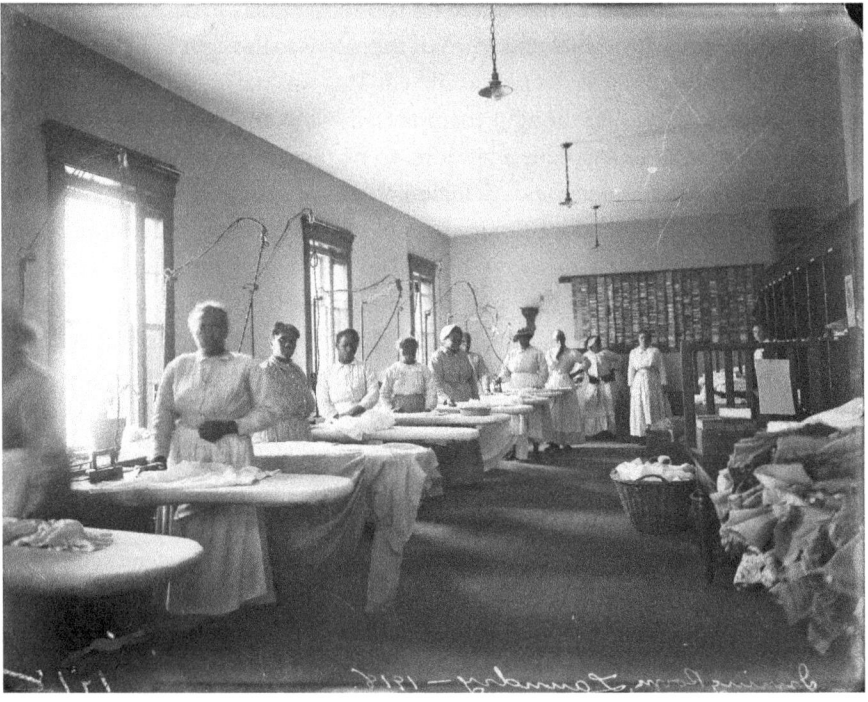

Black female patients iron garments and sheets in the hospital laundry in 1918. Although labor was considered to have a therapeutic value, it could also reduce the asylum's operating costs. One hospital administrator remarked, "The paid employees have been, and are being, replaced by patients wherever possible." *National Archives, photo 418-G-188.*

disease. He expressed concern to the staff that Mary was in her condition because of the action of "some evil person." Mary herself attributed her mental illness to being poisoned, according to her brother. "Now do tell me just what you think," Horace requested of the doctor, "if you think she will ever recover—or if you think her case hopeless—for I fear that she is under some evil affect."[45]

The mother of nineteen-year-old Mary C. was similarly tentative in explaining what may have led to her daughter's acute dementia, although what she suggested to the hospital staff was compatible with the cause listed in the register book: overwork. Mary was not a particularly sickly child, according to her mother, yet she had recently been experiencing irregular menstruation. During the summer of 1882 Mary, a public school teacher, began "complaining a little and was advised by friends to stop teaching and take a rest." Once the school year started back up in the fall, however, she was unable to resume teaching "on account of sickness." Though Mary's mother may have been unsure about what caused her daughter's mental illness, she wanted to make clear to the hospital staff that she expected them to take good care of her. She pointed out that Mary was a "girl of good caracter" and that she could produce references from "distinguished ladies and gentlemen," including the superintendent of the District's colored public schools. She also informed the staff that she was willing to pay the nurse "if she will give good attention" to Mary. In spite of this very confident posture, Mary's mother acceded to the medical authority of Godding and his assistants. "I have been advised by white and colored not to come," she wrote in a letter a few weeks after Mary's admission. "What ever you say is best I will do. If you say it will do her harm of course I will not come."[46]

The wife of John B. expressed a similar trust in the institution's staff. "While my anxiety is very great," J. A. Bowman wrote a Dr. Patterson, "my whole faith is in you." Bowman was particularly concerned, however, that her husband have enough warm clothes. She also conveyed to Dr. Patterson that John constantly requested to return home and she sought the physician's honest opinion as to whether he was ready for short stints away from the hospital. "Please give it a consideration and do what you can do for me," she entreated. "I am so anxious about him, and afraid, he will get worse again, as I know his disposition so well."[47] As these examples suggest, relatives of individuals who were committed to Saint Elizabeths sought to positively influence their treatment by offering their own knowledge about the causes of their illness as well as aspects of their temperament that might give the doctors a clue about how best to approach them therapeutically.

Relatives continued to take an active role in monitoring the treatment of their loved ones once they had become settled at Saint Elizabeths.[48] Many families requested that the hospital intervene to protect their institutionalized relatives from either harming themselves or being harmed by others. This latter concern was not limited to interactions that might exacerbate their illness or impede their recovery. It also encompassed the fear that individuals might try to take advantage of their mental condition. The father of nineteen-year-old William A., admitted in March 1885 after being diagnosed with acute mania as a result of malaria, requested that the hospital staff keep his son's friends from visiting him. "I have just heard that a party of my son's young friends propose going over to see him tomorrow," William's father wrote. "I don't want them to see him as I think it will do him more harm than good."[49]

Godfrey Smart, a male relative of Emma S., felt similarly. Emma was being visited so often that Smart thought it might "retard her recovery." He felt so strongly about this that he sought to interpose himself into the doctor-patient relationship. "If you did not allow person to see her, except on a note from me," Smart wrote to Godding, "if you should think it advisable, oblige me by doing so."[50] Retarded recovery was the least of the concerns of A. E. Winslow, the sister of John T., who was admitted in April 1878 after being diagnosed with chronic dementia. Her twenty-four-year-old brother owned a portion of a parcel of land in the District, and she was afraid that other family members might attempt to finagle him out of his share. Winslow was particularly concerned about an aunt, who she claimed "took brother out of the Asylum before and then let him wander all over the streets after she saw that she could not get control over his share of the property." In order to protect her brother from being the victim of inheritance theft, she requested that the hospital staff not release John into the custody of anyone without a court order.[51]

Family members sought to make their committed relative's stay at Saint Elizabeths as comfortable as possible, sending them clothing, reading material, and games; writing them with updates about goings-on at home; and making sure that staff members were keeping them well-fed and groomed. Some enlisted the assistance of their employers to give their inquiries about their relatives more gravitas. This was the approach of Mary B.'s sister, who was the cook of Samuel Jackson Randall, Democratic representative from Pennsylvania and former speaker of the House of Representatives. After learning about Mary's commitment in April 1882 with the diagnosis of acute mania—and most likely at the prompting of Mary's sister—Randall wrote to Godding to express his interest in her status. "If anything occurs which so [requires?] her sister's attention or knowledge—please let me know and I will at once give response," he informed the superintendent. "I need not add that we desire your considerate care for this woman, for we are sure she will receive it."[52] While it is possible that Mary B.'s sister understood the intricate internal workings of the federal government—the fact that the hospital was overseen by the Department of the Interior but received its funding from Congress—she surely understood the weight that a letter from a US congressman would have with the superintendent.

Some family members took additional steps to see that their relatives were productively occupied, even though they may not have shared Godding's perception of labor as a form of therapy. The mother of Mary H. demonstrated her own understanding of Mary's illness, as well as her own economic need, when she inquired as to whether Godding thought that Mary was "well enough to work in the Laundry as I want her to do something to employ her mind." Mary's mother's desire that she be put to work fit easily with the moral treatment model even as it most likely reflected her hopes that Mary be able to return to wage-earning once she was released.[53]

Henrietta F.'s sister was perhaps driven by the same motivation. The epileptic Henrietta was admitted to Saint Elizabeths for a second time in June 1884 with a diagnosis of acute recurrent mania. Approximately a year later, Henrietta's sister wrote to the hospital staff in order to get an assessment of her mental condition and to gauge her ability to work:

> I am in hopes that she will soon be able to come home soon as she request me to get her a situation & I have succeeded in geting her a place in the Laundry of the same place where I am. but it seem that she prefer being over there. there you will do me a great favor if you can give her a permanent situation in the Laundry or any place that may be vacant as she says she is feeling very well at the present I would like for you to try her for a while & any time she get tired she can come home.[54]

The sister's set of requests reveals a degree of comfort with Henrietta's institutional situation. Taking her cue from Henrietta's apparent satisfaction with being at Saint Elizabeths, the sister still wanted the staff to employ her in the type of work that she would most likely be limited to doing once she was released. The last line of her letter suggests that she thought of the asylum as more of a curative hospital than a custodial institution; she also perceived the asylum as a temporary refuge for her sister, one that could be entered and exited almost at will. A few years later, however, Godding disabused Henrietta's family of that notion. In response to her mother's request that Henrietta be allowed to return home for a short stint, Godding not only declined but gave a clear explanation of his rationale. "I have to inform you, as I did her brother sometime ago," he wrote, "that in the light of my past experience with Henrietta, I do not feel that I can conscienciously [sic] proceed in the matter as suggested by you, unless I know that she will be observed more closely than while at home upon a former occasion."[55] For all of the familial prerogative patients' relatives sought to exert in their interactions with Saint Elizabeths' staff, it could rarely overcome the medical authority of the superintendent, which was backed up by the power of the state.

As the case of Henrietta F. and her family illustrates, one of the principal ways families attempted to monitor the treatment of their institutionalized relatives was to get them home on temporary parole. They did so, moreover, in ways that reinforced the superintendent's medical authority as well as established their own sense of ownership over the care of their loved ones. John S. sought to take his wife, Julia, who had been committed in June 1888 with a diagnosis of chronic melancholia, home for a temporary stay to see if he could take care of her himself. "I wanted to see you on the regards of taking my wife out next month on a tryal," he wrote to Godding, "[and] if I can[']t manage her I will Bring her Back & if not I will keep her." John S. enlisted the assistance of employers and others to give him leverage with Saint Elizabeths. His August 1888 letter appeared on "House of Representatives U.S." stationery, although it is not clear with which congressman he had a relationship. John's request was successful, as Julia was discharged as "improved" two days after he wrote his letter.[56]

The family of Josephine F. similarly sought to take on some role in her treatment by requesting that she be permitted to leave the hospital for short periods. They did not want to completely sever her or their connection to Saint Elizabeths. "Of coarse," one daughter wrote in 1893, "I would not like to have you fully discharge her in case something might happen and might cause me a good deal of trouble." Hospital administrators complied with Josephine F.'s family's requests. Although the register book indicates that she was not discharged between her admission in August 1885 and her death in January 1908, she did spend some time away from the hospital. In 1901 another daughter wrote to Superintendent Alonzo Richardson requesting medical intervention. "[My mother] is very much excited and has been for several days," her daughter informed Richardson.

> She seems at times to realize her condition and tries very hard to controle herself but it is only for a little while. I should have been over to see you before but it is not convenient for me to leave home, as I have small children, and I do not think it wise to leave my mother long enough to come over and return but if you could or would give me something to give her to quiet her I would be more than gratful to you and will try and arange to come or send over for it please let me hear from you as soon as possible, as she is very noisy to day but we are not afraid of her. Of coarse the children are but they are kept away from her as much as possible.[57]

Josephine's daughter's communication is a clear indication of the commitment required to balance caregiving, the protection of other members of the household, and, most likely, the need to earn wages. The daughter's plea to Richardson also reveals the desire of this patient's family to develop a collaborative relationship with the hospital as they attempted to provide noninstitutional care for their mother.

For some, this sense of entitlement could evolve into a challenge to the superintendent's medical authority. This certainly was so in the case of Jesse S., admitted to Saint Elizabeths in June 1885 with the diagnosis of chronic melancholia as a result of typhoid fever and "night work." Within a month of his admission, Jesse's wife wrote to Godding to request that he be allowed to come home. He had appeared well to her when she visited, and a hospital attendant had apparently told her that "he had never had a bad spell." In her request to Godding, Jesse's wife suggested that everyone would benefit from his parole. "I would be glad to have him home," she told the superintendent, "it would be less trouble for me and it would be less expense for you." She requested that Jesse be allowed to stay with her for at least a week, but added, "If he gets worse at home may I have the privilege of sending him back again." It is unclear if Godding allowed Jesse to stay away from the hospital for such a long period, but by August he was being permitted to leave the hospital for day trips. On one occasion, Jesse's wife wrote to the superintendent to thank him for sending an attendant along for one of their rides as she "could not have got along without him." Having established what she felt was a coequal status in Jesse's treatment regimen, his wife became comfortable challenging Godding's decisions. "I should like to know why I cannot take my husband home for a few hours," she complained in a letter in September. "I will be responsible. Please give me a decided answer from yourself." Jesse's wife was finally able to get him discharged in October, after reiterating that a local physician would monitor his health and her brother would provide financial support until Jesse was able to work again.[58]

Other family members challenged the medical authority of the hospital staff even more brazenly. The husband of Emma O. refused to comply with Dr. A. H. Witmer's order that she be returned to Saint Elizabeths after a brief parole. "I find Her Different and is well as she will Ever be," Frank responded. He laid out for Witmer all of the steps he was taking to ensure that she did not have a relapse, including renting a large furnished room for her, making sure that she had enjoyable excursions such as a steamboat ride on the Potomac, and preventing her from being exposed to large Fourth of July crowds. Frank thanked Witmer for everything that the staff had done for his wife and ended his note with a very courteous, yet firm, declaration that she would not be returning: "You Can Come some time in passing and see Emma."[59]

Family members had to make an important calculus that took into consideration their relative's condition, their own ability to provide the kind of support their relative needed, the quality of care they perceived their relative received in Saint Elizabeths, and the overall level of comfort they had with allowing a potentially dangerous person into their home, their familial relationship notwithstanding. In some instances, the fear of permanent institutionalization outweighed the fear of being harmed by one's mentally ill relative. For instance, through an intermediary the mother of Ambrose W., a twenty-four-year-old epileptic who was admitted in January 1884, inquired about her son and the prospects of his returning home, despite the fact that Ambrose had "made a murderous assault upon his mother and undoubtedly would have killed her if she had not escaped from him." Nonetheless the intermediary, a local proprietor, informed Godding that "naturally she wants him released as soon as it is prudent to do so, but is fearful of a recurrence of the violent mania." Ambrose was released two weeks later, but it is unclear whether he returned to his mother's house.[60]

As this example suggests, there were families throughout the District and beyond who attempted to obtain the release of their loved ones, enlisting the aid of lawyers, employers, and other reputable citizens. There were just as many who, although distressed at the thought of their relatives residing permanently in an institution, felt that it was the best situation for all concerned. "It caused me great pain to bring my mother back to the Asylum," Josephine F.'s daughter wrote to Godding, "it was very unexpected. When I wrote to you she was very well and lively." Josephine's daughter requested that Godding send her information about her condition as soon as possible, as she "fear[ed] this [admission would] be her last."[61]

For the father of Walter J., admitted to Saint Elizabeths with a diagnosis of chronic epileptic mania, the safety of his son and other children was of paramount concern. Apparently a single father with at least four other children, Henry found it difficult to deal with an adult son with epilepsy. Within two years of his admission, however, Walter was returning to his home in northwest Washington for short periods of time. Henry thought these visits were good for Walter, but he became increasingly concerned about his ability to protect his other children—who were "nervous" during these visits—should Walter have a severe attack. Henry worked as a messenger at the Treasury Department and could not spend sufficient time at home to look after Walter. He also worried that he could not shield Walter from neighborhood derision. "I find it almost impossible to protect him from remarks calculated to disturb his nervous system and live in constant dread lest he would, in a moment, inflict some injury to some member of my family," he wrote to Godding. "He is harmless if not thwarted, but it is hard to impress those acquainted with his condition that they should humor him and utterly impossible to indicate the same to the boys in the street."

Ultimately Henry asked Godding to take Walter back, despite Walter's insistence that he remain at home. "At first he was very positive in declaring that he would not return," Henry wrote of his son, "but by judicious management he agreed to return. Mild restraint is what he requires, but my forced absence from home prevents me from exercising the necessary surveillance. I am more grateful for your kind attention which I have learned the past few days to appreciate more highly, if possible, than heretofore." Walter died three years later, in the custody of the staff of what Henry referred to as the "best humane institution on the face of the Globe."[62] Henry and his family were members of a small but growing black middle class. His wife, Catherine, was listed in the 1880 census as keeping house, and they employed a young female servant. Their neighbors included a white physician and a black carpenter. Although there is not a large enough sample to draw correlations between the class background of patients' families and their responses to institutionalization, it is certainly possible that Henry's federal employment made him even more inclined than others to embrace the federal institution as a solution to his domestic crisis.[63]

Henry's main concern was that if his son were not institutionalized, either Walter or his siblings would potentially be physically harmed. Other parents of Saint Elizabeths inmates expressed a concern about their inability to provide sufficient care if their children were released. One father conveyed this rationale to his son, a sailor who had been admitted to the hospital in August 1887 with a diagnosis of chronic melancholia as a result of intemperance. "I have written to you twice but have received no answer," Dennis M. reminded his son, Isaac. "You wrote last year that you wanted me to bring you home. The Government can take care of you much better than I can."[64]

Maria C., whose forty-year-old son, George, was admitted to Saint Elizabeths twice in the short span of three months, expressed a similar sentiment, although in a prickly letter to the hospital staff instead of to her son. George was initially admitted to the hospital in April 1885 suffering from acute mania as a result of an injury to the head. After being released in May, he ended up back in Saint Elizabeths in July. This time his diagnosis was paresis, or partial paralysis. In November, Maria wrote to one of the staff physicians inquiring about the health of her son. She herself was sick and hoped that he would not be released anytime soon. In addition, she expressed some concern about being alone with him in her house. One month later George apparently communicated to her that, after an examination, staff physicians had discussed the possibility of discharging him. This provoked a somewhat fretful letter from Maria, in which she offered her own assessment of George's health: "I think my self he is not well enough to come out for I am sick myself with the Rhumastism so that I can hardly get along myself. And please dont let him out here to run the street like he did before and I am not able to run after him and take care of him and if you think he is fit to come out you can let him out."[65] George was never released, and he died in the hospital in December 1886. We do not know whether Maria's assessment carried any weight with the asylum's physicians or, indeed, whether George was even being truthful about the physicians contemplating his release in the first place. Despite the syntax of the last line of her plea, within the context of the entire letter, it reads as if she was throwing down a gauntlet. The tone suggests she meant that if the staff at Saint Elizabeths felt that George was ready to be discharged, then they should maintain responsibility for caring for him. Of course, we will never know. What is significant here is that Maria, like many other relatives of inmates, felt entitled to communicate her beliefs and her desires with respect to her son's illness and how the hospital should deal with it.

Although it had some of the characteristics of a penitentiary—and some patients and their families may have perceived it as such—Saint Elizabeths was also seen as a resource for some members of Washington, DC's African American community. Whether it was a space for the provision of healthcare, a refuge from conniving family members, or, as some of the letters have suggested, a means of employment, many black Washingtonians considered the institution a potential asset to deal with problems within their families and communities. When African Americans interacted with Saint Elizabeths, they understood it to be more than a hospital. They understood it to be an arm of the federal government, an embodiment of the state. Whether it was Henry J., a federal employee drawing on another federal institution for assistance, or the father of Isaac M., who directly ceded the ability to care for his son to the "Government," black Washingtonians were not reticent about accessing the levers of the state. Furthermore, many attempted to maneuver those levers in a way that preserved their own autonomy and sense of responsibility for their loved ones. In doing so, they made claims on the state at a time when African American citizenship was under assault from all directions. These efforts might not have been a collective endeavor, but they demonstrate their sense of entitlement as citizens.

Race, Moral Treatment, and Conflicting Imperatives

The state of psychiatric treatment was on Godding's mind when he delivered his departing address as AMSAII president in 1890. The superintendent offered a grim assessment of the profession's current capacity to cure the mentally ill, even as he expressed a cautious optimism about the future. He emphasized the importance of making medical interventions in cases of acute insanity and pointed to potentially promising new therapies such as brain surgery, hypnosis, hydrotherapy, and the use of electricity. But his confidence in the curative possibilities of psychiatry was tempered by acknowledgment that the chronically mentally ill presented a challenge for the profession, and especially institutional psychiatrists. "It is undoubtedly true," he told his fellow superintendents at the Niagara Falls meeting, "that when all has been done a majority of those persons admitted to our hospitals as insane will remain permanent inmates." The best that his peers could do for this unfortunate class was to continue to provide moral treatment—ensuring that the hospital had a homelike atmosphere and that patients were "employed at something, industrial or other[wise]."

Unfortunately this therapeutic model was becoming less effective because of the overcrowding that characterized most state institutions. The excessively large patient populations not only militated against the tranquil environment necessary for moral treatment; they also impeded hospital staff's ability to adequately employ more active therapies in acute cases. "Day by day, year after year," Godding lamented, "I have seen the individualized treatment of special cases swamped by the rising tide of indiscriminate lunacy pouring through the wards, filling every crevice, rising higher and higher until gradually most distinctions and landmarks have been blotted out." Godding's criticism of the state of psychiatric treatment was shared by many of his colleagues. By the 1890s the increased number of the chronically insane in state institutions, the ascendancy of a neurological paradigm of mental illness that emphasized its hereditary and organic nature, and a growing concern that they were not keeping pace with other medical fields when it came to scientific advances contributed to a therapeutic pessimism among asylum physicians. In Godding's case, as in those of his peers, this pessimism was compounded by parsimonious government support and intrusive regulation.[66]

Despite the expansion of the hospital grounds during Godding's tenure, the institution was still experiencing overcrowding on the eve of his death in May 1899. In 1896 Saint Elizabeths had to stop admitting independent, or pay, patients because the existing buildings could barely accommodate soldiers, sailors, and indigent civilians. Godding lobbied for the Interior Department's purchase of Wilson Park, a plot of land on the southern border of the hospital, on the rationale that the federal government should make every effort to physically expand the hospital, especially given that members of the US Army and US Navy were returning from fighting the Spanish, "stricken with fever and bereft of reason." He thought it particularly negligent of the government to allow these soldiers and sailors to be treated in such close proximity to insane convicts and the criminally insane, a position that was shared by William Van Amberg Sullivan, Democratic senator from Mississippi.

In his support for the bill, Sullivan also broached the topic of race. The commingling of the white and African races in Saint Elizabeths was just as noxious, he pointed out, as the mixing of mentally ill military personnel and lunatics with criminal tendencies. "We have a case where the only question remaining," Sullivan told his colleagues, "apparently, is whether we are going to permit the present state of affairs to continue for the future—whether we are going to permit the criminal classes to be dumped in there and held there with the other classes of insane; whether we are going to permit the races to be mingled there the one with the other. No sane man would submit to the very same treatment to which the insane are—without their consent of course—subjected." Opposition to the bill came from numerous quarters, including congressmen who thought the asking price of $245,000 was too steep, and a local white neighborhood organization, the Congress Heights Citizens' Association, which feared that an expansion of the hospital would bring it too close to a newly built public school. In the end, opponents of the bill carried the day.[67]

A year after the bill to acquire Wilson Park was introduced, the hospital's annual report expressed concern about another class of patients that was rapidly increasing: African Americans. Despite the fact that between 1896 and 1900 the number of black patients as a percentage of the total inmate population had increased by less than 1 percent, the authors of the report felt it necessary to speak specifically to the substantial number of African Americans in the hospital. Perhaps it was part of a ploy to tap into Sullivan's and like-minded congressmen's concern about potential race-mixing, in a larger effort to pressure Congress into acquiring more land for the hospital. The Board of Visitors in fact proposed a major expansion of the hospital campus. The existing buildings were on the western side of a major thoroughfare called Nichols Avenue. In order to fully accommodate increasing numbers of patients, the board suggested that the hospital would have to begin constructing buildings on the eastern side of Nichols Avenue if the federal government did not purchase Wilson Park. From the board's perspective, expansion on the eastern side was less than ideal because it would encroach upon the hospital's farmland. Even though no one associated with the hospital had raised the specter of race-mixing as an argument for the acquisition of Wilson Park, the benefit of more rigid racial segregation did factor into the board's case for expansion. "If restricted to the land now belonging to the hospital it will be necessary to extend the building site to the east of Nichols avenue and to use for this purpose a considerable portion of the farm land of the institution," the board informed the secretary of the interior. "It has been suggested that the colored patients be all provided for on that side and also the more disturbed and untidy of the white males."[68]

By proposing that all of the black patients be sequestered alongside the most depraved white male lunatics on the eastern side of Nichols Avenue, some within the hospital's administration conflated blackness with disorder and, by correlation, whiteness with respectability. This was, in short, the application of the policy of housing African American male patients with the criminally insane in Howard Hall to the hospital as a whole. But it went further in that it ignored gender distinctions within the larger class of mentally ill African Americans. Hospital staff need not worry about effectively implementing segregation of the sexes within the African American patient population because the race had not achieved the same gender differentiation as more "civilized" whites in the first place. Conversely this policy rationale reaffirmed the respectability of white women—or at least the possibility of obtaining or regaining this status.[69]

It is not surprising that board members would float this proposal, especially given that black madness was construed within the medical profession as being particularly depraved and violent. Even the concession of Godding's primary assistant physician, A. H. Witmer, that insanity in blacks and whites was "essentially the same" did not dislodge the medical consensus regarding mental illness in African Americans. Indeed although Witmer allowed for the presence of melancholia among African Americans, he continued to advance the theory that the practice of suicide was exceedingly rare. The general idea that mentally ill African Americans were less likely than whites to become withdrawn or introverted influenced the hospital's inmate management practices.[70] The hospital administration subscribed to and reproduced a racial logic which posited that black insanity, regardless of its specific causes or symptoms, approximated the most pathological and violent forms of insanity among whites.

The proposed sequestration of African American patients on the eastern side of Nichols Avenue never materialized. Some board members had reservations about creating such a sharp division within the patient population, reservations that were shaped more by a desire to maintain operational efficiency than by an altruistic concern for the effects that more rigid segregation might have on the psyches or material conditions of African American patients. "Nichols Avenue is a busy thoroughfare," the 1900 annual report stated,

> the travel on which is annually increasing, and it is also occupied by a line of street cars with overhead trolley. To place several hundred of the population of the hospital on the side of this avenue opposite to the rest of the institution would, as we believe, seriously jeopardize their safety. There is of necessity frequent interchange among the different portions of the hospital, and if restricted to the colored patients alone, which will not be found possible, this would be very considerable. The chief amount of work now done by patients in the domestic departments, including the laundry and kitchen, is done by the colored female patients. This arrangement would necessitate their crossing this avenue at least four times daily.[71]

Although critics of the proposal did evince a concern for the physical safety of the black female patients, they stated their concerns within a larger set of assumptions about black women and work. For the hospital administration there was no doubt that African American female patients would perform the kind of labor that was associated with African American women outside of the hospital's walls. In this sense, the desire to more rigidly segregate patients on the basis of race conflicted with the desire to reproduce the social roles of racialized groups within the asylum.

As the hospital entered the twentieth century, then, race continued to figure into how the staff and administrators approached their understandings of insanity and implemented patient policy. The post-Reconstruction period had led to a rethinking of black mental illness, drawing on both biology and culture to explain its increase and its fundamental distinctiveness from insanity among whites. Even as hospital administrators continued to take seriously their responsibility for tending to the healthcare needs of mentally ill African Americans, they subordinated those needs to the needs of white patients. This dynamic continued into the early twentieth century as, beginning in 1903, William Alanson White assumed the position of superintendent and oversaw the modernization of psychiatric therapy at the hospital for the next three and a half decades.

5

"Mechanisms of the Negro Mind"

Race and Dynamic Psychiatry at Saint Elizabeths, 1903–1937

In October 1903 Dr. William Alanson White became superintendent of Saint Elizabeths. The forty-six-year-old New Yorker had been trained at Long Island Medical College, where his "total instruction in psychiatry," he recalled in his autobiography, was a professor's impromptu lecture inspired by a case of suspected malingering. He interned as a house and ambulance surgeon at the Eastern District Hospital in Brooklyn and on the staff of the Alms and Workhouse Hospital on Blackwell's Island. White developed an interest in psychiatry in the course of taking classes in psychology and philosophy, which were cognate fields in the late nineteenth century. After failing to obtain a position as assistant physician at the Utica Asylum in upstate New York, he secured employment at Binghamton Asylum on Long Island in 1892. He remained there for eleven years before assuming control of Saint Elizabeths.[1]

When he arrived at Saint Elizabeths, White found the practice of psychiatry there to be somewhat outmoded. Godding had instituted a pathology department during his tenure, but, for the most part, White was dissatisfied with the absence of the standard practices and procedures associated with European, particularly German, clinics. A few decades after taking the helm of Saint Elizabeths, White recounted his initial vision for the hospital:

> When I came to the Superintendency of Saint Elizabeths Hospital . . . I found an institution with all the traditions of humanitarianism and the Quaker ideas which had found their way from England but which had never assimilated the scientific aspects of the problem and was comfortably moving along in the old lines of a domiciliary institution. . . . It was my aim at that time to bring to bear in the Hospital the knowledge which had been developed very largely at that time in foreign countries,—the scientific understanding of this class of patients and the methods of therapeutically handling their individual problems,

to get away as far as possible from the oldtime mass handling of patients in large numbers to the individualization of the specific cases with a view to their understanding and with a view to helping them.[2]

Despite several challenges, White managed to shepherd the institution into the age of modern psychiatry, and in the process he modernized Nichols's dream by turning Saint Elizabeths into a model teaching and research hospital.

During his tenure, Saint Elizabeths established strong relationships with local medical schools; staff psychiatrists and physicians were on the faculties of these schools, and students took clinical courses routinely offered at the hospital. Under White's guidance, the hospital also initiated outpatient clinics, child guidance centers, and psychiatric social work services, projecting Saint Elizabeths' medical authority into the community with ever increasing regularity. The therapeutic regime was also transformed over the course of his superintendency. The nineteenth-century moral treatment model gave way to therapies aimed at curing mental illness through both physiological and psychological interventions. All of these were more invasive than moral therapy in their own ways, attempting to access the interiority of the mentally ill either by manipulating the blood, glands, and brain or by peering into the unconscious. With varying levels of support from the hospital administration, staff members began to research and utilize somatic treatments such as malaria fever inoculation, chemical- and electrical-based convulsive therapies, and prefrontal lobotomy. Moreover White was an adherent of psychoanalysis, and, as such, psychotherapy became an important tool in staff psychiatrists' armamentarium.

Central to White's modernization of Saint Elizabeths was his formal partition of the medical services and the laboratory research work, creating separate clinical and scientific departments, each overseen by its own director. The scientific department consisted of a pathologist, clinical pathologist, histopathologist, and psychologist. For White, the inclusion of a laboratory capable of conducting research into abnormal psychology was critical because it served as a bridge between the clinical observations of patients on the ward and the pathological findings of postmortem cases.[3] White also modernized the medical services by standardizing the clinical record and introducing the conference report. He directed the staff to examine patients no less often than once a month in their first year after admission and no less often than once every three months for patients considered to be in a chronic condition (except, of course, when acute medical crises required immediate attention).

Standardizing the clinical records required transitioning to the "folder system," whereby each patient's file was to be kept individually, as opposed to the earlier practice of accumulating massive amounts of patient data in bound volumes.[4] Utilizing this more comprehensive case record system, White instituted regular meetings six days a week in order to give staff physicians an opportunity to consult each other about particular patients' diagnoses, symptoms, and prognoses. In addition to utilizing the conference report in order to develop a consensus around what constituted recovery or improvement, the superintendent envisioned the report's having some value in the aftermath of a patient's death. That is, a close perusal of a detailed clinical report by the entire medical staff would potentially allow them to draw correlations between the clinical observations of patients while they were alive and the pathology reports that were produced from their autopsies.[5]

For all of its scientific and medical advancements, White's superintendency was plagued by some of the same problems that hounded his predecessors. Despite taking over the hospital after a brief period of expansion by his immediate predecessor, Dr. Alonzo B. Richardson, White continued to battle problems of chronic overcrowding, understaffing, and lack of resources.[6] These problems precipitated a congressional investigation in 1906 after the Medico-Legal Society of Washington, DC, a local organization of physicians and lawyers concerned with medical jurisprudence, issued an unsolicited public report on Saint Elizabeths. The society's report criticized the institution's administrative inefficiency, pointing out that although the death and recovery rates at Saint Elizabeths were comparable to other insane asylums, the hospital's per capita cost was $220, as compared to the national average of $78. The report also claimed that patients were routinely abused, including being strangled with wet towels, placed in straitjackets, strapped to beds, battered, and force-fed.[7]

That spring a congressional committee—consisting of three Republican and two Democratic representatives—questioned 287 witnesses, including "disinterested persons" such as superintendents of other insane asylums. Former and current employees and patients told the committee of instances in which patients working in the laundry were choked with towels; patients were straitjacketed and bound to trees; patients were coerced by attendants into assaulting one another; and at least one shirtless patient had his back flogged with a belt. Witnesses also spoke of unsanitary conditions and practices in the hospital's kitchens and the tactic used by staff to circumvent the Board of Visitors' monthly inspections by cleaning up the wards and making sure to take all of the ambulatory patients for a walk at the scheduled time of the board members' arrival.[8]

An important line of inquiry taken up by the committee was the hospital's practice of segregating patients—the criminally insane from the noncriminal insane, whites from blacks, and epileptics from nonepileptics. In his testimony, the first assistant physician, Dr. Maurice Stack, indicated that male "colored epileptics and homicidals" were housed in the same wards with nonepileptic and noncriminal African American men. White confirmed this during his own testimony, when he was asked if epileptics were separated from the general patient population. "All of them except the colored," White responded. "You understand," he continued, "the problem of segregation in our institution is particularly difficult, because we first have to divide them into male and female and then into black and white, and the difference between dividing into two sections and into four is not a difference of twice as much. It increases in difficulty by geometrical ratio." But White went further, making the point that the creation and maintenance of race-exclusive wards increased the overall cost per patient. In housing approximately a half-dozen tubercular African American male patients in a building that could accommodate at least thirty individuals, White confessed, "we are losing a good deal on that segregation."[9] Stack's and White's testimony revealed the paradoxes of the simultaneously arbitrary and dogmatic nature of segregation policy at the hospital. On the one hand, the lack of resources and a superficial perception of mental illness among African Americans led to the commingling of categories of patients who would otherwise be segregated according to the professional standards of the day. On the other hand, in his efforts to adhere to strict racial segregation, White drove up the per capita cost of running the institution, ironically one of the reasons the Medico-Legal Society criticized his administration.

And yet the presence of African American patients at Saint Elizabeths presented White and his staff with the opportunity to study the black psyche and what they presumed to be its fundamental distinctiveness from the white psyche. In the early twentieth century, psychiatrists were moving toward a dynamic conception of the field, one that went beyond contemplating the prognosis of mental disorders based on static descriptions of symptoms and, instead, stressed the importance of approaching whole individuals—including constitution, life experiences, conscious and unconscious memories—and their interactions with their social environments.[10] The necessity of developing a comprehensive physical, psychological, emotional, and experiential portrait of the mentally ill individual as a basis for addressing, and perhaps eliminating, their psychoses and psychoneuroses resulted in the increased use of psychotherapy on Saint Elizabeths' wards. But foundational to this psychotherapeutic regime was also the desire to discover the universal processes that contributed to—as well as undermined—the ability of a person to successfully adapt to his or her environment. In this sense, the "new psychiatry" that was practiced at Saint Elizabeths integrated research and treatment.[11] With respect to race, much of the clinical investigation during the White years was aimed at establishing a comparative psychology through which the psychiatric profession would be able to more fully comprehend white abnormal psychology. But even as the empirical data failed to support their theoretical premises, Saint Elizabeths psychiatrists continued to reaffirm the existence of a distinctive black psyche that operated by different mechanisms than did the white mind.

The Emergence of Dynamic Psychiatry

By the time White assumed leadership of Saint Elizabeths, the field of psychiatry was undergoing a significant transformation. This transformation had begun with the ascendancy of neurology in the late nineteenth century. In much the same way that the germ theory had revolutionized medicine by confirming the idea that many somatic diseases were specific entities caused by microorganisms, the field of neurology promised to advance understandings of mental disease by establishing a correlation between diseased or damaged sections of the nervous system and abnormal behavior. This scientific turn expanded the purview of the field beyond institutional administration to include laboratory study of mental diseases and the treatment of nervous conditions such as neurasthenia and hysteria. A greater understanding of brain anatomy and neural function led to the displacement of eighteenth-century faculty psychology—the belief that the mind was compartmentalized into areas that governed intellect, moral affect, and passion—that had underpinned the asylum physician's craft. As White wrote in the beginning of his influential textbook, first published in 1907, "The old psychology conceived of mind as composed of a number of cubby holes in each one of which was pigeon-holed a special faculty, feeling, thinking, volition, each one of which was quite as distinct from the others as this illustration implies. This conception has become inadequate and false." The acceptance of the interconnectedness of mental functions eventually contributed to the demise of the tripartite paradigm of mental disease that identified mania, melancholia, and dementia as the primary forms of insanity.[12]

The man who was most responsible for introducing a new classificatory scheme to replace the outdated trinity was the German psychiatrist Emil Kraepelin. Working at the renowned psychiatric clinic at Heidelberg University during the 1890s, Kraepelin employed a longitudinal approach to charting how psychosis evolved in individual patients as a step toward understanding the nature of mental illness. He was particularly concerned with cases in which dementia, which normally occurred late in the life cycle, afflicted people at an earlier age. His meticulous collection of patient data allowed him to construct a new diagnostic concept of—or, rather, elaborate on and develop a new way of thinking about—a form of insanity that some psychiatrists had begun noticing years earlier. Dementia praecox, the Latin term for precocious dementia (a dementia that occurred early in an individual's life cycle), typically surfaced between puberty and age thirty; was characterized by cognitive decline, although its manifestation might differ from patient to patient; and resulted in permanent, irreversible loss of mental function. Although the symptoms of dementia praecox sufferers varied, the progression of the disease and its pessimistic prognosis is what distinguished dementia praecox from other psychoses. In moving away from the emphasis on symptoms that were associated with mid-nineteenth-century forms of insanity and identifying a mental disease on the basis of its course and outcome, Kraepelin revolutionized the way the psychiatric profession classified mental disorders. A few years later he added another disease concept to the diagnostic lexicon of psychiatrists when he identified manic-depressive psychosis, a condition in which sufferers cycled through periods of mental excitation and depression with intervals of lucidity.[13]

By the first decade of the twentieth century, dementia praecox—which psychiatrists would increasingly refer to as schizophrenia in the interwar period—and manic-depressive psychosis had become the principal diagnoses of sufferers of mental illness, accounting for more than 50 percent of cases in some institutions.[14] Upon becoming superintendent, White quickly implemented a classification scheme that included dementia praecox and manic-depressive psychoses along with, among others, toxic psychoses, paranoia and paranoid states, paresis, and senile psychoses.[15] Although he acknowledged the overall contribution of Kraepelinian nosology to the field, like many of his American colleagues White recognized the limitations of its rigidity as well as its implications for understanding the nature of mental illness and how to treat it.

In the first edition of his textbook, for instance, published just two years after he introduced a Kraepelinian-dependent classification scheme into Saint Elizabeths, he informed the reader that the symptoms of the manic stage of manic-depressive psychosis could be misinterpreted as dementia praecox; as such, it was incumbent upon the psychiatrist to engage in long-term observation of the patient in order to identify other symptoms associated with the latter disease. However, he prefaced the entire textbook with an admission that the diagnostic criteria that formed the basis of the new psychiatry were roughly placed signposts rather than precise markers on some psychical map. "As a matter of fact our knowledge of insanity is altogether too limited at present to justify the expectation that the problem of classification can be solved," White wrote. "Any attempt at grouping mental disorders under separate heads must at present be but tentative and incomplete."[16]

White became even more doubtful about the Kraepelinian paradigm by 1920. Particularly with respect to dementia praecox, he wrote to a colleague, "On the diagnostic side I feel that we have no reliable criteria of diagnosis."[17] This skepticism also characterized White's and others' attitudes toward the influence that Kraepelin's classification had on the profession's understanding of the causes and prognoses of mental diseases. If there was murkiness between the diagnostic criteria distinguishing dementia praecox and manic-depressive psychosis, for example, then what did that mean for the therapeutic possibilities for patients caught in this confusion? The prognosis for manic-depressive psychosis was more optimistic than for dementia praecox in the sense that its sufferers did not experience permanent mental deterioration. Given that the grim prognosis of dementia praecox might make hospital superintendents inclined to provide minimal therapy, where did this leave manic-depressives who were misdiagnosed? Also, how were the spontaneous recoveries of those diagnosed with dementia praecox to be explained? The dire expectations of the outcome of dementia praecox exacerbated the atmosphere of therapeutic pessimism in mental hospitals in the late nineteenth and early twentieth century.

Dr. C. Macfie Campbell, an assistant physician at New York's Bloomingdale Hospital and a member of the Cornell University Medical College faculty, expressed his frustration with Kraepelin's disease construct in a contribution to White and Smith Ely Jellife's edited collection on nervous and mental diseases. "How can one treat a disorder with regard to the nature of which we have so shadowy a conception?" he asked. "The treatment, as outlined by Kraepelin, bears no direct relation to the hypothetical disorder of metabolism, but is merely directed toward maintaining the nutrition of the patient by the usual methods, procuring sleep, managing the excitement, and in the quieter phases furnishing suitable occupations."[18] Despite the purported advances in the diagnosis and classification of psychoses, Campbell regretted the persistence of what was essentially the moral management model associated with the nineteenth-century asylum.

Linked to Campbell's observation of the therapeutic cul-de-sac created by Kraepelin's new diagnostic category was his critical appraisal of the etiological theories advanced by the German psychiatrist. As Campbell pointed out, there was no "direct relation" between treatment and the "hypothetical disorder of metabolism" that Kraepelin posited as the causal factor in dementia praecox. For Kraepelin, psychoses were the result of abnormal physiological processes. Rather than attributing insanity to brain lesions—a hypothesis that animated, but ultimately frustrated, neurologists—he theorized that it was the product of the accumulation of toxins within the body. Whereas physicians in the nineteenth and early twentieth centuries had postulated that many somatic diseases were the result of autointoxication originating in the intestines, Kraepelin suggested that mental disorders emerged from the poisoning of the glands. The toxins emitted by the gonads, for instance, explained dementia praecox's typical onset during adolescence, when the sexual glands were becoming more active. The proposed somatic origins of psychoses, Kraepelin and like-minded psychiatrists believed, promised to elevate their discipline within the larger field of medicine in that they would now be able to draw correlations between their clinical observations and the gross and cellular pathologies they observed in the body's interior. They would, in other words, be able to specify mental disease by its origins (rather than solely through symptoms), much as physicians were able to specify somatic disease by identifying the responsible pathogenic microorganism.[19]

But there was resistance to Kraepelin's biological reductionism within the American psychiatric profession, not the least of which may have been caused by his emphasis on the glandular basis of psychopathology at a time before the field of endocrinology had fully matured.[20] Much of this resistance was led by Adolf Meyer, who happened to be the individual most responsible for introducing the Kraepelinian paradigm to the United States in the first place. Born in Switzerland and trained at the University of Zurich, Meyer immigrated to the United States in 1892 at the age of twenty-five. He served as the pathologist of Illinois Eastern Hospital for the Insane in Kankakee from 1893 to 1895, and then occupied the position of pathologist and clinical director at Worcester Lunatic Hospital from 1895 to 1901. It was at this latter institution where he implemented Kraepelin's diagnostic criteria. Meyer would go on to become the director of the Pathological Institute in New York City and, ultimately, the chief of Johns Hopkins University's Henry Phipps Psychiatric Clinic. These prominent positions, along with his teaching post at Johns Hopkins, gave Meyer an inordinate amount of influence on the development of American psychiatry. Along with his fellow Swiss émigré August Hoch, Meyer moved American psychiatry away from a crude somatism to a more ecological understanding of mental disease.[21]

Although he did not completely reject its biological aspects, Meyer advocated for an etiology of mental illness that was grounded in psychogenesis. That is, rather than viewing psychosis as solely the product of organic (i.e., anatomical or physiological) malfunction, psychiatrists needed to understand it as the result of an individual's maladaptation to his or her environment.[22] Psychoses could not be reduced to bodily processes, uniform symptom clusters, predictable courses, inevitable outcomes, and pathological specimens. Thinking about mental illness in this way resulted in a superficial approach to a patient's symptoms, a form of psychiatry that critics derided as "descriptive." Rather, Meyer and those influenced by him appealed for a more dynamic psychiatry, one that took into consideration the totality of the afflicted individual, including personality type, life history, and—for those who would eventually subscribe to psychoanalysis— repressed memories, which were the residue of internal psychosexual conflicts.

This approach to understanding and treating the mentally ill was a clear rejection of the materialist conceptions of insanity that underpinned nineteenth-century asylum medicine. Psychiatrists had to acknowledge that psychoses could originate, evolve, and subside in an individual independently of any physiological process that was going on in his or her body.[23] This did not mean that the corporeal was insignificant, however. Indeed practitioners of this new psychiatry rejected "psychophysical parallelism," an earlier doctrine in the field of psychology that posited a correspondence, but not an interaction, between the physiological and mental functions of the human body. Soma and psyche interacted in extremely important ways, and it was incumbent upon psychiatrists to understand how these interactions preserved mental health or precipitated mental disorder.[24] Further, the interrelated physical and mental processes occurring in the body shaped, and in turn were shaped by, the individual's environment. It was the psychiatrist's responsibility to investigate and determine how these multilevel interactions played out not only contextually but diachronically as well.

This framing of mental illness was captured in Meyer's use of the concept of "psychobiology." Meyer reasoned that mental illness was a combination of an individual's constitutional and temperamental predisposition as well as, over time, the "deficiency of critical and consecutive thought habits." He named this latter phenomenon "habit disorganization" or "deterioration."[25] But habit disorganization did not manifest identically in people; rather, the way this process developed was shaped by individual personality. Meyer purported to identify several different "reaction types" that would conduce to neurotic and psychotic disorders. Reaction types de-emphasized the static diagnostic concepts that underpinned Kraepelin's classification scheme and emphasized psychopathology's origins in an individual's adaptation to his or her surroundings. In order to effectively diagnose and treat the mentally ill, psychiatrists had to look beyond obvious signs and symptoms and decipher the more complex personality types and their reactions to environmental stimuli. Rather than being mere observers and classifiers, psychiatrists needed to engage in excavation projects.[26]

White, a prominent member of the Meyer camp, defined psychopathology and the psychiatrist's role in arresting it along these lines. "The mental symptoms of the psychoses can be spoken of as a disease only in the sense that, and in so far as, they represent failure on the part of the individual, a lack of capacity for efficient adjustment," he wrote in the tenth edition of his textbook, *Outlines of Psychiatry*. "And inasmuch as it is the individual's adjustment to the other individuals who make up his social environment that constitutes his reactions as essentially human, it is disorder at this level of adjustment, namely, the *social level* that essentially characterizes the psychoses."[27] What Kraepelin's conceptualization of psychosis had failed to do, White believed, was take into consideration the "entire life of the individual" as a contributing factor in the onset of mental disease. "Inasmuch as the symptoms must be explained by an uncovering of their past," White reasoned, "it follows that a psychosis is a form of reaction which can only be interpreted if we know the history of the development of the individual."[28]

The history to which psychiatrists needed to be attentive extended beyond the consciously recoverable experiences of the individual to include the interactions and experiences that had been expunged from his or her psyche.

The unconscious was a realm that dynamic psychiatrists had to be comfortable navigating. Psychoanalysis would become an indispensable tool for this navigation, and both Meyer and White incorporated the technique into their therapeutic repertoire. Neither man, however, became an inflexible follower of any particular psychoanalytical tradition. Meyer was instrumental in introducing psychoanalysis to the American psychiatric profession, although he increasingly became skeptical of Freudians' tendency to reduce the psychogenic origins of mental disorders to overly schematic notions of libido, instincts, and psychosexual conflict.[29]

White's embrace of psychoanalysis occurred fairly quickly. There was very little Freud in the inaugural edition of his textbook, and White mentioned the Viennese's work on hysteria only in the chapter on borderland and episodic states. Between 1909 and 1911 he published two articles and one book on psychoanalysis. The third edition of his textbook, published in 1911, expanded coverage of Freud's work on compulsion and anxiety neuroses; it also explicitly referenced psychoanalysis as a form of therapy. In a very cautious, balanced evaluation of Freudian theory in 1912, White credited psychoanalysis with being an effective tool for unraveling the "mental tangles" of their patients. However, he did not take a firm position on one of the criticisms of Freudianism—that is, its reduction of mental disorder to psychosexual conflict. "Whether an upset in the sexual sphere must always necessarily be at the bottom of a psychosis or a neurosis, is, upon theoretical grounds, a debatable question." By the seventh edition, which was published in 1919, the standard psychoanalytic lexicon filled the pages, with White speaking of introversion, transference, and projection. Nonetheless, like many American psychiatrists, White was an eclectic. He wrote to W. A. Robinson in 1917, "We have followed Professor Freud's work and are using his psychoanalytic methods, without, however, dogmatizing about it or allying ourselves with any special cult."[30]

One of the advancements of dynamic psychiatry and psychoanalysis, their advocates claimed, was that they offered more hope to those afflicted with mental disorders than the somatic-based approaches associated with the Kraepelinian paradigm. Rather than analogizing psychoses to somatic diseases—with their specifiable origins, generalizable symptoms, and predictable outcomes—dynamic psychiatrists emphasized the individualistic nature of mental illness. Kraepelin had made the mistake of attempting to develop a singular portrait of the psychosis sufferer, they argued. "If we are to understand the psychosis we must understand the individual," White declared in the first edition of his textbook. "We must study not only his origin and development but his adjustment to conditions. We can not understand a psychosis by subjecting it to cross-section for the purpose of defining its content at a particular point, or by subjecting it to longitudinal section for the purpose of tracing the beginning and the end of symptoms. Such subjection to the narrow field of an optical section will not do—it must be studied as a life history. Our patients must be considered as individuals who under certain conditions have reacted in certain ways."[31] In their gathering of information about psychopathology in general, dynamic psychiatrists were also committed to developing and perfecting new therapeutic techniques. As such, dynamic psychiatry ushered in a therapeutic optimism that displaced the pessimism that had settled among asylum staffs dominated by hereditarian theories and neurological models of mental disease.[32]

But what did it mean to articulate this view of mental illness—and the prospect of recovery—in an institution and larger social and cultural environment in which African Americans were seen less as individuals and more as an undifferentiated racial group? There were, in fact, limits to dynamic psychiatry's individualizing of mental illness, limits that were in part the product of a stubborn collective—if occasionally wavering—belief in racial difference. To be sure, those committed to a dynamic conception of psychopathology were skeptical of hereditarianism for a number of reasons, including the racial implications that fueled anti-Semitism in Europe and underwrote eugenics policy in the United States.[33] The inherent tension between embracing a dynamic understanding of the mentally ill individual and adhering to the idea that there were racial psyches that could constitute the subject of comparative study contributed to a muddled and retrogressive approach to insanity among African Americans.

"Broken Fragments of the Primitive Life": Psychodynamic Research and the Idea of the Black Psyche

In April 1916 White attended the annual meeting of the American Medico-Psychological Association, as the AMSAII was renamed in 1892.[34] At the meeting, Dr. E. M. Green, the clinical director of the Georgia State Sanitarium, presented a paper on the existence of manic-depressive insanity among people of African descent. Along with dementia praecox, manic-depressive insanity had become one of the most commonly diagnosed mental disorders in the early twentieth century. Because of the pioneering clinical work of Kraepelin, psychiatrists were less inclined to think of mania and melancholia as either discrete mental diseases or variants of a singular psychosis; rather, they increasingly understood them as mental states that, when cycled through by an individual, constituted manic-depressive illness. This new conception unsettled earlier associations of mania and melancholia with levels of cognitive development and led to some debate over the extent to which people of African descent suffered from this newly identified psychosis.

Based on an examination of the records of close to three thousand black men and women admitted to his hospital between 1910 and 1915, as well as the annual reports of four mental hospitals that admitted African Americans, Green's study offered some conclusions that were contrary to many of his colleagues' assumptions about the black psyche. Whereas many psychiatrists—particularly northern psychiatrists, according to Green—drew correlations between susceptibility to manic-depressive insanity and an advanced level of social or civilizational advancement, Green asserted that the prevalence of the disorder among southern blacks confounded its conceptualization as a largely white, middle-class psychosis. "The negro is generally looked upon as having a more primitive type of mind than the white," he pointed out to his audience, "but the present study shows, nevertheless, that he exhibits the manic-depressive reaction type rather more frequently than does the latter." Although he was skeptical of any racially reductionist theories that posited fundamental distinctions in the ways that blacks and whites responded to psychical stress, Green did construct a profile of manic-depressive psychosis within the African American population that contained residual elements of earlier medical thought about black insanity. He suggested that the data confirmed certain assumptions regarding the racial inflection of the disorder, namely, that among African Americans "depressions are comparatively uncommon" and that the disorder "would more frequently be manifested in the manic form."[35] Thus, despite his openness to a race-blind conception of the psychosis, Green satisfied for many a desire to see racial differences in the mental illnesses exhibited by blacks and whites.

White was the first person to respond to Green's presentation. He commended the study but went on to lament the profession's overall lack of research with mentally ill African Americans. "We have a considerable number of negro patients in the public institutions of this country, and until very recently there has been no effort at all made at a comparative study of their psychic disturbances," White told his colleagues. "I presume this is particularly due to the fact that institutions exist for negroes alone, and but few for the white and negro together; hence the comparison is not thrust upon the attention of the medical officers, and also because many of you have never had any experience with this race." White went on to point out that, outside of the research being conducted by Green and Dr. George H. Kirby at Manhattan State Hospital in New York, Saint Elizabeths was the only mental hospital in which significant work was being done in an effort to ascertain the "racial peculiarities" of mental illness.[36]

The same year that Green presented his research, an assistant physician at Saint Elizabeths named Arrah Evarts published an article in the newly launched journal *Psychoanalytic Review*, entitled "Dementia Precox in the Colored Race." Evarts's research was based on her work with African American female patients at the hospital. In a footnote at the beginning of the article, the journal's editor remarked upon the importance of Saint Elizabeths having a racially heterogeneous patient population. "The existence side by side of the white and colored races in the United States offers a unique opportunity," he maintained, "not only to study the psychology of a race at a relatively low cultural level, but to study their mutual effects upon one another." The editor was most likely White, who, along with the prominent New York psychiatrist Smith Ely Jelliffe, founded the *Psychoanalytic Review* in 1913.[37] White's endorsement of the kind of work being done at Saint Elizabeths and his trumpeting of the hospital's privileged status in the area of race psychology research was no small aspect of his professional identity. He and his psychiatry staff engaged in research that aimed at both contributing to the field of comparative psychology and, in the case of African Americans, as he would put it a few years later, "classify[ing] disorders from the standpoint of a special racial standard."[38]

White laid the groundwork for clinical research in 1914 by creating a clinical psychiatry position, a position that would be staffed by a person who was trained in psychoanalysis, who was expected to psychotherapeutically treat patients, and who was encouraged to do laboratory-based research. The first person to occupy this position was Edward J. Kempf, a midwesterner who trained at Western Reserve Medical School in Cleveland and, unlike most American psychiatrists at the time, did not travel to Vienna or Zurich to study with the leading psychoanalysts. Nonetheless he became a convert to psychoanalysis and was actually fired from his post at the Indianapolis State Hospital in 1913 for using it to treat some of the patients suffering from dementia praecox.[39] Kempf held the position at Saint Elizabeths until 1920. The clinical psychiatry staff grew over the following decade. In 1923 Nolan D. C. Lewis became head of clinical psychiatry. A graduate of the University of Maryland's medical school, Lewis did postgraduate work at Johns Hopkins and spent a year studying at the University of Vienna. Under his stewardship, the clinical staff grew to four physicians—three of whom were trained in psychoanalysis—and one psychologist. The centrality of psychoanalysis to the hospital's identity was characterized by Jelliffe, who, in a 1929 letter to Sigmund Freud, summed up White and Saint Elizabeths by stating, "His whole hospital from the nurses up is all analytic."[40]

Kempf took great advantage of his new position to engage in clinical research. In his reminiscences of his early career, he remarked that at Saint Elizabeths he "had complete freedom to think out any problems in psychopathology and psychotherapy and select any male and female cases out of over 3,000 for analysis."[41] During his six years at the hospital, Kempf published a number of articles and two monographs. Conducting research using both primates and Saint Elizabeths patients, Kempf sought to develop a theory of psychosis that would blend Freudian psychogenesis with a physiological or neurological mechanism. Rejecting psychophysical parallelism in favor of an integrated nervous system, he theorized that the visceral body produced particular affective cravings—hunger, sex, and fear, to name a few—that the conscious mind had to gratify with minimal effort. This "continuous dynamic pressure" determined "the evolution of organic structure, of personality, behavior and achievement."[42] Psychoses developed, Kempf theorized, when the ego struggled to keep cravings from emerging into one's consciousness. The conflict between the ego and "the not quite socially justifiable or utterly unjustifiable cravings" was responsible for an individual's psychopathology.[43]

As his invocation of the "social" suggests, Kempf placed mental illness and mental health in a psychobiological framework. Normal adjustment to one's social environment required a balance between the healthy expression of the libido and a resistance to excessive sexual morality. "Man is a biological creation," he averred, "and only exists as a healthy, happy, constructive force so long as he lives in harmony with the self-refining tendencies of Nature and avoids both the castration tendencies of the prude and the degenerating exploitation of the vulgar." Kempf's understanding of psychopathology bore the imprint of Meyerian clinical psychiatry, which refused to reduce mental disease to either somatic or psychological causation. He had, in fact, been on Meyer's staff at the Phipps Clinic before taking his position at Saint Elizabeths.[44]

Unlike some of his fellow psychiatrists at Saint Elizabeths, Kempf was not particularly interested in the question of comparative psychology. In the introduction to his study of psychopathology, he clearly evinced a universalist conception of the psyche when he claimed that the data "demonstrated that all peoples tend to suffer from similar affective difficulties and that similar adjustments to similar cravings produce similar psychoses, no matter what country or race they come from." Yet Kempf's universalism was belied by assumptions about the white psyche and concerns about racial degeneracy. Of the ninety-four patients who were the subjects of his study, only one was of African descent—a thirty-nine-year-old man whose paranoid dissociation Kempf attributed to an acute homosexual panic. There was no hint of a belief in racial distinctiveness—at least in a narrow black/white sense—in his discussion of the case. Elsewhere in the study, however, Kempf expressed some apprehension about the possibility that the psychic conflict between the ego and affective cravings would become routine in "the more highly developed families of the race," given their stricter adherence to moral and social conventions. As abnormal responses to cravings—ranging from autoeroticism to homosexual eroticism—became more common in this group, Kempf asserted, the prospect of the "American people" being eclipsed by the "more primitive European immigrant" increased.[45] The American people whom Kempf imagined when he raised the alarm about race suicide and promoted race conservation most likely did not include people of African descent. Even as he purported to advance a universalist understanding of the mind and mental illness, his theory of psychopathology both assumed and reified the white psyche as the norm.[46]

But many of Kempf's colleagues and those who followed him at Saint Elizabeths explicitly rejected a universalist conception of the psyche and attempted to map out an African American mind that was at least inherently different from the white mind, if not altogether inferior to it. Between 1914 and 1933 at least ten studies on psychoses among African Americans or the distinctions between blacks and whites were authored and published by psychiatrists at Saint Elizabeths. Although most of them were published in White and Jelliffe's journal, a few appeared in the flagship journal of the American Psychiatric Association (which had changed its name from the American Medico-Psychological Association in 1922). The psychiatrists worked with different subsets of the African American patient population and were concerned with different research questions. They also employed different research methodologies, such as case series studies based on analyses of patient histories as well as clinical observations, including dream interpretation and word association; aggregate data studies based on analyses of patient histories and observations of the correlation between race and diagnoses; and psychoanalytic case studies. While Saint Elizabeths psychiatrists shared some fundamental concerns with academic comparative psychologists—including the effects of evolution on mental function and the relationships of organisms to their environments—understanding the connection between mental processes and behavior in nonhuman animals was not on their research agenda.[47] Ultimately, the conclusions they drew and, perhaps more important, the premises from which they started reflected an a priori belief in a distinctive black psyche. Moreover, inasmuch as they were producing psychiatric knowledge about people of African descent, their published research worked to reaffirm the white psyche as the norm and the fundamental abnormality of the black psyche.

Research into the black psyche trafficked in such stock ideas that we might consider the published work as rising to the level of genre.[48] Like the medical literature produced in the postemancipation period that attributed rising rates of insanity among African Americans to their release from bondage, the studies conducted by Saint Elizabeths psychiatrists drew on and reproduced certain truisms that presupposed racial difference. There were, however, a few things that distinguished the knowledge produced during the White era from the postemancipation period. One difference was that the former was based much more on actual clinical observation. Another significant distinction is that White's clinical staff used very little of the degeneracy discourse that characterized the postemancipation literature. Even though Saint Elizabeths psychiatrists used the same images of the negro and the same language as the earlier generation of physicians commenting on race and insanity, they did not

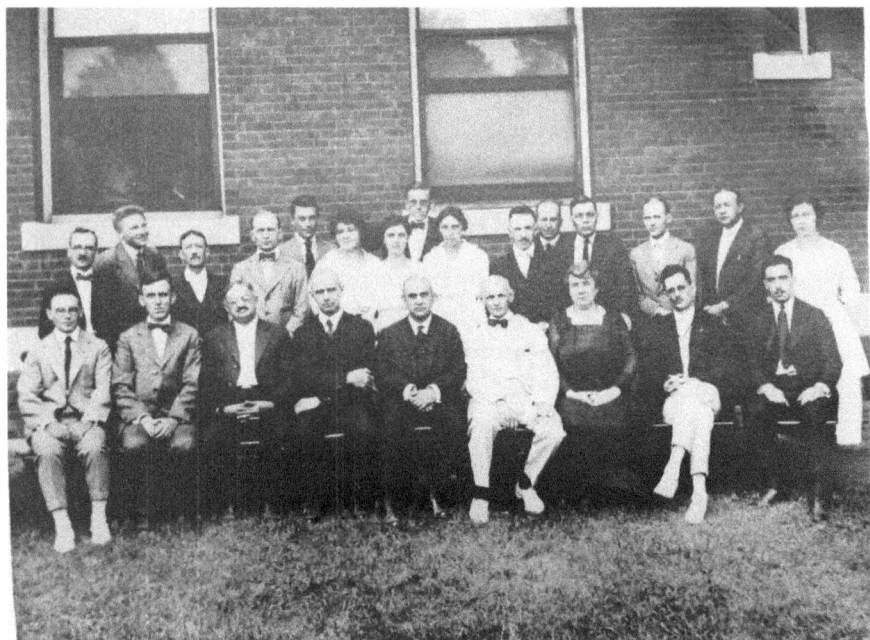

Some of Saint Elizabeths' clinical staff posing for a group photo shortly after World War I. Superintendent William A. White (fifth from left, front row) encouraged many of the hospital's psychiatrists—including John E. Lind (second from left, front row), Mary O'Malley (seventh from left, front row), and Lois Hubbard (seventh from left, back row)—to conduct research into the psychological differences between blacks and whites. *National Archives, photo 418-P-394.*

raise a red flag about the imminent extinction of the black race. This is not surprising. African Americans themselves, especially elites and intellectuals, had been combating ideas about black degeneration for decades. And any rational person could see that the African American population was not declining in number; in fact, with the massive migration of blacks from southern rural areas to northern and midwestern cities in the 1910s and 1920s, it may have appeared to whites that the race was growing exponentially.[49]

Nevertheless there were important holdovers from the earlier medical literature. One was the persistence of impressionistic judgments. Even though they might ground their empirical claims in individual case studies, aggregated data, or statistical profiles, Saint Elizabeths psychiatrists incorporated other forms of knowledge into their research, especially historical and ethnographic studies of people of African descent. Arrah Evarts, for instance, spoke of the necessity of understanding the "race history" of African Americans in order to comprehend the prevalence and pathology of dementia praecox within the group. Among other sources, she drew on such disparate representations of African history and culture as the work of Liberian intellectual Edward Wilmot Blyden and the safari chronicles of Theodore Roosevelt. According to the article's editor, Evarts's work was as much an "anthropology of the negro" as it was a study of dementia praecox.[50]

Similarly, John E. Lind—a senior assistant physician and at one point the chief medical officer of Howard Hall—cited extensively from the work of Alfred Burdon Ellis, a British military officer who wrote three books on Yoruba language and culture, and Robert Hamill Nassau, a Presbyterian missionary who published a book on fetishism in West Africa. Lind was particular about the sources that he drew from, rejecting banal diaries and travelogues for books "written by men who have spent their lives among the Africans and studied their languages, customs, religious beliefs and laws carefully."[51]

Evarts and Lind, along with many of their colleagues, insisted on the importance of situating African American mental illness within an evolutionary framework that considered their distance from—or, as it turns out, their proximity to—their ancestral past. "In endeavoring then to find a phylogenetic origin for the symptoms shown in the psychoses of the American Negro," Lind declared, "it would seem that we must look to the racial characteristics, religion, laws, customs, etc., of the true Negro, especially as he is seen in the region about the west coast [of Africa]."[52] Lind's reference to phylogeny in an article published in 1914 reflected the endurance of recapitulation theory, one of the principal nineteenth-century theories that elaborated the mechanisms of evolution. First articulated in the biogenetic law developed by German zoologist Ernst Haeckel, recapitulation theory held that as an individual organism matured, it passed through all of the developmental stages that composed the evolution of the species to which it belonged. Although the axiom "Ontogeny recapitulates phylogeny" referred broadly to all biological development, it was quickly taken up to explain the evolutionary pace of distinct races and the civilizational distances between them.

One of the most prominent American intellectuals to utilize recapitulation theory was the psychologist and president of Clark University, G. Stanley Hall. Concerned that the combination of an increasingly modern society and a repressive Victorian sensibility was creating a generation of weak-willed white American men, Hall advocated for the cultivation of savage behavior in young white boys. His advice was based on the premise that white youths were recapitulating the behavior of their race at its more primitive stage of evolution. They needed to be allowed to complete this phase of their development; if remnants of their ancestral behavior were arrested at this earlier stage, they, and ultimately the race, would cease to continue to evolve. The corollary to Hall's use of recapitulation theory was that the "lower races," including African Americans and Native Americans, had long ago stopped evolving, making the adults of these groups the developmental equivalent of white children.[53]

Interestingly enough, at a time when Hall was refining his use of the theory, it was being discredited by the emergence of genetic approaches to evolution. Recapitulation theory rested upon the Lamarckian concept of acquired inheritance—that is, traits and characteristics that were acquired could be passed on directly to one's offspring. In this sense, Hall's pedagogical philosophy posited that direct intervention in the lives of children and adolescents could produce the necessary traits and characteristics that would benefit each succeeding generation. Lamarckism, however, was displaced by the germ plasm theory of August Weismann, which held that traits were passed intergenerationally through the germ cells—sperm and ova—rather than the cells that made up the rest of the body, or somatic cells. As such, biological evolution occurred over the span of generations; the characteristics that one acquired in one's lifetime could not be directly bequeathed to one's offspring. Even as recapitulation theory was becoming a less suitable paradigm for understanding biological evolution, however, it remained a usable framework for psychiatrists to explain the phylogenetic dimensions of mental illness.[54]

It persisted in muted form, for instance, in the genetic psychology that Hall, and later White, posed as a fundamental concept in the study of mental processes. Genetic psychology assumed that the individual psyche was shaped by the cumulative history of the individual's "species" (or race) as much as it was by the individual's more immediate interaction with his or her social environment. "Genetic psychology," White wrote in his textbook, "gives the same value to mind that anatomy and physiology do to the body and like them recognizes that present forms can only be explained by the past. In other words the mind has a history just as the body has: it has its embryology and its comparative anatomy, and a study of the development of the mind in the individual, and its degree of development, likeness and differences in different races throws the same sort of light upon psychological facts as does the study of embryology and comparative anatomy upon the facts of anatomy and physiology."[55] As this passage suggests, for White, genetic psychology presupposed the existence of comparative psychology, an area in which he hoped Saint Elizabeths staff would contribute pioneering research.

Some of these very same staff members' attempts to oblige White explicitly utilized recapitulation theory as a lens through which to investigate mental illness among African Americans. Evarts began her article on dementia praecox with a succinct definition of recapitulation theory, concluding the first paragraph by stating, "Again and again do we see an individual, struggling against the awful onslaught of a psychosis, reverting to progressively lower and lower strata of the formation of his race." Dr. W. M. Bevis, an assistant physician at the hospital in the post–World War I period, began a 1921 article by pointing out, "[The] negro race evinces certain phylogenetic traits of character, habit, and behavior that seem sufficiently important to make the consideration of these peculiarities worth while." The "fact" that people of African descent were less evolved than whites and that this developmental disparity contributed to how each group experienced mental illness was so self-evident, Dr. Mary O'Malley stated in the introduction to her 1914 article, "that it requires no further discussion."[56]

Yet it did. Despite the fact that presumptions of racial difference shaped the research questions posed and the methodologies employed by Saint Elizabeths psychiatrists, the collective histories of their subjects confounded any neat correlative or causal relationships between race and group-specific psychopathology. Given the history of race-mixing in the United States, the question of what actually constituted the phylogenetic nature of the negro hung over the research conducted by the psychiatrists. This question produced a particular meme that ran through many of the articles published by Saint Elizabeths staff: that of the pure African versus the mixed-blood negro. John Lind felt that it was necessary to qualify his study of the function of dreams among African Americans, for instance, by acknowledging, "Perhaps only a small percentage, or it may be none, of the negroes whose dreams are recorded below, were of pure African blood." O'Malley, a senior assistant physician, likewise counseled her readers, "The race under consideration does not belong to the pure type of its ancestors, but has a greater or less degree of Caucasian blood intermixed with that of its own ancestry." She went on to note that the degree of miscegenation taking place in the nation's history made it "difficult to determine definitely what part either race plays separately in any patient or to determine the proportion of white and colored blood in an individual under observation."[57] These caveats, however, did not prevent them from moving forward in making sweeping claims about the influence of racial difference in the development of psychoses among African Americans.

At least one psychiatrist provided a class-based interpretation of miscegenation, thereby casting suspicion upon the racial credentials of race-mixing whites while confirming assumptions about the innately inferior psychological character of people of African descent. Bevis pointed out that miscegenation posed the potential for the evolutionary advancement of the "mulatto." However, given that "the white man by whom this fusion of blood starts is most often feeble-minded, criminal, or both," the typical offspring of mixed-race unions inherited the undesirable traits of both races. In the end, most Saint Elizabeths psychiatrists who acknowledged the impact of miscegenation on the historical development of the African American population resolved the intellectual problem by arguing that the influence of blacks' ancestral past was too powerful to play a secondary role in the evolution of their psyche. Lind, for instance, simply pointed out that, despite the extensive race-mixing that occurred in the United States, the African American patients with whom he worked showed "psychological aspects quite similar to those of the savage."[58] Although they did not use language with implications of racial extinction, the studies published in the 1910s and 1920s shared with the postemancipation literature a narrative of black racial atavism—the idea that African Americans were reverting to their savage ancestral past.

There was ample evidence of this reversion, according to the Saint Elizabeths psychiatrists. The evidence appeared in both the general observations they made of African American life as well as the specific signs and symptoms they observed in their African American patients. Blacks' propensity toward superstition and belief in witchcraft, for instance, were echoes of African paganism that shaped their interpersonal relationships and made their religion more an exercise in emotional catharsis than a set of moral standards. Although blacks kept their superstitious selves concealed from whites out of fear of being shamed, according to O'Malley, their innate belief in the supernatural surfaced in their delusions and obsessions.[59] Saint Elizabeths psychiatrists spoke of other primitive behaviors that connected African Americans to their African ancestors, including their inability to think beyond the immediate, their capriciousness, their natural duplicity, and their fear of darkness. Lind acerbically expressed his opinion regarding the degree to which the black psyche had failed to evolve: "Because he [the American negro] wears a Palm Beach suit instead of a string of cowries, carries a gold-headed cane instead of a spear, uses the telephone instead of beating the drum from hill to hill and for the jungle path has substituted the pay-as-you-enter street-car his psychology is no less that of the African."[60]

But when Lind and others spoke of the primitive nature of African Americans, they were not just referring to a biological or cultural atavism; they were also thinking about the role of the unconscious in contributing to their psychoses. The primitive remnants of their African past, submerged within the race's collective unconscious, broke through in moments of psychic crisis, shaping the form and content of the mental disorders to which individuals succumbed. In this sense, Saint Elizabeths psychiatrists' understandings of mental illness among African Americans drew on the concepts of genetic psychology. Yet they were just as likely to utilize the Freudian concept of the primitive unconscious and the Jungian concept of the racial unconscious, both of which contained elements of recapitulation theory and Lamarckism.[61] American asylum psychiatrists were generally more influenced by the ideas of the Swiss psychoanalyst Carl Jung than they were by the ideas of Freud. In part, this was due to Jung's experience working with institutionalized patients in Zurich and his published work on dementia praecox, which was translated into English in 1909.[62] Saint Elizabeths psychiatrists certainly had more opportunity to interact with Jung. Unlike Freud, who visited only once, in 1909, Jung spent more time in the United

States, including at least two visits to Saint Elizabeths—once in 1909 and again in 1925—where he analyzed some of the African American patients.⁶³

White was certainly influenced by both Freud and Jung. In 1919 he confessed to Meyer, "I find myself in considerable harmony with Jung's attempt at defining a social consciousness, although I confess I have not read his paper fully."⁶⁴ Two years later White published an article on dementia praecox that bore the imprint of both psychiatric luminaries. Acknowledging that dementia praecox was a form of psychosis that entailed a regression of the personality, he sought to elaborate on the disorder's psychogenic mechanism. White asserted that all regression psychoses (including manic-depressive psychosis) were the result of intrapsychic conflicts in the unconscious. However, whereas it was easier for the psychoanalyst to comprehend the exhibited symptoms of the conflicts that played out in the unconscious that was formed in the infantile stage of the life cycle (the "individual's personal psychological history"), it was much more difficult to understand symptoms that were expressions of a deeper unconscious, of an unconscious that preceded an individual's birth ("archaic" or "phylogenetic material").

The psychic conflict at the root of dementia praecox reached into the deepest reservoir of the unconscious, which explained, for White, why the manifestations of that psychosis were so "alien" to psychiatrists. "We are not able," White wrote, "to feel ourselves into the position which the praecox patient occupies with relation to the world; we do not understand what he says; we do not comprehend the meanings of his symbols; he seems to us outside the plane of our experience. This is," he continued, "because his symptoms hark back to a period of which we have no recollection." White's use of the terms *archaic* and *phylogenetic* to describe the collective unconscious was most likely informed by his reading of Freud, who used the same terms in his 1900 book, *The Interpretation of Dreams*. Yet although he did not directly reference Jung, the symbols emerging in the praecox patient's delusions and hallucinations—including fire, "mythological animals," "the heavenly bodies, particularly the sun"—were clearly evocative of Jung's universal archetypes.⁶⁵

Four years later White published another article in which he more explicitly acknowledged Jung's influence on his thinking about the "malignant psychoses," especially dementia praecox. White drew clear distinctions between the Freudian concept of the personal unconscious and the Jungian concept of the racial unconscious, which he defined as the "philogenetic [sic] background upon which the rest of the psychic material is erected, so to speak, as a superstructure." He emphasized the importance of "differentiating material in the end result which is contributed as personal experience of the individual, that which is beneath his personal experience, which is unconscious and is contributed by the race."⁶⁶

The idea of a racial unconscious undergirded Saint Elizabeths psychiatrists' research into the psychoses of African Americans, regardless of whether they paid fealty to Freud or Jung. They believed that the cumulative cosmologies, cultural practices, and experiences of a race indelibly imprinted the psyche of an individual; in periods of psychic conflict, that deep racial history, those aspects that characterized the race at an earlier stage of evolution, emerged for all to see. Evarts eloquently articulated this understanding of the psychogenesis of mental illness. "In studying the mechanisms of those mentally deranged, we have learned to recognize and appreciate the constant outcrop of the phylogenetic memories in their words and actions," she wrote. "These are but broken fragments of the primitive life, isolated peaks, as it were, standing above the smooth sea of ordinary life and convention[,] enveloping the rugged mountains built of the age-long life of humanity."[67] When Evarts invoked "the primitive," she meant the antecedent stages of every race, not just those races that were still considered *to be* primitive in the early twentieth century. Yet this psychoanalytic concept took on different significance when it was used to discuss mental illness among African Americans, who were thought to be closer to their evolutionary forebears than European races were.

In fact it is possible that the presumed primitiveness of African Americans—or their perceived cultural and developmental proximity to Africans—contributed to the psychiatric consensus that they were more likely to be afflicted with dementia praecox than with any other psychosis or neurosis. In the 1910s and 1920s dementia praecox tended to be the most frequently diagnosed mental disease among institutionalized African Americans. In his 1921 survey of public mental institutions in the South, W. M. Bevis concluded that blacks were diagnosed with the disorder at a "considerably higher percentage" than whites. This diagnostic pattern characterized admissions at Saint Elizabeths as well. For instance, in 1926 and 1928 dementia praecox represented a plurality of the diagnoses of African Americans admitted to the hospital for the first time, at 29 percent and 32 percent, respectively.[68]

Although some psychiatrists were still influenced by Kraepelin and inclined to stress the constitutional determinants of dementia praecox, others undoubtedly found it easier for a psychogenic model of the disease to accommodate their presuppositions about the primitiveness of African Americans.[69] This psychogenic model, which incorporated the idea of a racial unconscious, allowed these psychiatrists to begin constructing a comparative psychology. Evarts, for instance, explained African Americans' predisposition toward dementia praecox as a function of their slower evolutionary development compared to the European races. O'Malley similarly attributed the prevalence of the psychosis to the "primitive order of intelligence of the colored race and the near approach of the general make-up of the individual to dementia precox types." Whereas for O'Malley it was the typical African American's "characterological indifference to environmental influences" that approximated the dementia praecox personality type, for Evarts it was African Americans' barely submerged primitive past. Either way, African Americans' "characterological" or developmental proximity to dementia praecox—their "normal abnormality," as it were—shaped how psychiatrists approached diagnosing them, evaluating their symptoms, and assessing their chances of recovery.[70] Furthermore, psychiatrists contemplated these relationships against the backdrop of what they considered constituted a normal psyche and a normal culture, both of which were racialized as white.

In a paradoxical way, from Saint Elizabeths' psychiatrists' perspective, African Americans' level of evolutionary development, combined with their level of social development, made it more challenging for them to identify sufferers of dementia praecox. Given that black culture was supposedly more primitive than white culture to begin with, the obvious premonitory signs of dementia praecox in whites—which would appear as regressive behavior—might be misinterpreted as normal behavior among African Americans. "Because the colored patient already lives upon a plane much lower than his white neighbor," Evarts claimed, "actual deterioration in the individual must be differentiated from the supposed loss of a racial period he has not yet attained." While this statement reflected a belief in the influence of the race's evolutionary history, Evarts also suggested that more immediate social conditions—the race's more recent history in the United States—posed a problem in diagnosing African Americans in the early stages of the disease. Referring to black women who worked as domestic servants, but implying that this was true of the race in general, Evarts suggested that as long as the manifestations of the disease did not affect their "ability to earn [their] daily bread," it was unlikely that they would be brought to the psychiatrist's attention. She illustrated this point with anecdotal experience: "Many colored servants come to us from white families, and their mistresses, in speaking of them, will say, 'We knew that she had been queer for a long time, but her work was not changed.'"[71] The distance—both evolutionary and sociological—separating whites and blacks created a yawning gap between psychiatrist and patient that needed to be traversed in order to provide treatment, but it also presented an opportunity to produce knowledge about racial psychological differences.

Assumptions about the racial differential in the level of evolutionary advancement shaped how Saint Elizabeths' psychiatrists evaluated the symptoms of African Americans once they were diagnosed and institutionalized. In assessing the dreams and delusions of his African American patients, for instance, Lind emphasized their resemblance to particular aspects of the presumptively more primitive cultures of their African ancestors. He was careful to acknowledge that "the primitive" also emerged in the delusions of whites afflicted with psychoses, but he reaffirmed the scientific "fact" that there was a natural racial distinctiveness in the psychopathologies of whites and African Americans. "I believe that in the white patient," he suggested, "the appearance of such symbolisms is indicative of a regression relatively to much lower levels than in the case of the Negro." The more primitive nature of African Americans, Evarts asserted, meant that they engaged in less disturbing practices, at least when it came to what was considered to be more degenerate behavior, such as masturbation and playing with feces. Since Africans were more libidinous to begin with, she surmised, African Americans had fewer "buried complexes" around sex and sexuality. As such, their psychoses did not manifest in "sexual perversions" to the same extent as in white patients. Even the apparently more prudent behavior of mentally ill African Americans was reframed as indicative of their lack of civilizational advancement. There was a particularly rich irony in Evarts's attributing a perceived sexual restraint among black patients to a presumed hypersexual phylogenetic past.[72]

But from Evarts's perspective, the developmental and cultural proximity of African Americans to their ancestral past presented the opportunity for recovery. To the extent that dementia praecox was a regression to a more primitive stage of the race's evolutionary history, African American sufferers did not have as great an expanse to cover as white sufferers did in order to get back to the point where they could assimilate these "broken fragments" back into their "ordinary life." "Because the patient has not so very far to climb back to her original estate," Evarts counseled, "she can usually return to her former sphere of life, take up her work where she dropped it, and show practically nothing of the storm through which she has passed, although a recurrence of her trouble is liable to follow another strain." Despite Evarts's optimism, the idea that black dementia praecox sufferers might be more prone to recovery precisely because of their more primitive nature did not translate into robust therapeutic efforts by Saint Elizabeths' staff.[73]

Any pursuit of effective treatments was fundamentally bound up in Saint Elizabeths' psychiatrists' efforts to conduct comparative psychology research using African American patients, research aimed at delineating the outlines of the normal and abnormal psyche. In 1913 Lind published one of the first studies on mentally ill African Americans that was actually based on clinical observation. Using the psychoanalytic method of dream interpretation, Lind sought to elaborate on the distinction that Freud made between the dreams of adults (as complex manifestations of psychosexual conflict) and the dreams of children (as simple wish-fulfillments). After providing a cursory interpretation of the dreams of seventeen African American male patients and judging them as simple wish-fulfillments, Lind concluded that African Americans were psychologically on the same level as children. But equally important, he ended his article with the following provocation: "Although Freud has recommended the study of child psychology as a valuable aid to the understanding of abnormal adult psychology, it must be remembered that in his country there is no such race as we have here whose psychological processes are simple in character and so readily obtainable. Perhaps to the American investigator, the negro might prove as valuable and more accessible than the child."[74]

Close to two decades later, another psychiatrist at Saint Elizabeths, Philip Graven, published an article on psychoses among blacks using quite a different methodology. Graven attempted to use psychoanalysis on one African American male patient but admitted in the article that the process had come to "a complete standstill and the procedure had to be abandoned." Nonetheless Graven went on to provide a detailed discussion of the patient's background and symptoms. Some of the same tropes of the earlier literature characterized Graven's study as well, although he was more attentive to the social differences within the race. He highlighted, for instance, the fact that the patient was a young professional, the son of a federal employee. Still, Graven characterized African Americans similarly to the way Lind had done some seventeen years earlier. "So it may be said that while we are, on the one hand, actually dealing with a colored man, age thirty-two, a practicing physician, yet, on the other hand, we are psychologically dealing with a child, perhaps at the age of eight," Graven indicated. "This aspect of the case would tend to emphasize the general view held regarding the childlike character of the negro."[75]

Unlike Lind, when Graven infantilized African Americans, he was not issuing a blunt challenge to his colleagues that they conduct research on this group as a means of further understanding the abnormal white psyche. He did, however, tout Saint Elizabeths for its "excellent facilities for studying the negro." Yet in the conclusion of his article, Graven admitted that "nothing characteristically 'negro,' such as race inferiority, can be deduced from this case. The type of conflict and reaction could equally well have been found in a 'white' case."[76] Graven's was not the first such admission. Mary O'Malley had drawn a similar conclusion in her article on comparative psychiatry sixteen years earlier. Despite all of the assumptions about racial difference that littered her study, she filed a very telling disclaimer early on: "Yet when all of the features are given due weight one is surprised to find how little divergence in the two races there is in their mental activities in health and disease." She tersely reinforced this conclusion at the end of her article: "The mental mechanism in the given psychoses does not essentially differ in the two races."[77] This admission did not stop O'Malley and her colleagues, with the enthusiastic support of White, from pursuing a research agenda aimed at delineating the "mechanisms of the negro mind" and illustrating how they differed from the mental processes of whites.

Throughout the White superintendency, the clinical staff at Saint Elizabeths was the most prolific producer of psychiatric knowledge about people of African descent in the United States. The backdrop of this activity was the general shift from a descriptive psychiatry—characterized by somatic theories of causation, symptom-based classification, and therapeutic pessimism—to a dynamic psychiatry that was defined by psychogenic theories of causation, an emphasis on the interaction between the person and the environment, and a therapeutic method based on the importance of ascertaining the *meanings* of individual symptoms. But there was hardly a neat transition between these two psychiatric paradigms. The profession made room for both approaches and individual psychiatrists could move between these different conceptualizations of mental illness or hybridize the two.

Emblematic of this particular approach was Nolan D. C. Lewis. In 1923, the same year he became head of clinical psychiatry, Lewis published a study on the biological dimension of the etiology of dementia praecox. His research, however, was not based on actual clinical encounters with Saint Elizabeths patients. Rather, his was a retrospective study that evaluated the records of 601 autopsied patients and sought to correlate their anatomical abnormalities and pathologies with their clinical symptoms. Lewis concluded that the organic or constitutional factors that contributed to dementia praecox were an underdeveloped circulatory system—manifesting mostly in a smaller than normal heart and aortic vessel—and metabolic imbalance, a reverberation of Kraepelin's autointoxication theory that Lewis encased in the new field of endocrinology. That is, he identified the abnormal production of particular glands, especially the thyroid, adrenal, and gonads, as responsible for the onset of the disease. In establishing the somatic foundation of the disease, Lewis rejected the assumption of racial difference when he observed that the "two outstanding organic features . . . are apparently as universally present [within sufferers of dementia praecox], regardless of race, age, size."[78]

But Lewis also acknowledged that dementia praecox was the product of psychogenic processes. "The knowledge of the presence of these fundamental organic peculiarities composing the soil in which the disordered mental habits arise," he advised, "should in no way interfere with the dynamic conceptions of the mental disease nor discourage the all important studies on mental mechanisms." In classic psychobiological fashion, Lewis pointed out that as long as the personality types that were predisposed to dementia praecox were kept in a "protected environment"—meaning the nurturing home—it was unlikely that the disorder would develop. It was only when they were released from this environment that "an additional strain upon the organs of the body, particularly upon the circulatory, glandular, and nervous system," would precipitate the psychosis.[79]

Even though Lewis's characterization of the psychogenic dimension of dementia praecox resembled the postemancipation discourse around black insanity, his discussion of both the organic and psychical origins of dementia praecox was devoid of any explicit racial content. Nonetheless his nod to psychogenesis allowed him to incorporate the primitive meme into his discussion of the disease among African Americans, even though, unlike his Saint Elizabeths colleagues, he did not argue for the importance of the racial unconscious. For instance, Lewis's identification of all of the autopsied black patients as African—as opposed to Negro or colored—worked to reinforce the cultural and developmental proximity of African Americans to their ancestral past. Moreover, in the very first case he discussed, that of a thirty-two-year-old black bellboy, Lewis used rhetoric that explicitly invoked "the primitive": "The life of this individual shows maladjustment with an early arrest in development at the level of savagery and inability to stick to an occupation, from an early period until his commitment to an institution for the mentally disordered."[80] Lewis's discussion of this particular research subject contained residual elements of recapitulation theory, with the individual repeating the evolutionary history of the race and becoming stagnant at the undeveloped stage of savagery. Even as he denied the existence of racial distinctiveness in terms of the biological substratum that provided the foundation for dementia praecox, then, Lewis rhetorically reaffirmed the "racial peculiarities" of people of African descent when it came to the psychogenesis of mental disease.[81]

Lewis's claims notwithstanding, the dynamic psychiatric viewpoint that undergirded the research conducted on African American patients at Saint Elizabeths failed to achieve White's vision of establishing the "racial peculiarities" of mental disease, let alone developing any theoretical models that explained how the presumed primitive psyche of the negro might shed light on the pathological white mind. Perhaps this was inevitable, the result of the inherent contradiction between dynamic psychiatry's emphasis on the *individual* nature of mental illness, on the one hand, and comparative psychology's emphasis on the *group* as the unit of analysis, on the other. The tension between the particular and the universal—or the individual and the type—had certainly been a preoccupation since the nineteenth century of scientists and clinicians who were concerned about the psyche.[82] Perhaps the indeterminacy of these studies is evidence of the paradigmatic shift itself from a psychiatry rooted in nineteenth-century biological theories of mental illness—which fit nicely with older ethnological models of race—to a psychiatry that took into consideration a number of variables, including environment, culture, and interpersonal relations, in its quest to diagnose and treat a universal psyche. Or perhaps it was due to the inchoate nature of psychoanalytic theory and research, along with the fractured state of the psychoanalytic community.[83] There is no indication that there were major epistemological or methodological disputes between the Saint Elizabeths psychiatrists who were engaged in comparative psychological research. Even as they grappled with changing ideas about what constituted mental illness, they shared an impulse to see racial difference as a constant.[84]

Ultimately the comparative psychology research conducted by Saint Elizabeths' psychiatrists ended up being a refurbishing of old, postemancipation discourses of black insanity in the new language of dynamic psychiatry. And yet Saint Elizabeths' psychiatrists told themselves that their encounters with African American patients were motivated as much by the goals of treatment as they were by any research agenda. Exhibiting a great deal of pride in the existence of a racially mixed population at the federal hospital, White ended his comments on E. M. Green's 1916 conference presentation by predicting that more research along comparative psychology lines would "be of great service to us in throwing light upon many of the difficult questions concerning the colored race."[85] In their quest to understand the black psyche, however, Saint Elizabeths' psychiatrists did little more than reaffirm the white psyche as the norm. This racialization shaped the therapeutic optimism that accompanied dynamic psychiatry.

6

"He Is Psychotic and Always Will Be"

Racial Ambivalence and the Limits of Therapeutic Optimism, 1903–1937

With its emphasis on the individualized nature of mental disease, dynamic psychiatry held out the promise of the development of effective therapies. If psychiatrists could get beneath the surface of patients' symptoms and understand their "meanings and values," then they stood a better chance of facilitating mentally ill individuals' readjustment to their social environments.[1] The methods of treatment associated with dynamic psychiatry rendered the primary therapeutic model of the nineteenth-century asylum obsolete. William Alanson White trumpeted the advances of the new psychotherapy of the "modern hospital" over the "old asylum's" moral treatment regimen—which he identified as occupational or industrial therapy—in a 1921 article on dementia praecox. "Many have come to believe, and this applies to the laity solely," he argued, "that the be all and end all of therapeutics for the mentally ill is kindness, sympathy, and work, the work taking very largely the form so familiar to you in the recent development of occupational therapy: basket-making, bead stringing, leather tooling, modeling, needle work, toy-making, etc." Although he acknowledged that the remnants of moral treatment still had some practical value in "socializing" the mentally ill into "useful occupations," White considered the older therapeutic model subsidiary to the intensive psychological work that psychiatrists needed to do with their patients.[2]

To be sure, elements of moral treatment persisted at Saint Elizabeths. In addition to occupational or industrial therapy, the hospital continued to subscribe to the therapeutic possibilities of recreation and leisure, providing patients with a well-stocked library; encouraging patients to contribute to an in-house newsletter, the *Sun Dial*, which was started in 1917; and expanding the auditorium in Hitchcock Hall in order to accommodate larger audiences for motion pictures and patient-staged shows.[3] The administration also continued to provide for the spiritual needs of the patients, employing chaplains from five different Protestant denominations who each spent two months of the year conducting services in the hospital's chapel. Catholic patients were able to regularly attend Mass on the hospital grounds.[4] The core principle of moral treatment—the imperative of creating as normal a social environment for the patient as possible—permeated everyday life at Saint Elizabeths, even if the staff no longer explicitly referenced it as a therapeutic modality.

By the 1910s and 1920s Saint Elizabeths' psychiatrists were able to employ a broader array of therapies. They expanded the use of hydrotherapy, which had been in operation at the hospital since the last decade of the previous century. A few years after World War I, White authorized several of his staff members to begin conducting malaria fever inoculation therapy experiments on Saint Elizabeths' patients, a form of treatment aimed at curing general paresis, a neuropathological condition that resulted from tertiary syphilis. As an increasing number of members of the clinical staff were trained in dynamic psychiatry, psychotherapy was employed with greater regularity on the wards. Not all patients were considered appropriate subjects for psychotherapeutic intervention, however. In general, psychiatrists believed that once a psychosis had progressed to the point that an individual needed to be institutionalized, it was less amenable to clinical approaches such as talk therapy. Even though White did not share the "pessimism, voiced for example by Freud, as to the impossibility of improving the Praecox by treatment," he was hardly optimistic that psychoanalysis could be an effective form of mass treatment, especially given the high patient-to-staff ratio at the hospital.[5] The limited use of psychotherapy is illustrated by the statistics: in 1932 and 1934 staff psychiatrists worked with, respectively, a monthly average of twenty-five and eighteen "selected patients."[6]

White and others did not explicitly use race as a criterion in defining the ideal target for psychotherapy, nor did they provide racial breakdowns of the overall statistics of psychotherapeutic treatment in the hospital's annual reports. An examination of the case files of black patients between roughly 1905 and 1935, however, does reveal that Saint Elizabeths' psychiatrists psychotherapeutically engaged African Americans, and in ways that revealed both a concern for their mental well-being and a deep sense of racial antipathy. They rarely did the kind of intensive psychoanalytic work that was central to dynamic psychiatry's treatment model. But they did do a kind of nonintensive psychotherapy that was aimed at assessing their patients' present state of mind and evaluating their progress. Staff psychiatrists were generally more concerned with the surface manifestations of blacks' psychoses than they were at getting at the roots of the complexes that caused their psychoses. This may have been a product of the overdiagnosis of dementia praecox among African American patients, a psychosis that was generally still considered to be intractable from a psychoanalytic perspective. Likewise, to the extent that dementia praecox was seen as a reversion to the primitive stage of the race's development, some psychiatrists believed that it was easier for African Americans to recover given that they were not as evolutionarily advanced to begin with, making intensive therapy unnecessary. Regardless of the underlying assumptions of their psychotherapeutic approach to African American patients, Saint Elizabeths' psychiatrists continued to demonstrate a belief in racial difference in their professional discussions of treatment and in their everyday interactions. For all of its progressive potential, then, the therapeutic model associated with dynamic psychiatry represented little improvement over moral treatment for African Americans.

African American patients were not merely objects of medical scrutiny and targets of institutional discipline, however. They interacted with physicians, nurses, and attendants in ways that challenged the staff's authority to not only determine the clinical encounter but to establish particular truth claims about black insanity as well. Yet they also interacted with the staff in ways that reaffirmed their own identities as sufferers of mental illness. Everyday life for African American patients in White's Saint Elizabeths consisted of negotiating the multiple dimensions of power—the medical power to define illness and health, the social power to define race, and the inherent power to define one's own identity—that suffused the institution.[7]

Constructing the Treatable Patient

The new therapeutic regime that dominated Saint Elizabeths during White's superintendency both facilitated and was dependent upon the collection and preservation of enormous amounts of personal and medical information about patients. Indeed the case history, made possible by the vertical archiving of data about individual patients, was indispensable, especially for psychotherapists. By constantly assembling fragments of the "organism-as-a-whole"—family history, early behavior that was indicative of a reaction type, events precipitating institutionalization, state of mind at various points, character of interaction with people and the environment—into a case file, staff psychiatrists possessed a tool that could be used to navigate a patient's psyche and evaluate how he or she was responding to therapy.[8] Medical historians and other scholars for some time have approached case files not as objective representations of clinical facts but as literary forms in which medical professionals construct disease and illness experiences through narratives.[9] They also construct the identities of patients, in the process discriminating between the salvageable and the unsalvageable in ways that reflect their assessment of the clinical facts and the cultural assumptions embedded in their own worldviews. While the narrative quality of the medical record has often provided the basis for humanitarian action, it is critical to recognize that these narratives could also facilitate medical inaction.[10]

The first step in the process of converting the sufferer into a patient involved the intake procedure.[11] The reception of individuals also commenced their categorization, as they were initially processed in departments according to their race, gender, civil status, and, in the case of service members, rank. White males were received in the west side department, for instance, with active-duty and retired military officers in a different ward within the department. Along with black and white District and federal prisoners, the admission of all African American men, regardless of their civil status, began in the Howard Hall department, albeit in different wards. Black and white women were received in separate wards in the east side department. Upon their entrance, individuals' personal clothing and belongings were confiscated and inventoried. They were also bathed and physically examined—for the purpose of detecting any signs of somatic disease or trauma but also for purposes of recording any distinguishing marks or physical stigmata. Ideally, within two days the patient underwent a mental examination by a staff psychiatrist. An assistant physician then "worked up" the patient, assembling into a case file material from the mental and physical examinations, any additional laboratory tests—including Wasserman results in order to detect the presence of syphilis—and the patient's photograph. In some instances, the patient was presented at a preliminary conference of several staff members, during which they rendered a diagnosis and proposed a therapeutic approach.[12]

The staff constructed a patient's profile out of information gathered through a number of exchanges, including a visual scrutiny of the body and its interior spaces, an interview of the patient, and a survey of the family. Since dynamic psychiatry's approach to understanding mental illness was based on the concept of maladjustment, it was "of the highest importance to have, as fully as possible, a conception of the individual before he became afflicted, so that we may understand the symptoms which are the expressions of this reaction," White counseled psychiatrists.[13] Saint Elizabeths' staff routinely gave questionnaires to the families of patients in an attempt to get a fuller picture of their medical history and to assess the personality types of their relatives.

Typical of this procedure was the list of questions sent to the stepmother of Charles T., a twenty-two-year-old black Washingtonian who wound up in the hospital after injuring his head attempting to escape from the DC Reformatory, where he had been serving a five-year sentence for burglary. Among the sixteen questions were queries about Charles's early childhood, his emotional life, and his sexual history. "From conversation with him and observations of him," the staff wanted to know, "how would you describe his personality make-up and the traits that lead [sic] to his maladaptation?" The questionnaire ended with the request that Charles's stepmother share any letters that she had ever received from him. The assistant physician who sent the questionnaire expressed sympathy for Charles's stepmother and sought to bolster her confidence in the hospital's efforts to treat her son. "I appreciate of course how unpleasant, even distressing it is for you to speak on this subject, for it concerns your intimate life," the physician wrote, "but I am making an effort to study the peculiarities and character make-up of your son in the hope that a more complete knowledge of the same will enable me to understand better how to direct his future life; for his is not at all a hopeless case; he is young and plastic and I believe something worth while may still be done for him, and thus perhaps save you a son and a citizen to the community." The physician may have been particularly attentive to Charles's stepmother's apparent reluctance to fill out the questionnaire and taken pains to empathize with her because of her class position. Charles clearly came from a middle-class background, as his father was identified as a graduate of the University of Rochester, a government clerk, and a minister.[14] His parents were cooperative with the staff, providing extensive information about Charles's youth, family background, and their own opinions about the cause of his mental illness. His father, for instance, related Charles's childhood tendency to complain of "ill-treatment whenever he was corrected." He also speculated that Charles was "born abnormally" and that his congenital deficiency was made worse by his indulgence in masturbation during adolescence.[15]

For every clinical interaction indicating that staff psychiatrists had the same respect for the psychological and emotional lives of African American patients as they did for whites, there were arguably more that betrayed a fundamental indifference, if not antipathy, toward the black sufferer of mental disease. The ways that white psychiatrists evaluated the symptoms of black patients and assessed their prospects of recovery were shaped by the social and cultural distance that separated them from African Americans and the larger racial order that produced distorted representations of blackness. The inclination to filter the symptoms of mentally distressed African Americans through preconceived notions of what constituted black psychology and culture is perhaps best illustrated by John E. Lind, a staff psychiatrist who authored a primer in 1914 on how to conduct mental examinations of black patients. Reflecting the general consensus within the psychiatric profession regarding the underdeveloped nature of the negro, Lind cautioned psychiatrists and general practitioners to take this into consideration when examining them. "It is not surprising that when an isolated individual is observed by one not familiar with the psychology and prejudices of his race," Lind argued, "characteristics normal to the individual are sometimes mistaken for symptoms of a psychosis." In other words, African Americans' presumed normal abnormality posed the potential problem of misdiagnosing them as insane. All of those signs and symptoms that might signal regression and mental deterioration in a white person—a capriciousness to the point at which orientation toward time and place was of no concern, sexual looseness, inattention to family, a propensity to experience hallucinations, superstitious paranoia—were, in fact, consistent with the negro's character and temperament.

Lind was careful to acknowledge that he was "speaking only very generally," but it is unlikely that he did not expect and hope for his concluding advice to be followed in every clinical encounter involving an African American:

> To sum up, then, it might be said that there are two things to be kept in mind especially, in the mental examination of the negro, one is, not to jump to conclusions, the other is, not to take what he says at its face value. Examine each statement carefully to see whether he actually means it as he says it or not. Remember that his vocabulary is limited, that he does not speak your language. After you have decided that he actually does mean the statement as it is given, consider whether or not it is in accord with his psychology, his superstition, his prejudices, and his theology, in short, if it is what you would expect of a person whose great grandfather was perhaps a cannibal; and finally remember that, if after you have made a careful mental examination of a negro, and there is a doubt in your mind as to whether he is crazy or not, he probably is not.[16]

Presumptions about the essential nature of the negro and the ways in which it was determined by biological underdevelopment, cultural stagnation, and collective history, then, shaped the mental examination, that most fundamental and intimate aspect of the clinical encounter.[17]

The collective history of African Americans and contemporary racist representations of blackness characterized the way many on Saint Elizabeths' staff constructed the identities of black patients. In working up the clinical records of older patients, for instance, psychiatrists were known to ask some whether they had been enslaved and, if so, to name their master. It is highly unlikely that this information was being sought for psychotherapeutic purposes because the age of these patients and the duration of their institutionalization made them unlikely candidates.[18] Black patients' identities were often constructed in the clinical record in ways that rendered them two-dimensional racist caricatures. Maria W., in the hospital for twenty-eight years after being admitted with a diagnosis of chronic dementia, became a "quiet good-natured darkey" in the eyes of the observing physician. After his examination of William T. in 1921, Dr. Lane characterized him as "very intelligent for one of his kind." Mary J., admitted in 1882, was described by Dr. Alexander after an examination in 1911 as "the old type of colored mammy."[19]

The medical examination, however, was a dialogical encounter and opened up the possibility for black patients to claim their own identity as well as to challenge the psychiatrist's medical authority.[20] Ten months after sixty-five-year-old George S. was admitted to Saint Elizabeths for acting erratically and having auditory hallucinations, he was examined by Dr. Benjamin Karpman. Although he was characterized as being "rather angry," George was fairly forthcoming about his family and personal history, including the kind of work he did, his marital history, and his previous illnesses. When it came to discussing his sexual history, however, he became quite obstinate, as indicated in Karpman's notes: "Denies masturbation. Denies perversion. Will not give any information about his sexual life."[21] Several things might explain George's reticence. It may have been a product of his age or his own sense of respectability that prohibited him from discussing such matters publicly, much less with a stranger. It may have been prompted by his desire to keep the most personal aspect of his life his own. And then it may have been a combination of these factors and more that prevented him from cooperating with Karpman in this particular area of inquiry. In preserving some sense of a private self that was closed to the psychiatric gaze, moreover, George undermined racist notions about the hypersexual nature of blacks.

Other patients used the examination to more directly challenge their own institutionalization and the legitimacy of the psychiatrists to authorize it. Annie R., admitted in 1905 with a diagnosis of recurrent mania, became uncooperative in her encounter with Saint Elizabeths' staff in ways that sought to establish an identity that countered the one imposed on her by the institution. In an examination in August 1919, she admitted to having previously experienced auditory hallucinations, but she denied that she continued to do so. At one point, according to Dr. Thompson, she refused to cooperate. Annie "will not permit further physical examination," Thompson reported, "because this is a hospital for the 'crazy, the blind and those who have lost limbs and those who have come out of the river,' and she is none of these."[22]

Margaret Ann B. displayed similarly disputatious behavior in her initial mental examination. The fifty-three-year-old cook from New York had been on her way to visit relatives in North Carolina when she was sent to Saint Elizabeths in April 1920. The circumstances surrounding her arrest and commitment are unclear, but the two District physicians who certified her mental condition indicated that there was evidence of "mental deterioration" and that she "hears voices." Saint Elizabeths' staff were able to find out from her husband that she had been admitted to a Long Island hospital several times over the past decade after becoming "suddenly disturbed." Unlike Annie R., Margaret Ann resisted the institutional designation of insanity in somewhat more indirect ways. Although she answered no when asked whether she was sick, at other points in the examination she responded to the psychiatrist's queries with a particular indignation that questioned her examiner's authority to medically scrutinize her in the first place. When Dr. Rawlings asked her to list the days of the week and months of the year forward and backward in order to assess her cognitive ability of association, Margaret Ann responded, "If you will refer to your calendar it will tell you all about the months and days of the year. Business folks should have a calendar." To Dr. Rawlings's attempts to ascertain the beginnings of Margaret Ann's psychosis, she replied, "Oh God, there you go again—have you got good sense woman, are you delirious, or what are you [?] (rambled on)."[23] Between questioning the psychiatrist's own state of mind, on the one hand, and her professionalism, on the other, Margaret Ann made it clear that, although her current situation was being dictated by Saint Elizabeths' staff, they were not the only ones capable of evaluating others in the clinical encounter.

Occasionally patients would challenge the medical authority of psychiatrists in ways that might actually confirm the profession's characterizations of black insanity and, in turn, facilitate the reproduction of those characterizations. William T., the patient whom Dr. Lane described as "very intelligent," was admitted to the hospital in June 1888 with a diagnosis of chronic melancholia. He had been in the hospital for twenty-five years before a case file was generated. William certainly exhibited symptoms that were characteristic of some form of psychosis, including his belief that his body was suffused with a "mysterious fluid" which had the same properties as electricity and was administered by the navy. Although his comments during various mental examinations about the collusion of psychiatrists and attendants or his records being kept in a centralized location on the hospital grounds were not on their face irrational, they were recorded by the staff as evidence of his obstinacy. In a mental examination conducted in March 1915, for instance, Dr. Wender reported on William's recalcitrance: "An attempt to obtain a history from the patient failed on account of lack of cooperation of latter. He stated that he is supposed to be insane and the physician being a hired official ought to recognize all diseases and tell everybody's history on inspection." During the same examination, William expressed frustration with the process in ways that reflected recognition of the power differential that existed between doctors and patients as well as whites and blacks. "When an attempt is made to interview him," recorded Wender, "he refuses to discuss his various persecutory delusions, stating that the physicians are working hand in hand with the attendants and he being only an ordinary negro, is not a reliable person and his word is not taken for anything."[24]

Although psychiatrists were entirely used to patients developing rhetorical strategies to evade their probing questions, when William invoked race it placed the exchange in a different clinical and political register. William offered a critique not just of the paternalism that structured the doctor-patient relationship but of the racism that existed in American society. His point that whites were not inclined to accept the fact that blacks may be telling the truth challenged the belief held by many psychiatrists that the *natural* duplicity and obtuseness of African Americans created almost insurmountable barriers for the psychotherapist.[25] On the other hand, the guardedness that any patient might have had when being examined by a psychiatrist, when exhibited by an African American such as William no doubt served to confirm racially inflected theories about the inaccessibility of the black psyche.

Although they rarely did so with an eye toward employing it psychoanalytically, staff members routinely documented the behavior and mental states of African American patients. Keeping clinical records allowed the staff to monitor patients and their responses to different treatment modalities—both longer-term psychiatric treatment as well as treatment for more acute medical crises. As such, African American patients found themselves objects of extensive medical surveillance and scrutiny, even though there is little evidence that Saint Elizabeths' psychiatrists attempted to use their delusions or repetitive actions to ascertain the complexes underlying their psychoses or to engage many of them in talk therapy. But neither did staff members think about their black charges solely as irredeemable lunatics. They tended to their somatic illnesses and psychic wounds in ways that were certainly rooted in a desire to heal. However, the questions of who was considered to be a treatable patient and what was considered effective therapy were very much shaped by a persistent belief in racial difference.

Somatic Therapies and the Disciplining of African American Patients

Members of the clinical staff at Saint Elizabeths were intimately involved in the development and regularization of two radical somatic therapies in the second quarter of the twentieth century, although the therapies themselves engendered very different levels of support from the hospital administration. The neurologist Walter Freeman, the American popularizer of lobotomy—a psychosurgical procedure, developed by the Portuguese neurologist Egas Moniz, that destroyed portions of the brain's prefrontal lobes—began his professional career at Saint Elizabeths. However, he did not begin doing the surgery on a regular basis until he had left the hospital and started a private practice in Washington. White expressed skepticism of lobotomy and did not allow the operation to be performed at Saint Elizabeths. Although some lobotomies were eventually conducted at the hospital after White's death, they were done so sparingly and, according to White's successor, "only as a last resort."[26]

White was much more open to malaria fever inoculation therapy, a fairly radical treatment for general paresis. Fever therapy was pioneered by the Austrian physician Julius Wagner von Jauregg, who, in the late-1880s, noticed that the symptoms of some of his mentally ill patients subsided when they developed typhoid fever. After 1900 he began focusing on treating individuals suffering from general paresis. Over the next several years, Wagner von Jauregg experimented with various fever-causing agents in the treatment of paretic patients before achieving moderate success with malaria during World War I. In 1922 White allowed several of his staff members to begin conducting malaria fever inoculation therapy experiments on their patients.[27] Although they represented only a quarter of first admissions between 1925 and 1930, African American men and women made up more than 40 percent of patients diagnosed with general paresis.[28] As such, they were as likely to receive this form of treatment as white patients were.

Undoubtedly the most frequently used somatic therapy during White's superintendency was hydrotherapy.[29] Psychiatrists used hydrotherapy hand in hand with nonintensive psychotherapy to manage the acute psychotic crises to which many patients succumbed. Hydrotherapy was actually introduced to Saint Elizabeths in the early 1890s, when the staff began treating patients who were suffering from general paresis, melancholia, and acute mania. The most frequently used methods were baths of varying temperatures, depending on the patient's mental condition; cold douches; and the wet pack, in which patients were tightly cocooned in cold or hot wet sheets and blankets, effectively immobilizing them for hours at a time. Opinions varied as to the physiological effects of hydrotherapy, ranging from the facilitation of the release of toxins from the body to the regulation of the cerebro- and neurovascular systems to the direct stimulation of the cortex. At a minimum, hydrotherapy relaxed the patient. "After a time it was observed that a majority of the patients went to sleep in the pack with a considerable regularity," the hospital reported in 1898. "Their rest was better at night, so that hypnotics came to be less and less used, while the wards were practically undisturbed by noise from the inmates at night."[30]

By the time of White's superintendency, the hospital staff was administering Scotch douches and continuous baths. In a Scotch douche, a patient stood in the middle of four pipes that converged overhead to form a showerhead. Nozzles on the pipes sprayed the patients with water along the entire length of their bodies. Some feet away, an attendant worked another hose, spraying cold water mainly at the spinal column. Continuous baths were a bit more coercive than their innocuous name sounds. Patients were placed in tubs, which were then covered by canvas or similar material. A hole allowed for the patient's head—the only part of the body not submerged beneath the water—to lean against the back of the tub. Attendants and nurses regulated the temperature of the water in accordance with the physician's prescription. Patients could remain in the tub anywhere from a day to several weeks, sleeping and taking their meals in this position. In 1907 White proudly announced to the Board of Visitors that he had installed a continuous bath room, which he was confident would "materially aid us in dealing with excited and disturbed patients."[31]

In an article for *Popular Science Monthly*, John Lind expressed some skepticism about hydrotherapy's ability to cure insanity, but he was convinced that it was a much better means of managing patient behavior than earlier forms of mechanical and chemical restraint.[32] White shared this sentiment. In the 1906 congressional investigation of Saint Elizabeths that had been prompted by the Medico-Legal Society report, he responded to intensive questioning about mechanical restraint at the hospital by informing the committee that he had discontinued the use of the bed saddle—a form of restraint in which patients were secured to the bed by ankle and wrist straps—and created two new hydrotherapeutic rooms. "The use of packs and other hydro therapeutic

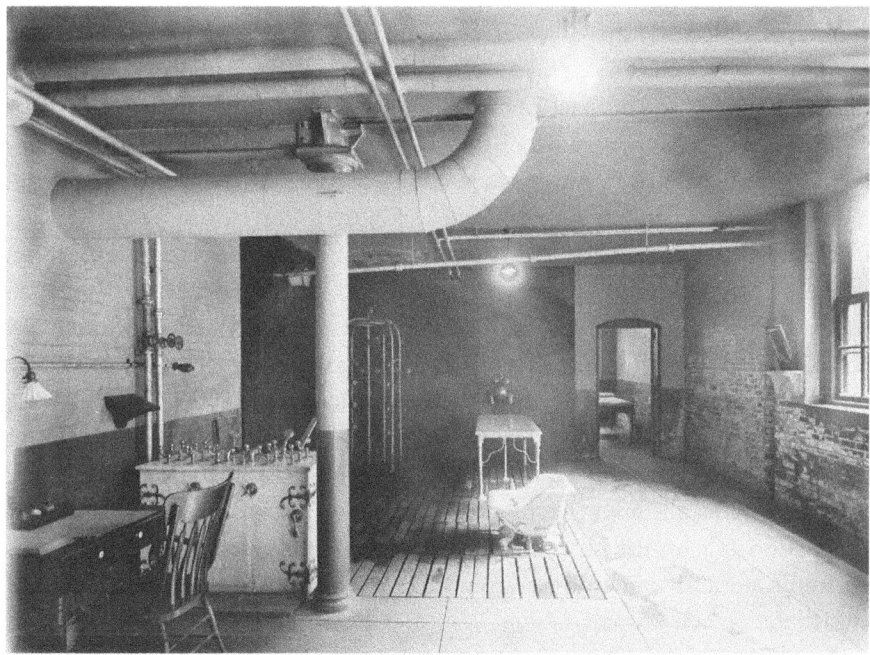

One of the hydrotherapy rooms, which includes a table for cocooning patients in wet sheets and a Scotch douche (rear), a shower consisting of four vertical pipes with nozzles that converged overhead to form a larger showerhead. Hydrotherapy contained elements of both treatment and discipline, yet the lack of hydrotherapeutic facilities for African American men due to lack of space meant that they were not subjected to this form of patient management until the late 1920s, even though they were figuratively and literally lumped in with the "criminally insane." *National Archives, photo 418-P-633.*

means," he assured committee members, "is the best possible way to do away with mechanical restraint."[33] Although he posed them as antagonistic—or, rather, as opposite poles of an evolving standard for treating patients—White's coupling of hydrotherapy and mechanical restraint actually reflected a prevailing approach among institutional psychiatrists that assessed mental health largely through patients' capacity for respectable self-comportment. As such, staff often conflated the control of unruly behavior with treatment of mental illness.[34]

Restraint and seclusion, as forms of patient management couched within a therapeutic paradigm, were prevalent throughout White's superintendency. Hospital policy did mandate that no mechanical restraint could be used without the consent of the attending physician.[35] The annual reports in the immediate years following World War I reveal interesting patterns in terms of how restraint and seclusion were deployed within the hospital. The reports do not clearly distinguish between the instances of restraint and seclusion, on the one hand, and the number of patients who were restrained and secluded, on the other. So, for instance, when the 1919 report indicates that there were eight seclusions of white females during that year, it is impossible to tell if there were eight different women secluded or if there were two women who were secluded four times.

Despite this lack of specificity, what does emerge from these reports is the disproportionate use of these methods on African American patients. In 1919, 1921, and 1922 there were disproportionately more instances of restraint and seclusion among African American male and female patients than among white male and female patients (see tables 6.1, 6.2, 6.3). The closest parity between black and white men was in 1919, when there was a recorded restraint for one of every 150 black male patients, as opposed to one for every 231 white male patients. In every other category in all three years, however, when we take into consideration the difference in absolute numbers, the hospital staff used these methods at least twice as much on African American men as it did on white men. Among women patients, the difference in usage rate was even starker. Other than in 1919, when white women were slightly more likely to be secluded than African American women, hospital staff employed restraints and seclusions disproportionately on the latter—the greatest disparity occurring in 1921, when African American women were seven times more likely to be restrained and secluded than white women.

Seclusion, in particular, was a technique used for disciplining or managing the behavior of disruptive patients as much as it was used to protect patients and staff from psychotic individuals. The hospital staff considered Ada R. to be a particularly troublesome patient and often responded by placing her in a secure isolation cell. "This patient escaped today from the laundry and went to Q Building, saying that she wanted to see Dr. O'Malley," Dr. Arrah Evarts noted in December 1912. She was most likely secluded for this reason, as a week later Dr. DeWitt wrote that

Table 6.1 **Restraints and Seclusions, 1919**

Total number of patients under treatment during year ending June 30, 1919	Restraints	Percentage	Seclusions	Percentage
White males 3,473	15	0.43	37	1.06
White females 711	0	0	8	1.12
Colored males 600	4	0.66	15	2.5
Colored females 393	0	0	4	1.01

Source: Report of the St. Elizabeths Hospital to the Secretary of the Interior for the Fiscal Year Ended June 30, 1919 (Washington, DC: Government Printing Office, 1919).

Table 6.2 **Restraints and Seclusions, 1921**

Total number of patients under treatment during year ending June 30, 1921	Restraints	Percentage	Seclusions	Percentage
White males 2,836	56	1.9	105	3.7
White females 750	3	0.4	7	0.93
Colored males 670	27	4.02	53	7.9
Colored females 411	21	5.1	51	12.4

Source: Report of the St. Elizabeths Hospital to the Secretary of the Interior for the Fiscal Year Ended June 30, 1921 (Washington, DC: Government Printing Office, 1921).

Ada "has been confined in the strong room, and now promises to conform to the rules of the hospital." In January 1914 Ada's actions warranted another seclusion. Along with fighting with other patients, she escaped from the ward in an effort to see White. "She visited the occulist [sic] one day for a pair of glasses," Evarts stated, "but became incensed that she had to wait a little while, so she left the building, scolding loudly, and in spite of her nurse went to the Superintendent's office to lay her grievance before him." Over the next few months an exasperated

Table 6.3 **Restraints and Seclusions, 1922**

Total number of patients under treatment during year ending June 30, 1922	Restraints	Percentage	Seclusions	Percentage
White males 2,803	22	0.78	62	2.2
White females 746	3	0.4	34	4.5
Colored males 698	14	2	33	4.7
Colored females 431	7	1.6	50	11.6

Source: Report of the St. Elizabeths Hospital to the Secretary of the Interior for the Fiscal Year Ended June 30, 1922 (Washington, DC: Government Printing Office, 1922).

Evarts reported that Ada tried to get other patients to stop doing ward work and disobey orders from the nurses; additionally, she often held closed the door to the ward, "not admitting the physician upon her rounds." Dr. Bogle, in July 1915, recorded Ada's explanation for the kind of behavior that led to her frequent isolation: "She says she is not crazy but that the other patients pick fights with her and follow up so that she is compelled to fight them. Then she gets locked up for her misdemeanors and this makes her so angry that she behaves badly in her room. She is quite plausible in her ingenuous explanation."[36]

Ada displayed a range of emotions and engaged in a number of actions that staff members considered to be so disruptive that the only way they could manage her was to separate her from the hospital's general population. That she was the target of this kind of management for behavior that contested the institution's control over her, as much as for behavior that was potentially dangerous to her fellow patients, might explain the disproportionate use of this technique among African American women. Resistive behavior from a population considered to be naturally docile and tractable not only challenged the medical authority of the hospital staff; it also defied the expectations that staff members held regarding the presumptive identities of black female, particularly elderly female, patients.

Some African American patients were placed in mechanical restraints or secluded in isolation cells because they posed a genuine physical danger to themselves or others. A black sailor, Samuel J., had been in the hospital since 1878, after being diagnosed with acute mania as a result of having been struck in the head by a pin used to fasten a ship's rigging. In the first decade of the twentieth century, when the staff began keeping a clinical record on him, the diagnosis was provisionally changed to dementia praecox, catatonic type. Samuel exhibited marked dementia and engaged in very disturbed behavior, according to his physicians, including assaulting attendants and stripping off his clothes. But these violent episodes were interwoven with periods of calmness, if not lucidity. "Became violent and had to restrain him and keep him in his room most of the time," a physician reported in September 1902. "Sam will go on theas [sic] spells about every two weeks when not on spell, he is quiet and obedient." According to the staff member examining him in August 1905, Samuel was neither oblivious to his disorder nor indifferent to the potential danger it posed to himself and others. "Has rather frequent attacks of destructiveness," the physician said of Samuel. "Seems to [be] aware of approch [sic] of mental storm and will ask attendant to put muffs on him."[37]

Lavinia M. similarly was reported as having cyclical periods of sufficient mental clarity that allowed her to work in the laundry and violent, destructive behavior that forced staff members to restrain or seclude her. "Physically patient is doing well," a physician noted in September 1907. "Mental condition not so good. Disturbed at intervals. Uses very profane language. Frequently strikes nurses and patients. Has been secluded several days this month. Habits very untidy Bowels regular. General Diet. Goes to Hydroroom daily for bath."[38] As Lavinia's clinical record indicates, staff used hydrotherapy along with restraint and seclusion to manage intractable patients.

Even though there was a disciplinary aspect to hydrotherapy, it was not predictably deployed in ways that were consistent with larger cultural assumptions about blackness and professional assumptions about black insanity.[39] For instance, despite the late nineteenth- and early twentieth-century psychiatric consensus regarding the predisposition of mentally ill blacks toward mania—a consensus that contributed to the decision to house and, later, process African American male patients in the hospital's department for the criminally insane— African American men were not regularly given hydrotherapeutic treatment. With the installation of a hydrotherapy room in Oaks B in October 1904, White reported that the hospital now had hydrotherapeutic facilities for black women, in addition to the ones for white men and white women. In fact, as late as 1913 it does not appear that African American men were receiving any hydrotherapeutic treatments. That year's annual report listed the average number of patients treated per month broken down by race and gender: white men (87), white women (59.2), and African American women (39.7). African American male patients were not even mentioned.[40]

By 1917 hospital administrators were expressing dissatisfaction with the lack of facilities for African American men. "Howard Hall has at present no hydrotherapy outfit for their colored patients, and it is highly desirable to provide an outfit of this character," the annual report stated. The report also indicated that the staff administered hydrotherapy to an average of 141 white men, 67 white women, and 58 black women per month. This time African American men were mentioned, but the figure listed was zero. This demographic discrepancy in the use of hydrotherapy is most starkly illustrated in the hospital's 1919 annual report. In that year 12,642 treatments were given to 1,176 white males; 470 white women received 12,270 treatments, and 453 black women were given 10,072 treatments, suggesting the disproportionate use of this therapy on women as a whole. In contrast, over the course of the same year only one African American male patient was treated with hydrotherapy (fifteen times).[41]

Even in the absence of an explicitly stated rationale from White or his staff, accounting for the massive gap between hydrotherapeutic treatment for African American males and everyone else is not especially difficult. Although African American men were not diagnosed to any large degree with the disorders White and his staff considered the most responsive to hydrotherapy—manic-depressive psychosis and alcohol-related psychoses—neither were African American women, yet they were given hydrotherapeutic treatments at similar rates to whites.[42] And while the staff administered hydrotherapy to many black female patients, in part, to manage their intractable behavior, surely African American male patients occasionally exhibited the kind of excitable behavior that would have warranted a trip to the hydrotherapy room had there been one available to them.

The demographic disparity in the application of hydrotherapeutic techniques was simply the result of the lack of resources. Staff psychiatrists could easily have ignored professional standards regarding the separation of male and female patients and utilized the Oaks B hydrotherapy room for both African American women and men. This would have been consistent with other segregation practices outside of the hospital, such as not providing separate ladies' cars for black women or having only unisex lavatories on Jim Crow train cars.[43] Insistence on maintaining both racial and gender segregation within the institution's therapeutic facilities forced Saint Elizabeths' staff to make important decisions about which populations to serve with the meager resources they had. The professional imperative of separating the sexes overrode the racist logic that fundamentally did not recognize the gender difference between black men and women to begin with.[44] As a result, ironically, African American male patients were not subjected to the therapeutic discipline of hydrotherapy even as they were figuratively and literally lumped in with the criminally insane. Instead difficult black male patients were more likely to be subjected to mechanical restraint and seclusion.[45] It was not until 1927 that the hospital had hydrotherapeutic rooms capable of serving white and nonwhite male and female patients. In that year the administration installed a hydrotherapy room in the Grey Ash Building within the Howard Hall department. Grey Ash accommodated black male veterans and convalescents. It is not likely that these facilities were state of the art, however. The buildings within the Howard Hall department housing African American male patients, in general, were described by the US comptroller general as being "of the old type of construction ... dark and poorly ventilated ... without proper bath and toilet facilities."[46]

The hospital administration ceased regularly reporting the annual number of hydrotherapeutic treatments in 1924, and it had stopped breaking this number down in terms of race as early as 1921. Thus it is impossible to determine how, if at all, hydrotherapy was applied differently to African American and white patients from the mid-1920s on. In fact the more important axis of difference in terms of the use of hydrotherapy at Saint Elizabeths is gender. In 1921, for instance, 302 female patients accounted for almost three-quarters of the 75,634 hydrotherapeutic treatments given by the staff. These women were subjected to an average of 178 treatments in the fiscal year 1921, as opposed to an average of 35 treatments for the 615 male patients who underwent hydrotherapy.[47] By 1932 women patients alone were given 74,279 treatments. Even though that year's annual report did not indicate how many patients were treated, if we assume that all 1,677 female patients under care during the 1932 fiscal year were given treatment (which is unlikely), then they would have found themselves in the hydrotherapy room an average of forty-four times.[48] One historian of somatic therapies has found that psychiatrists in several California mental hospitals were more inclined to perform lobotomies on female than male patients. This largely was a result of the rationale that the female mind was fundamentally governed by the body, and therefore women's mental disorders were more susceptible to corporeal manipulation.[49] Although there was little by way of medical literature that expressed the same sentiment, it is certainly possible that this rationale was at play in Saint Elizabeths' staff's use of hydrotherapy.

When it came to the use of hydrotherapy among African Americans, and especially African American women, another rationale seems to have been at play. While the staff may have thought women were more responsive to hydrotherapy because of some biologically essentialist notion about the female body, they may have been inclined to use this particular therapeutic procedure on women who challenged essentialist notions about the black body. That is, as African Americans, and particularly women, were thought to be naturally docile—an inheritance from their ancestors' "natural state" of slavery—those women who burst out of this externally imposed identity were subjected to a procedure that was both therapeutic and disciplinary. Staff used hydrotherapy to calm the agitated mind and to control the recalcitrant body. That this procedure was deployed within a larger context suffused with white assumptions about black servility, on the one hand, and black patients' contrarian behavior, on the other, illustrates the racial dimension of the clinical relationships that existed at Saint Elizabeths.

"A Maze of Unintelligibility": Psychotherapy and African American Patients

Assumptions about racial difference permeated the psychotherapeutic relationships between black patients and white staff members as well. Psychotherapy was a broad category of treatment that encompassed many different strategies. It included talk therapy based on psychoanalytic theory, but it went beyond this. Indeed White separated discussions of psychotherapy and psychoanalysis in his textbook *Outlines of Psychiatry*, and he pointed to the psychotherapeutic benefits of a particular form of hydrotherapy. "The continuous bath, in spite of all that has been written about its physiology," he asserted, "to my mind accomplishes its results psychotherapeutically, it is a concession to the regressive tendency minus the harmful effects of narcotic and sedative drugs."[50] White also expected the *Sun Dial* to have psychotherapeutic benefits; more than a mere "news organ," it would be a vehicle for "a new literature addressed to the mentally ill by the physicians, which will be of direct assistance to the patient in enabling him to understand the sort of thing that has gone wrong with him." The translation of specialized psychiatric knowledge into usable information for patients was only part of the psychotherapeutic process, however. White hoped that these articles would be the catalyst for some patients to initiate a relationship with the psychiatrists. "To that end," he informed the Board of Visitors, "I expect to ask the psychotherapists (there are now two of them on the staff of the hospital) to take a dispensary room at a certain hour on dispensary day, and receive patients from all parts of the hospital who wish to talk over their problems, size up the situation, and if apparently it is one that looks favorable make arrangements for regularly meeting the patient and trying to help him."[51]

For White, the potentially most efficacious form of psychotherapy was psychoanalysis. He felt it was superior to the most commonly used form of early psychotherapy, suggestion, because the latter addressed only the superficial manifestations of mental illness. Like many of his colleagues, his embrace of the more scientifically grounded psychoanalytic methods over suggestion was also an attempt to distance himself from the forms of psychotherapy associated with the Christian Science, New Thought, and mind cure movements of the late nineteenth century.[52]

Psychoanalysis was more rigorous, White believed, and required greater commitment from both the physician and the patient. The relationship between the two began with an "initial talk" in order to "orient [the psychiatrist] with regard to the general make-up of the personality" of the patient. Once it was determined that the individual was a good candidate for psychoanalysis, the psychiatrist needed to schedule regular sessions (what White called séances) in order to probe his or her unconscious. This was done through a number of procedures, including free association, word association, and investigation into the patient's "dream life." The environment in which the psychoanalytic encounter occurred was extremely important. The patient needed to be protected from external distractions, making it easier for any internal complexes to be detected as the patient spontaneously responded to the psychiatrists' queries and cues. But perhaps most important was that these sessions took place over the course of months. The intense plumbing of the psychic depths required that a strong rapport exist between the psychiatrist and the patient. The development of this rapport was dependent on the psychiatrist's approaching the patient from a nonjudgmental and empathic position. This rapport-building, or transfer, took a considerable amount of time but, once effected, made "for a more wholesome, a more robust philosophy of life, and finally when all the submerged complexes and mechanisms of the symptoms have been uncovered our patient emerges literally born again."[53]

By World War I psychotherapy was a sufficiently regularized treatment modality at Saint Elizabeths to warrant a mention in the institution's annual report. Between July 1918 and July 1919 there were 111 patients who were given "special psychotherapeutic attention"; interestingly, a majority of them were identified as dementia praecox types. To be sure, this was a paltry number compared to the 2,100 patients who were given hydrotherapy treatments and the approximately 3,500 patients who resided in the institution during the same time span.[54] The fact that such a small percentage of overall treatments ended up being reported to the institution's oversight department reflects the extent to which White considered psychotherapy to be central to Saint Elizabeths' identity as a modern psychiatric hospital.

In addition to the individualized sessions that White described in his textbook or that he envisioned taking place on dispensary day, an early form of group therapy emerged in the postwar period. The superintendent reported to the Board of Visitors in 1919 that one of his staff members had begun "a new experiment along these lines by grouping patients who have the same type of mental difficulties and giving them psychotherapeutic talks in classes of a dozen or twenty as a preliminary if necessary for more individual work."[55] Edward Lazell did not organize these gatherings as interpersonal therapy sessions. However, he was convinced that following lectures on such concepts as the fear of death, libido fixation, infantile wish-fulfillment, hallucinations, and homosexuality, the patients continued to discuss the ideas with each other, thereby "adding to the force of the talks." In a 1921 article for the *Psychoanalytic Review*, Lazell reported that he was amazed "to see patients who have been mute and apparently inaccessible make a rapid adjustment and ask the psychotherapist for further individual help."[56] By the end of the war, more and more patients were clearly being drawn into a new psychotherapeutic regime.

African American patients came within the purview of the psychotherapeutic gaze, but in ways that reinforced the white psyche as the norm. Perhaps most illustrative of this dynamic was the fine line psychiatrists walked in distinguishing between delusions and stereotyped behavior as symptoms of psychosis, on the one hand, and unusual revelations or bizarre practices as examples of the presumed innate superstition of the negro, on the other.[57] One of the ways this particularly manifested was in the phenomena of seeing ghostly figures and catching witches. While an inclination toward the supernatural might be interpreted as a sign of mental illness in a white patient—a reversion to a more primitive stage of the race's past, which was embedded deep in his or her unconscious—the same inclination exhibited by an African American patient became a more complicated puzzle to solve.

Dr. Arrah Evarts, an assistant physician at Saint Elizabeths from 1912 to 1918, attempted to work out this puzzle in a study on the relationship between the phylogenetic (racial) and ontogenetic (individual) dimensions of psychoses as they afflicted African Americans. Evarts claimed that while some white patients evinced a belief in the supernatural and magic, it was much more common in blacks. "This may be because the colored race is so much nearer its stage of barbarism," Evarts surmised, "or it may be because they are expressing much that is still an active factor in their everyday lives." To the extent that a magical paradigm for understanding the world and seeking to control it was reflective of an earlier racial history out of which modern civilization had evolved, Evarts claimed, residual elements of that thought and practice in African Americans were indicative of the group's slower evolutionary development as much as they were evidence of an individual's psychic regression. Evarts used the example of a black female patient who spent much of her time on the ward engaging in stereotyped actions aimed at catching witches in order to illustrate the phylogenetic factor in mental illness. "We have but to recall our own childhood with its belief in witches," Evarts argued, "their tricks and their slavery to whoever knew the proper motions and spells, to understand that this little brown woman has reverted not to a childhood like ours, to be sure, where there would be a questioning unbelief of these things, but to the early life of her race, where belief in witches was positive and means taken to control them invariably effective."[58] Evarts not only attributed this woman's belief in the existence of witches to a distinctive racial past. By explicitly using the term "our," she also amplified the patient's "otherness" by juxtaposing her racial unconscious against the unconscious of a white collective with which Evarts personally identified.

Yet Evarts also suggested that because African Americans as a whole had evolved at a slower pace than more advanced races, the "savage customs" of their ancestors were more present in their actual lives. There was always a possibility, then, that this inclination toward the supernatural was a product of the individual's immersion in a "primitive" culture more than a remnant of some distant past that had emerged from the racial unconscious. Indeed Evarts claimed this to be the case. Referring to the "so-called hallucinations and delusions" of her patients, she concluded that "while the phylogenetic element was undoubtedly present to a large extent in their production, the ontogenetic element was much the greater factor."[59]

The line between superstition and psychosis could be quite distinct at times and blurred at others. The physician observing Jane V. in 1909 and 1910, for instance, dismissed Jane's claim that she could see spirits through keyholes. "Can ascertain neither delusions nor hallucinations but she is very superstitious," she recorded in the clinical notes. The fact that Jane had been admitted in 1862 with a diagnosis of chronic dementia and was diagnosed upon her death in 1910 as an imbecile is perhaps one of the reasons why the psychiatrist attributed her claims about spirits to superstition rather than psychosis.[60] Yet the same psychiatrist was more apt to believe that the visions of another elderly black woman, Judy B., similarly admitted with a diagnosis of chronic dementia, were evidence of psychosis. "This patient has hallucinations of sight and hearing," the physician reported in January 1910. "She walks around restlessly, grasping at imaginary witches."[61]

While the psychiatrists observing Jane V. and Judy B. drew clear distinctions between superstition and psychosis, it was less obvious to the physicians who were monitoring Annie R. From 1920 to 1930 different physicians remarked on Annie's practice of rubbing salt over her body, including under her nails, in order to ward off witches. In consecutive observations in April and July 1920, Dr. Gertrude Davies and Dr. Lois Hubbard, respectively, commented on this behavior in particularly disinterested language, refraining from speculating about its roots in Annie's psychosis and even refusing to describe it as a response to hallucinations or delusions. In some ways, this matter-of-fact documentation rendered the practice as normal to Annie as the need to eat or sleep. Ten years later Hubbard recorded an observation of Annie that provided a more thorough, if somewhat ambiguous, attempt to explain her symptoms. "She is uncommunicative as to her mental content but seems to be absorbed in fairly satisfactory phantasies," Hubbard wrote of Annie. "Her behavior indicates delusions in that she will wrap herself in rags or in shawls or otherwise show that she is influenced by bizarre notions which may be merely the superstitions of the colored race."[62] The discrepancies between the ways physicians talked about Annie's behavior may have been the result of a number of factors: the different opinions of the physicians, the temporal distance between observations, the changing nature of the behavior, and the evolving ideas of the physicians themselves, among other things. That there was so much uncertainty as to what actually constituted psychosis and its symptomatology in African Americans not only made diagnosis difficult but also created confusion around therapeutic approaches and the ability to evaluate their efficacy. Moreover the fact that some African American patients continued to articulate vernacular ideas about disease and engage in certain folk healing practices—practices considered to be superstition by Western biomedical standards—after being institutionalized further muddied the clinical waters.[63]

The presence of alternative medical epistemologies among the patient population, too often perfunctorily recorded by the staff as symptomatic of psychosis or derided as superstition, also confounds any easy historical interpretation of the utterances and actions of African American patients. There certainly were African American patients whose responses to the psychiatrist's question "Why do you think you're here?" demonstrated that they themselves had internalized the terms, if not the precise language, of the profession's definitions of mental illness and mental health. Twenty-one-year-old Mary W. had been admitted in the 1880s with a diagnosis of acute mania and remained in the hospital until her death in 1936. When the staff began routinely recording their examinations of her in 1906, the temporal distance from her admission and the effects of long-term institutionalization produced divergent accounts of the circumstances leading to her commitment. In her first examination in June 1906, for instance, she attributed her commitment to the fact that she became "very much frightened after being told that her baby was being burned." Over the next twenty years, however, she admitted her insanity was the result of, variously, "intermittent fever," "a fall from a window," and being "shocked by a thunder and lightning storm."[64] Although these precipitating causes were more consistent with nineteenth-century understandings of insanity, they suggest that Mary comprehended her mental condition within a biomedical framework.

Ada R. and Ellen N., admitted in 1889 and 1920, respectively, reflected the internalization of a different conception of mental illness, one that was consistent with the psychiatric profession's turn toward psychogenic etiology and the internal emotional crises of the individual. Ada, admitted when she was twenty-two, was originally diagnosed as an imbecile as a result of a childhood illness. In 1911 she was examined by Dr. M. Edith Conser, who asked if she was insane. "I might be a little bit," Ada answered. "I do not think I have all that belongs to me." When Conser asked her why she was brought to Saint Elizabeths, she responded, "I was sick, I was bad and sick together. I had children and wasn't married." Ellen did not attribute her mental condition to her own moral failings, but rather those of her husband. In her initial workup in 1920, the physician summarized the circumstances of her mental breakdown thus: "Since February 1920 (about four weeks ago) this patient has been feeling nervous. She says she became easily frightened because she would hear voices of men and women talking to her saying that they were going to watch where she was going so they could kill her—also said her husband was going with other women." In a later interview, she confessed to being a "little too sad" on account of her husband. Unlike Mary W., who reflected a nineteenth-century paradigm that understood insanity as a mental phenomenon grounded in physiological processes, both Ada and Ellen, admitted some thirty years apart, are interesting examples of how, by the 1910s and 1920s, the dynamic psychiatry paradigm had become dominant within the profession and influential in society as a whole.[65]

There were, of course, African American patients whose utterances and stereotyped actions might reasonably be interpreted by contemporary psychiatrists and historians as evidence of their detachment from reality. Thirty-six-year-old Richard B., admitted in 1881 with a diagnosis of acute mania as a result of exposure, underwent an extensive examination in October 1913, during which he expressed the belief that he had "died several times, either by poison, or trauma." Ward notes on Charlotte T., admitted in 1874 with a diagnosis of acute homicidal mania, indicated that she "at times thinks somebody is trying to poison her." When twenty-seven-year-old Lawrence B., an army veteran who was diagnosed with dementia praecox while convalescing at a northeastern US Public Health Service hospital, was transferred to Saint Elizabeths in 1920, the staff observed that he "thought people were talking about him, that they were trying to poison him and influence his mind."[66] These were most likely delusions that were the product of these individuals' psychoses. There were certainly instances, too, in which claims about poisoning were less the manifestations of a damaged mind than expressions of an alternative way of understanding mental distress.

That their illness and institutionalization were the result of the malevolent actions of another individual was not an uncommon claim by African American patients. As John E. Lind wrote of his experiences examining African Americans, "Negroes have frequently been sent to the Government Hospital for the Insane, with some such statement as this: 'He thinks people are against him. Thinks people are putting a spell on him and trying to hoodoo him. Says some man burned some powder and this causes pain in his limbs.'" When Annie R. was admitted in January 1905, the staff member who initially observed her remarked that she "imagines she has been poisoned." Six months later Annie claimed that "her brother put her in here for spite," an accusation that the staff member chalked up to her delusional state of mind.[67] But what the physician recorded as a symptom of Annie's psychosis may in fact have been a vestige of a folk cosmology of health and disease that had its roots in slavery and traditional African belief systems.[68]

As much as early twentieth-century urban African Americans may have attributed mental illness to neurological damage or social stress, some also understood mental illness to be an affliction caused by individuals schooled in the practice of conjure. Alternately known as hoodoo, mojo, tricking, or fixing, conjure was an amalgamation of African, European, and Native American beliefs in the supernatural and magical practices. Conjurers sought to harness the spiritual powers present in the objects of everyday life—herbs and minerals, bodily byproducts, household items, graveyard dirt, and so forth—in order to protect or harm individuals, give assistance to someone in the pursuit of love or economic prosperity, and divine the desires and intentions of humans and spirits.[69]

One of Arrah Evarts's patients, an African American woman named Viola whom Evarts described as "of the criminal rather than the insane type," related a set of experiences involving another black female patient she believed to be a practitioner of conjure. "'Maggie has been telling me,'" Viola informed Evarts,

> every time I write my dreams for the doctor that the doctor gives me snake dust to throw over her head to keep her from going home, and she will have the spell turned back on the negroes and white people too. Every morning when Maggie is scrubbing and gets near my door she makes a cross on the floor at my door, puts her hand all over her head and face and makes signs and she says "Oh, my God, let the spells go back on Viola and the white people too." She says I sit and read her mind, then write to the doctor what she is thinking about and that the doctor gives me a hoodoo to throw around so it will fall in her path and cause her to fall and break her leg so she will have to stay here all her life.[70]

Viola's anecdote is interesting on several levels. For one, it reveals that the staff employed psychoanalytic techniques with some African American patients. Her anecdote also illustrates that some African American patients comprehended their illness and institutionalization within a medical epistemology that blurred the boundaries between the scientific and the supernatural. That is, Viola potentially subscribed to the therapeutic rationale of dream interpretation even as she believed in the power of conjure. It also suggests that there were multiple interpretations of the psychiatric procedures that went on in Saint Elizabeths. Even as the staff may have attempted to utilize psychoanalytic techniques to ascertain the nature of patients' psychoses and to provide therapy for them, these efforts were not always understood in the same way by the subjects of these techniques.

Viola's recounting of her interactions with Maggie also reveals that the persistence of folk thought about health and disease could create conflict between patients. According to Viola, Maggie "wanted my right foot stocking sole and a piece of hair from my head and she said she would make me bark like a dog and have me fixed so that I will never get out of here."[71] Since the power of conjure rested on the belief in contagious magic—or the idea that an effective spell required that the conjurer possess or manipulate some item that had been in contact with the target of the spell—Viola probably took steps to prevent her personal belongings or bodily residuum, such as hair and nails, from falling into Maggie's possession. To the extent that this became perceived as a repetitive act, it could evolve into a symptom of her psychosis in the eyes of staff members.

Patients' practice of concealing trash or accumulating it on their person was regularly remarked upon by physicians. One staff member observed in September 1909 that Mary W., admitted in 1881 with a diagnosis of rheumatic fever–induced chronic mania, "collects trash and secretes it about her body." According to the physician who conducted an examination of Lavinia M. in September 1913, she "collects up trash and carries it around in her stocking." This kind of behavior could lead to a great deal of tension between patients as well as between patients and staff. In April 1913, for instance, Evarts recorded the following observation of Mary K., a fifty-six-year-old woman who had been in Saint Elizabeths for over two decades after being admitted with a diagnosis of puerperal mania: "This patient is collecting a great deal of trash and keeping her room filled with it. She is so disagreeable that it is hard to get another patient to room with her, and is growing irritable when one tries to persuade her to any mode of action other than her own."[72] These stereotyped actions may very well have been the symptoms of these patients' mental illnesses. However, it is possible that this behavior, in at least some cases, reflected a belief in conjure, which further reflected an alternative medical epistemology that cannot be reduced to the simple label of "superstition." In this sense, what physicians were apt to identify as delusion or stereotyped movement—an indication of the patient's detachment from reality—may in fact have been these patients' attempts to explain and control the circumstances of their reality.[73]

But psychiatrists often reduced patients' expressions of what they perceived to be reality to a nonsensical distortion that was inconsistent with the facts viewed from their own professional perspective. The transformation of patients' perception of reality into a psychiatric definition of delusion emerges with particular clarity in the ways that psychiatrists characterized patients' descriptions of the hospital and their experiences within it. Staff members may have considered septuagenarian Julia Ann R. to be a lifer when she underwent an examination in July 1910. Thirty years old at the time of her admission in 1869, Julia Ann had spent most of her life in Saint Elizabeths. When a staff psychiatrist asked her to name the institution, she responded, "I ain't ever know. It is a starving place." In a conference report made a year and a half after her death, Evarts described Julia Ann "to be disoriented, and to entertain hallucinations and delusions, to be amnesic, demented, but with some reasoning and judgment." Many of her answers indicated poor memory at best and full-blown dementia at worst. Nonetheless the fact that she answered one question about who her master was with "Jule Terror" suggests that she was entirely capable of conveying a feeling that was authentic to her own experience, thus placing her comment about the severe nature of Saint Elizabeths in a different light.[74]

Other patients emphasized the carceral nature of the institution. When Dr. Isaac Kelly attempted to ascertain Richard B.'s orientation to place by asking him where he was, Richard replied, "Washington County Jail." Edmund T., a Floridian who was convicted of murdering his wife and daughter, had been in Saint Elizabeths since 1891. When asked a question aimed at determining his orientation for person in a November 1910 examination, he responded by calling the nurses "keepers of the prison."[75] Richard's and Edmund's responses certainly may have been manifestations of a clouded consciousness, and in both cases it is difficult to tell how the physicians interpreted them, as they merely transcribed the interviews without offering any medical opinions. And yet these same responses clearly conveyed Richard's and Edmund's sense of the disciplinary nature of the hospital and the power relations that existed within it.

In other instances, psychiatrists were more direct in characterizing the utterances of patients as evidence of their psychosis, even though the clinical record leaves room for ambiguity. For instance, what may have been Maria W.'s observations about the practice of surveillance at the hospital was reduced to a delusion when Dr. Edith MacDowell wrote in her case file that "she always imagines that men are watching her."[76] In the conference report following Richard B.'s death in 1914, Dr. Herman Maul distilled from the clinical notes the patient's hallucinations and delusions: "Patient thought he was being persecuted, that people choked him, knocked him down and put green poison into his mouth." It is entirely possible that Richard was relating an experience in which he had been manhandled by attendants and forced to take medicine, yet Maul rendered Richard's recollection as a figment of his distorted imagination.[77]

The possibility that Maul's own conclusions were the result of a hasty examination or an overdetermined reading of statements *as* symptoms becomes more apparent if we consider the exchange between Dr. Reeves and Richard B. a year earlier:

> REEVES: Did you ever hear strange noises?
> RICHARD: No.
> REEVES: Do people speak to you or about you?

RICHARD: Sometimes they speak to me if there is any work to do.
REEVES: What do they say?
RICHARD: Nothing as I know of.
REEVES: Do the voices call you bad names?
RICHARD: Not as I know of.
REEVES: Do these voices sound natural or spiritual?
RICHARD: The voices I hear, sounds all right.
REEVES: Are they telepathic messages?
RICHARD: Not as I know of.
REEVES: Do they come from God?
RICHARD: I could not tell you.[78]

In working up his patient, Reeves either construed every intelligible thing Richard said as evidence of his mental illness or he engaged in a line of questioning that presupposed Richard's insanity. Unwittingly or not, Reeves transformed the people who spoke to Richard into voices; in doing so, he recorded a fairly innocuous answer ("Sometimes [people] speak to me if there is any work to do") as a symptom of Richard's psychosis.

The kind of nonintensive therapy applied to African American patients had the effect of reaffirming their diagnosis of insanity as much as it did of gauging their improvement or assessing their prospects for recovery. But the mental examination and therapy session (to the extent that there was one) posed an epistemological problem for Saint Elizabeths' psychiatrists, challenging them to parse out the differences between utterances and actions that were expressions of the negro's natural character and those that were symptoms of psychoses. Regardless of what determinations they made, clinical staff constructed African American patients' perspectives and responses to institutionalization as fundamentally irrational. In doing so, they also reinforced the white psyche as the norm. While the black psyche was framed as largely inaccessible—due to the absolute cultural foreignness and the natural duplicity of the negro—white sufferers of mental illness were presumably, deep down, desirous of cooperating with the psychiatrist's attempts to probe their innermost emotional selves, despite conscious and unconscious resistance. The "maze of unintelligibility" was ultimately more navigable when it was in a white person's mind than when it belonged to a negro.[79] To be sure, white patients were not exempt from the kind of superficial therapy that predominated on African American wards. Given the sheer size of Saint Elizabeths' patient population, it would have been impossible to provide intensive psychotherapy to anything but a small fraction of whites. The engagement between psychiatrists and patients took on a particularly racial cast, however, when it came to the role of labor in the hospital's therapeutic regime.

"Worked Nearly to Death": Resisting the Therapeutic Rationale of Labor

As the exchange between Reeves and Richard B. reveals, Richard cognitively processed questions aimed at assessing his mental condition through the very material relationship that he had with the institution: work. Indeed in one mental examination conducted by Dr. Kelly in November 1910, Richard told the physician that he was "not crazy but is worked nearly to death."[80] Work—both on the wards as well as in the general facilities—was not just an important realm in terms of the daily operation of the institution and the management of inmates. It was also a key aspect of the clinical relationship that psychiatrists developed with their patients. The ability and willingness to work became one of the ways in which physicians measured the overall physical and mental health of their patients. Work also became one of the areas in which patients could contest their institutionalized existence. When African American patients did just that, cultural assumptions about blacks' "natural" relationship to certain types of labor allowed staff members to frame their unwillingness to work as a symptom of their mental disquiet.

Staff members commented on the capacity and inclination of African American patients to do work with far greater regularity than they did for white patients. In the ward notes of randomly selected case files of African Americans admitted between 1869 and 1905, references to work appear in 77 percent of the cases, as opposed to 45 percent of randomly selected case files of white patients admitted between 1869 and 1897.[81] What emerges from these ward notes is the racialized labor regime that operated at Saint Elizabeths in the early twentieth century and the meanings that psychiatrists assigned to their African American patients' relationship to work. For instance, while black and white patients assisted with work done on the ward—presumably making beds, dusting furniture, sweeping floors—ward notes indicate that black women were more likely to work in the laundry, black women and men were more likely to work in the kitchen, and white men and women were more likely to work in the dining room.

The frequency with which staff members recorded the work done by African Americans and the ways they described it reveals that labor became an important lens through which they evaluated their black patients' mental conditions. "This man is totally out of touch," Dr. Joseph Gilbert wrote of William S. in 1927. "Is unable to reply to any questions, only shakes his head or utters some incoherent phrase. Nothing can be learned regarding the possibility of delusions. He is apathetic and indifferent; takes very little interest in his surroundings. Does no work. Physical condition good." Initially admitted in 1895 with a diagnosis of acute mania, Alice G. was described by Dr. Anita Wilson in 1916 in language that associated her with the shut-in personality type that characterized dementia praecox: "She takes no interest in her personal appearance, frequently leaves her dress open, and stockings down but at times when asked to work she will assist without showing any interest in it." A week after she was recorded as doing well, a staff member updated Lavinia M.'s worsening condition in terse language that drew a tight relationship between her mental state and her capacity to work. "Patient disturbed does not go to laundry," the staff member succinctly noted.[82] It is not at all unusual that these psychiatrists would have used quotidian activity as one of the criteria by which they determined clarity of consciousness, assessed the ability to interact socially, and measured progress. The fact that work was so consistently used as a criterion for African American patients, however, reveals the assumptions that psychiatrists made with respect to race and labor.[83]

But work was also an institutional relationship through which some African American patients contested the staff's medical authority and power to define their identity as mentally ill individuals and to dictate the conditions of their existence in the hospital. When staff members began keeping records on fifty-five-year-old Landro B. in 1900, he had already been in the hospital for eighteen years, having been admitted for a second time in 1882 with a diagnosis of acute melancholia. The very first clinical note on Landro indicated that he had "extravagant ideas" that he was employed by the government and receiving a salary for "valuable service, such as drawing of battleships." Five years later Dr. James Toner noted in Landro's case file that he continued to have delusions about "patents and inventions" and that he had made so many drawings of battleships that the staff had to destroy the boxes in which they were contained because they posed a fire hazard. There is much evidence in his clinical record that Landro suffered from some form of psychosis, although for some examining physicians the most telling sign—Landro's insistence that he not be identified as colored because he was born to white parents and only became darker through his contact with a black wet nurse—loses some of its definitive power given that he was listed as a mulatto in the 1880 census.[84] Nonetheless Landro was considered sufficiently functional to have parole privileges, often leaving the hospital on Sundays unattended.

The belief that he was not receiving pay to which he was entitled plagued Landro throughout his confinement in Saint Elizabeths. In one examination in 1911 that had a psychotherapeutic dimension to it, Dr. Solomon asked Landro if anything was annoying or troubling him. "Only one thing—that back pay," was his response. There were also times when Landro conflated the relationship he imagined he had with the government and the very real material relationship he had with Saint Elizabeths, working in the hospital's tailor shop during much of his institutionalization. "He continued to believe that he was allowed a salary by the government and that this accumulated for him," John Lind wrote. "On several occasions during the many years he was here he became somewhat irritable on account of not receiving this money and would quit work for several days, but always got over this and returned to work."[85]

Other African American patients resisted the staff's expectations that they work. Jesse Owsley, who had served with the all-black 8th Illinois Infantry in Cuba during the Spanish-American War, was transferred to Saint Elizabeths from the Soldiers Home in Danville, Illinois, sometime after his honorable discharge. He was one of the few black witnesses who testified in the 1906 congressional investigation, during which he was questioned about the staff's handling of patients. Owsley related an incident in which he was ordered by an attendant to sweep the floor and he refused. When the committee chairman asked him why he objected, Owsley responded, "Because I was not sent there to sweep floors, and one thing [or] another. I was sent there as a crazy man." His next statement revealed something of the charged atmosphere when African American patients refused to conform to certain expectations whites had about black labor. The attendant "called me a black * * * and he says: 'You will sweep the floor; I will see that you do,'" Owsley recalled, "and he knocked me down." Owsley's resistance to work was born out of a sense of entitlement accompanying his service in the military. Soldiers' and sailors' refusal to labor, the summary of the investigation reported, was motivated by their belief "that they are entitled to a life of entire ease and freedom from work, as they would be were they in entire possession of their mental faculties and inmates of a Soldiers' Home."[86]

While the committee attributed military patients' idleness to their sense of government entitlement, they suggested that civilian patients' reluctance to work was animated by an entitlement of a different sort. Both black and white patients avoided "voluntary labor" because of its particular racial valence. "The white people who go to the institution from the District of Columbia are averse to performing anything in the nature of manual labor, as they are inclined to think that such labor should be performed by the colored inhabitants [of] the institution," the committee reported. "On the other hand, the colored inhabitants of the institution are averse to performing labor because they feel that all labor is entitled to pay."[87] Both of the rationales behind refusing to work reflected a distinct, racialized understanding of social membership. For white patients, their racial affinity with the dominant culture and the hospital's staff naturally protected them from occupying the same position as African Americans in the social hierarchy. Their designation as mentally ill and their institutionalization, in other words, should not compromise their racial membership in the dominant culture. For African American patients, voluntary labor was reminiscent of slavery and economic exploitation more broadly. As such, demanding compensation or complaining about the lack of it—as Landro B. repeatedly did—revealed their self-identification as citizens who were entitled to the same rights and status held by white Americans.[88]

This sentiment is expressed in many African American patients' case files. Annie R.'s response to a staff member's demands was so indignant that it warranted a remark in her clinical record. "Patient are troublesome silly and disobedient meddlesome at all times[;] will run in the office when it is open," the staff member reported. "Refuses to help about the ward says that she didnt come he[re] to work and she was not going to work that the Government could keep her without her working." Annie's resistance to labor, at least on one occasion, resulted in a particularly coercive use of hydrotherapy. According to her case file, "Patient was ordered to go to Laundry all day Has been irritable for some time to nurses Refused to go to Laundry, But finally went, Seemed to think 'Mrs Klug Nurse' at Laundry was to blame for her having to go, got so angry with her that she upset clean clothes on floor and started to fight Struck nurse with wet gown in her face Broke her glasses and had to be brought back to ward. Kicked Nurses and Patients that came near her was ordered sent to O B [Oaks Ward B]. Cold Pack given for 30 minutes."[89] Staff administered the wet pack in order to calm down a particularly excitable and combative patient. But looking at its use within the larger context that this entry reveals affords a glimpse into another dimension of this therapeutic practice. Annie became annoyed and began exhibiting disruptive behavior after she was "ordered" to work in the laundry. Although those around her legitimately saw her as a physical threat, Annie's resistive posture to a labor regime that itself masqueraded as therapy was interpreted by the staff as a manifestation of her mental disorder that needed disciplining through another kind of therapy. In this sense, it is important not to underestimate the potential for hydrotherapy to be used in a punitive manner.

Whereas Annie voiced her opinion that she should not have to work in exchange for staying in the hospital, Mary K. claimed that the government was obligated to compensate her for the work she did for the hospital and for short periods of time would occasionally refuse to provide her labor. But one remark that she made to Dr. Wilson in 1914 placed the work that she did—and her institutionalization more broadly—within a far more racially fraught historical context. "[Mary] says she is . . . tired, not able to work, and is kept locked up for nothing," Dr. Wilson noted. "That she might just as well live in slavery times, because she works all the time, and gets nothing for it, not even enough to eat."[90] As these examples suggest, many African American patients were not inclined to internalize the therapeutic rationale that Saint Elizabeths' staff associated with work. Even as some psychiatrists continued to tout the effectiveness of menial labor for a certain subset of the patient population—and interpreted their refusal to engage in labor as a sign of their lack of well-being—African American patients challenged these expectations on a regular basis. Staff members were not the only ones who filtered their expectations about therapy through a racial screen—employing black female patients almost exclusively in kitchen and laundry work, for example; the patients themselves interpreted the staff's directives to labor through their own ideas about what constituted appropriate management of their bodies.[91]

When Mary K. invoked slavery as a marker by which to judge her confinement in Saint Elizabeths, the racism that pervaded the nation's past and present pierced the veil of objectivity that shrouded the clinical encounter. These kinds of ruptures are few and far between, but there is still tantalizing evidence that overt manipulations of racial codes occasionally surfaced in the relationship between white clinical staff members and African American patients. Dr. Mary O'Malley referenced slavery in a general observation she made about patient management. "In the hospital the colored patient is much more submissive and amenable to discipline than the white," she wrote in a 1914 article for the *American Journal of Insanity*. "As slaves they were docile, tractable and subordinate, and these instincts of obedience which have been transmitted from their immediate forefathers remain with them."[92] Ward notes indicate that these assumptions about the tractability of blacks were shared by other staff members. One physician illustrated the marked mental deterioration of William B., who had been admitted in 1877 with a diagnosis of acute mania, by noting the following in his clinical record: "He is simple and childish at all times. He will do anything you will tell him to do. For instance if you want him to Dance he will [do] so at any time."[93] It is impossible to be completely sure of the motive for asking William to dance, but the racist connotations of the act could not have been lost on the staff member doing the asking.

Playing on blacks' presumed natural docility was the strategy of one staff member who was concerned about a patient's health. In doing so, she manipulated the former enslaved woman's delusions that she could still see and communicate with her owners. "[Judy B.] will sometimes refuse to eat—but—if told Marse Hugh of whom she so often speaks would like her to eat it she will do so," the staff member reported in 1913. Interestingly, like Mary K., Judy used slavery as a marker against which to judge her institutionalization, but in a way that contrasted the two and reflected Judy's disdain for the hospital. According to a staff member observing her in 1914, Judy had become excited when she overheard a new nurse on the ward say that she was from Virginia. "I came from old Verginny to Orange Co. lived with Marse Hugh, Miss Sallie, Miss Hattie and all dem white ladies," Judy was reported as having said, "and I'se going back too just as soon as I get out of this Prison."[94]

The staff's occasional deployment of the memory of slavery notwithstanding, African American patients regularly disrupted assumptions about their natural docility; sometimes they did so in ways that revealed their own racial contempt.

Julia Ann R., a staff member observed in 1910, was generally "very pleasant until slightly crossed then she is very quarrelsome calls every one Miss Ann."[95] By labeling the psychiatrists, nurses, and attendants—and perhaps other patients—with the term that figuratively represented imperious white womanhood and racial privilege, Julia Ann expressed her discontent in a way that criticized the racial codes and racist strictures of white supremacy. Although it may have seemed nonsensical or arbitrary to the staff, her use of "Miss Ann" held important meaning for Julia.

It is true that the clinical relationship between white psychiatrists and African American patients was not solely one of friction and indifference. Even though few African Americans were subjects of intensive psychoanalytic treatment, this does not mean that the staff was not concerned about their mental and emotional well-being. In a 1914 article about dementia praecox among African Americans, Evarts made an interesting statement about the importance of race in the clinical encounter: "The race sense, if so we may call it, is so integral a part of the psychiatrist himself, that often he sees without seeing, and understands without understanding, when his patients are those of his own race. When, however, he is dealing with those of another race, this conformity of experience is lacking, and must be consciously made a factor in the equation before its final solution will be satisfactory."[96] While in some ways this reads as a forerunner to the late twentieth-century idea of cultural competency—and Evarts may have intended it to operate as such—the exhortation to Saint Elizabeths psychiatrists to become hyperconscious of the history and culture of African Americans ended up, ironically, reinforcing the very conceptions of racial difference with which they entered the clinical encounter.[97]

Race fundamentally shaped the therapeutic rationale that Saint Elizabeths' psychiatrists applied to African American patients. Rather than an effort to plumb the depths of the mind and ascertain the origins of their psychical conflict, the use of hydrotherapy, labor, and nonintensive psychotherapy was aimed more at managing patients and preparing them to resume their lives presumably as unskilled laborers and service employees should they eventually be deemed improved or recovered and released from the hospital. Given the sheer size of the hospital, most white patients also had the same therapeutic rationale applied to them, although, like white patients at other institutions in the early twentieth century, the various forms of therapy were most likely administered with the goal of allowing them to replenish their nervous energy.[98] For African American patients at Saint Elizabeths—like black inmates at other state hospitals and schools for the feebleminded throughout the South—the therapeutic regime that barely represented advancement over nineteenth-century moral treatment amounted to little more than efforts to rehabilitate them as laborers.[99] As much as Saint Elizabeths' psychiatrists' approach to African Americans was limited by the blinders of race, however, some developed an appreciation for the complex emotional interiority of blacks and generally sought to calm, if not heal, their disturbed minds. Even if staff members had wanted to relegate them to the figurative "back wards" of the hospital, the daily actions of their African American patients forced them to acknowledge that they were dealing with people who, regardless of their mental condition, were determined to shape the condition of their existence at Saint Elizabeths.

Therapeutic Pessimism Redux

In August 1922 several of Saint Elizabeths' psychiatrists convened a conference to discuss the case of Charles T., the young convicted burglar who was admitted to the hospital in 1918 after injuring his head while attempting to escape from the DC Reformatory. Charles had been discharged in 1919 despite a diagnosis of prison psychosis, a paranoiac state thought to be produced by imprisonment, and returned to the reformatory. He was readmitted in September 1920.[100] During his two separate commitments to Saint Elizabeths, the staff did seek to identify the roots of his psychosis by consulting his family and engaging him in talk therapy. The staff convened the conference because Charles's sentence had expired and he expressed a desire to go home. John Lind presented Charles's case, reporting on his family history and the history of his illness before concluding that he had a psychopathic personality of the criminal type. Lind recommended, however, that Charles be transferred from Howard Hall and that he be given ground parole and employed on the hospital campus. Although all of the doctors present agreed with Lind's recommendation, some offered up different diagnoses. Dr. Benjamin Karpman proposed a diagnosis of constitutional psychopathy with epileptic neurosis. Although this diagnosis suggested a somatic etiology, Karpman qualified it by pointing out that he thought Charles's psychosis had a "large psychogenic element." Suppressed homosexual feelings were most likely responsible for it, Karpman argued, noting that Charles was "very effeminate and shows many homosexual trends, but he is very inaccessible on that point." For Dr. Nolan Lewis, Charles's case resembled a "so-called psychosis of degeneracy."

Despite these variant diagnoses, the consensus was that Charles should not be discharged. The dire prognoses advanced by some at the conference took on a particular racial valence. Lind suggested that Charles's "biological inferiority" would prevent him from ever returning to his precommitment "economic level" again. Although the biology to which Lind referred might have pertained to the constitutional deficiency of the psychopath, Lewis left no room for ambiguity in his remarks. "It is hard to say in a negro whether he has recovered from his mental disease," Lewis pondered. "My impression is that he will never be rid of his mental disease. I think it is inborn, inherent growth. I think, if it is, one may say he is psychotic. He may have had a few weeks of acute episode such as we see in these people. I think he is psychotic and always will be."[101]

Charles was hardly alone in being denied his release from the hospital. During the 1922–23 fiscal year, only 19 of the 707 African American men receiving treatment at Saint Elizabeths were discharged as either recovered or improved. This 1.8 percent discharge rate was well below that of white women (37 of 777, or 4.7 percent), white men (182 of 2,960, or 6.1 percent), and even black women (32 of 483, or 6.6 percent). That year happened to be an anomalous one for African American women, as their recovered/improved discharge rates throughout the 1920s averaged 2.8 percent.[102] In general, white male patients were much more likely to be discharged as either recovered or improved than any other category of patient, including white women. The higher discharge rates for white men were undoubtedly linked to the preponderance of soldiers and sailors among them. As military personnel suffering from shell shock, or war neurosis, were admitted to Saint Elizabeths following the war in ever larger numbers, psychiatrists' changing theories about mental illness being the product of maladaptation to environment and not solely an organic or hereditary disease were increasingly confirmed. Approaching mental illness from this dynamic perspective produced a great deal of optimism among psychiatrists that they could, in fact, successfully treat individuals suffering from psychogenic disorders. Many of the white male patients who were discharged as either recovered or improved were the beneficiaries of this optimism.[103]

This therapeutic optimism, however, did not, by and large, extend to African American patients. Indeed African American men and women (and, to a lesser degree, white women) were much more likely to be removed from the hospital's rolls either by being discharged as unimproved or by death. Though there were a few years in the 1920s when unimproved discharges and deaths accounted for close to 66 percent of the total number of white men removed from the hospital's rolls, they typically averaged only between 40 and 50 percent in any given year.[104] By contrast, unimproved discharges and deaths routinely made up 75 percent of the removals from the hospital's rolls for African Americans, a predominantly civilian population. In 1927, in fact, 85 percent of African American male patients who were removed from the rolls were either discharged as unimproved or died.[105]

It was in this year that the staff convened another conference to evaluate Charles. He had continued to demand his release, and staff members found it necessary to consider whether he was sufficiently improved, or even recovered, to warrant a discharge. Lind presented the case again and, although he did not change his original diagnosis of psychosis with psychopathic personality, he did recommend that Charles be discharged as recovered. Charles was present at this conference, and staff members examined him. Dr. Arthur P. Noyes, the first assistant physician, the second highest clinical position in the hospital, offered a different diagnosis upon concluding his examination. "This boy held his lips in a constrained position, strongly suggestive of a precox mechanism," Noyes observed. "His general manner was stilted, he was silly and his replies were given in a low, soft and somewhat affected tone. He recognized that he had been suffering from mental disability when he entered the Hospital but declared he was now well." The majority of the physicians at the conference agreed that the correct diagnosis for Charles was dementia praecox rather than psychosis with psychopathic personality. And while they quibbled as to whether he was recovered or merely improved, they agreed to discharge him as improved. Noyes, however, captured the overall pessimism of the staff in rendering its collective decision. Given that his sentence had expired and he had not gone through another legal process adjudicating his mental condition, the hospital could not justify keeping Charles, even if Noyes himself believed that he would continue to exhibit "antisocial behavior" once he was released. "I think we will have to let the man go," Noyes soberly noted, "and we should acquaint his relatives with the situation and I would be inclined to tell them we did not consider him entirely well and ask them if they wish to do anything about having him sent to Gallinger and sent around through with a hearing before a jury."[106]

Charles's conference reports are emblematic of the clinical ambiguity and ambivalence that characterized the relationship between the hospital staff and African American patients. Staff members' assumptions about racial difference and their occasional racist behavior marked the clinical encounter between Charles and Saint Elizabeths' psychiatrists, as evident in Lewis's speculation about the racially determined permanence of Charles's psychosis and several of the physicians' references to the twenty-seven-year-old as "boy." Staff members brought their socially embedded notions and expectations regarding the constitution, temperament, and culture of people of African descent into what they considered to be the objective, dispassionate, and analytical space of the ward. And yet Saint Elizabeths' psychiatrists did not completely abandon their African American patients or their families. Noyes's suggestion that Charles's family be informed of the reservations of the staff and counseled about the resources available at Gallinger Hospital, the District's public hospital, reflected a different relationship between Saint Elizabeths and the community than had existed earlier in the century. Ever since the hospital's founding, superintendents and staff physicians had maintained communication with the families and friends of their patients. By the 1920s, however, they were much more active in working with families and community institutions to facilitate discharged patients' readjustment to society. These efforts, in the form of outpatient clinics and psychiatric social work service, were influenced by the mental hygiene movement of the post–World War I period.

7

Mental Hygiene and the Limits of Reform

Saint Elizabeths in the Community, 1903–1937

In the summer of 1930 William White delivered an address on mental hygiene on WMAL, a Washington radio station. Informing his audience of all of the strides that the psychiatric profession and mental hygiene movement had made in preventing and curing mental illness, White reminded them that no one was immune from it. Indeed he suggested that the exponential increase in the number of beds in public mental hospitals over the previous fifty years meant that most people listening to his talk had either been afflicted with a mental disorder or knew of someone who had been. Toward the end of his lecture, White challenged his listeners to remain vigilant in their awareness of the dangers of mental illness. "You are in every conceivable way closely affected by this great menace," he declared, "and it is for you to assist all who are making the effort to minimize the ill effects that flow from this source as far as possible, to assist the mental hygiene movement, which has as its ultimate goal the prevention of mental disease, to help secure the adequate care of those who are ill at the earliest possible moment so as to insure the greatest number of recoveries, and in every way to spread that knowledge of mental disorder and that desire for mental health which is calculated to counteract it."[1] In rallying the audience to his cause, White pointed out that their tax dollars were funding the expansion of public hospitals. As such, to the extent that it would preempt the institutionalization of individuals, early intervention in the "neuroses as well as the more serious mental sicknesses" would redound to the personal welfare of the psychically distressed and would also reduce the financial burden on the larger society.[2]

White's address reflected a professional consensus on the importance of approaching mental illness in ways that relied less and less on the brick-and-mortar institution. Beginning in the midst of Progressive reform in the early twentieth century and certainly in full flower by the mid-1920s, variations of a broadly defined community-oriented psychiatry began to shape the relationship between mental hospitals and the populations they served. The mental hygiene movement was spearheaded by Adolf Meyer, the dynamic psychiatrist who developed the psychobiological paradigm of mental illness, and a former institutionalized patient, Clifford Beers, among others, and driven organizationally by the National Committee for Mental Hygiene. It arose in response to the growing belief that institutions had become warehouses in which the insane were crammed and ill-treated. Mental hygiene advocates presumed that the best way to treat mental illness was to prevent it from developing to the point that an individual needed to be institutionalized. This required the psychiatric profession to interact with those most vulnerable to mental diseases in more meaningful ways outside of the hospital. But it also required a more expansive purview of what warranted psychiatric intervention. Whereas the missions of asylum physicians and neurologists had been primarily to diagnose, determine the internal mechanisms of, and perhaps cure insanity, dynamic psychiatrists were as interested in preserving mental health. To the extent that they understood mental illness to be the manifestation of an individual's maladaptation to his or her social environment, the personal relationships that constituted that environment were subject to investigation and remediation.[3]

By the time that White gave his address, a number of local institutions included the maintenance of mental health in their core missions. Gallinger Municipal Hospital had a mental hygiene clinic, in which a psychiatrist and a psychologist examined adults and children who were referred by the District's Board of Welfare. Three other institutions had more direct links to Saint Elizabeths even though they were, by and large, privately run and received little government funding. In the summer of 1929 a number of prominent Washington citizens formed the Washington Institute of Mental Hygiene and appointed White as its president. The institute served as an umbrella association with the goals of educating the broader public about the importance of mental health, coordinating mental hygiene efforts across the city, and establishing new clinics in the District. Falling under the auspices of the institute was the Life Adjustment Center, a mental hygiene clinic that was launched by a Congregationalist minister in December 1928 and, as such, predated the institute itself. Also predating the institute but coming under its influence was the Neurological Clinic of the Children's Hospital, a private hospital in Northwest Washington that received some federal funding. The institute had a more direct role in opening the Washington Child Guidance Clinic in November 1930.[4]

Along with its connections to mental hygiene clinics in the District, Saint Elizabeths projected its psychiatric authority into the community in a number of other ways. These included its advocacy for reforming the legally cumbersome commitment process in the District in a way that would strip the process of its carceral undertones and the stigma that was associated with it. Saint Elizabeths officials also argued for a change in the District's lunacy laws that would make it easier for mentally distressed individuals seeking psychiatric care to voluntarily admit themselves to the hospital. Further, inasmuch as the preservation of the mental health of the noninstitutionalized and the amelioration of the conditions of the institutionalized were two sides of the mental hygiene coin, the hospital administration sought to alleviate the overcrowded wards by discharging more and more patients but providing follow-up care through its outpatient clinics and psychiatric social work services.

But Saint Elizabeths' mental hygiene crusade penetrated only so far into black Washington. To a large degree, professional assumptions about a distinctive black psyche that influenced the prospects for mentally ill African Americans' recovery continued to shape Saint Elizabeths' psychiatrists' assessments of their black patients. As a factor in their mental hygiene efforts, however, this was less significant than the overall racist environment of Progressive-era and post–World War I Washington, DC. The nation's capital saw increasing discrimination against black federal employees during the "New Freedom" era of the progressive president Woodrow Wilson; the fortifying of segregation in residential areas, private businesses, social services, and public space; and a four-day race riot that involved African American residents, local whites, and white soldiers and sailors in July 1919. The intensifying segregationist culture of the District in the 1910s and 1920s cannot be disentangled from the limited vision of southern Progressive reformers, who, like the psychiatric profession, prioritized the well-being of whites over African Americans.[5] But the mental hygiene efforts of Saint Elizabeths were also shaped by the intended objects of reform. As in the postemancipation period, in both subtle and overt ways African American patients and members of their social networks sought to manage their therapeutic experience by collaborating with the hospital in a manner that they believed to be in their own best interests. At other times, they directly challenged Saint Elizabeths' medical expertise and institutional power.

"A Progressive March": Reforming the District's Lunacy Laws

Although White consistently crowed that the therapeutic, research, and teaching strengths of Saint Elizabeths made it a thoroughly modern mental hospital, he also lamented that the antiquated commitment laws of the District of Columbia undermined the institution's stature. The laws had not changed significantly from those that governed admission in the mid-nineteenth century. The most recent law, passed in 1904, authorized the Metropolitan Police to detain anyone suspected of being of unsound mind without having to obtain a warrant, as long as that individual had been apprehended in a public place. Police were required to notify the spouse or nearest relative or friend about the detention. The police could also enter private residences and businesses without a warrant to arrest and detain a person suspected of being insane if two "respectable residents" of the District made affidavits to the effect that the person harbored "homicidal or otherwise dangerous tendencies" and should not be permitted to remain at large. In these cases, the police also needed medical certifications of two physicians who had examined the individual. If they believed psychiatric treatment was necessary, the District's Board of Commissioners could commit the individual to Saint Elizabeths for no more than thirty days.[6]

The 1904 law applied specifically to indigent residents and nonresidents in the District, although there is no evidence that the police applied it this strictly. The Board of Commissioners certainly had every incentive not to commit individuals whose families were capable of paying for private care so as to avoid having to fund their stay from the municipal coffers. But it is unlikely that Metropolitan Police would have made these fine distinctions when confronted with individuals who were exhibiting erratic behavior, especially given that they routinely had to deal with people who came to the District, seat of the national government, under a delusional belief that they could influence public policy or that the government had personally wronged them.[7] On the other hand, some detentions of black Washingtonians engaging in erratic or disruptive behavior were the result of, at best, expedient and unreflective decisions and, at worst, racist assumptions about black culture. Dr. Mary O'Malley, senior assistant physician at Saint Elizabeths, observed that the Metropolitan Police's practice of apprehending and detaining African Americans on the assumption that they were insane was not particularly uncommon. "Colored individuals are occasionally arrested for drunkenness and disorderly conduct or for an unusual display of emotional reactions, singing, dancing, etc., or talking in an excited manner with one of their neighbors," she wrote in a 1914 article, "and when they are admitted for observation they are found to show no psychotic symptom."[8]

The 1904 law allowed for the discharge of temporarily committed individuals as long as the superintendent of Saint Elizabeths sent a certification to the Board of Commissioners attesting that they were either not insane or had recovered. If Saint Elizabeths' psychiatrists concluded that a temporarily committed person required further detention and treatment, however, they had to initiate a formal commitment procedure. The *writ de lunatic inquirendo* occurred in the Supreme Court of the District of Columbia's equity court and required a jury trial. It was this legal process that perturbed the hospital administration. "There is absolutely no reason or necessity for this, and it can only have the effect of humiliating both the patient and the patient's relatives," the administration declared in the 1904 annual report. "It is time that in this community, at least, insanity should be appreciated for what it is—a form of illness—and legal requirements that place a sick man on the same level as a common criminal have no place in an enlightened community."[9] Opposition to this aspect of the lunacy law was grounded in an ethos of mental hygiene, which itself reflected the convergence of dynamic psychiatry and Progressive reform.

Dynamic psychiatry's emphasis on curing mental disease by engaging the "organism as a whole" required a rethinking of not only the mentally ill individual but of the relationships among the individual, his or her social network, the physician, and the institution. Effective psychotherapeutic engagement necessitated an honest, open relationship between the psychiatrist and the patient as well as between the psychiatrist and the patient's family. Subjecting a mentally ill person and his or her family to a commitment procedure that resembled a criminal trial potentially undermined the level of comfort they had in seeking psychiatric help or cooperating with the institution. Moreover, to the extent that psychiatric care could increasingly be provided outside of the hospital's walls, maintaining a commitment process that was associated with incarceration violated psychiatrists' self-image as modern, science-based practitioners. A related concern that psychiatrists had with the jury trial was that it removed decision-making authority from those who were best equipped to wield it and invested it in a group of twelve randomly selected laypeople. They argued that commitment should be based on a diagnosis, not a verdict.[10]

Critics described the District's lunacy law as "barbarous," "archaic," and "ancient" and considered it more of an obstacle to, rather than a facilitator of, proper psychiatric care. In 1911 the secretary of the interior convened a special committee to consider the current operation and long-term needs of Saint Elizabeths, and at the top of the committee's list were the deficiencies of the District's commitment law. The committee pointed to states that had changed their laws in such a way as to make "hospitals for the insane easily accessible, so that they might extend their relief to the entire community, not only in cases of direct necessity, but early at the onset of mental disorder, and therefore be in a position to do maximum good." The committee ended up drafting a bill that it hoped Congress would consider. Although it kept the commitment procedure within the equity court, the proposed bill revised the process by vesting the authority to adjudicate an individual's mental state in the judge rather than a jury. After a commitment petition was submitted to the court, two physicians licensed to practice in the District and who had no connection to either Saint Elizabeths or the person in question would examine the individual and testify to his or her mental condition. The judge, or a relative or friend of the person whose sanity was being questioned, could request a jury trial. In the event that there was no jury trial, if the person was judged to be insane, that person or someone acting on the person's behalf could appeal within ten days of the hearing.[11]

The committee's main rationale for doing away with the mandatory jury trial was that the removal of the criminal taint from the procedure would make mentally distressed individuals and those who cared about them more willing to approach Saint Elizabeths for psychiatric care. Couched in this rationale but not expressly stated in the proposed bill was the idea that those seeking help should be able to enter the hospital of their own free will without having to go through a legal commitment process. Frederick A. Fenning, a prominent Washington lawyer and advocate for veterans, shared this sentiment, publishing an article in support of voluntary admission in the *Journal of the American Medical Association* in 1912. The District was behind the curve in its jury trial requirement, Fenning pointed out; many states had lunacy laws that allowed for voluntary admission. Fenning acknowledged the concerns that some had with the concept of voluntary admission: mainly the question of whether someone who was in need of psychiatric care could actually freely enter into a contract—which self-commitment amounted to—and the question of whether in doing so individuals forfeited their right to leave the hospital whenever they desired.

These would remain thorny issues, but Fenning pointed out that states which provided the opportunity for voluntary admission did not have any greater incidence of habeas corpus cases brought by patients against hospitals. Voluntary admission was a more enlightened approach to mental illness, one that was particularly beneficial for "persons with border-land and early stage cases." It allowed for a more humane, collaborative psychiatric intervention. "The laws permitting voluntary commitment have done a great deal toward assisting medical men in giving to those afflicted with mental disorder the advantage of our latest methods in the hope of not only alleviating suffering," Fenning claimed, "but with the larger and broader purpose of restoring the disturbed mind to its normal condition." It was well past time, the Washington lawyer advised, for the District to join other states in the "progressive march" of mental hygiene.[12]

The need to reform the District's lunacy laws remained a perennial concern for the hospital administration, appearing regularly in Saint Elizabeths' annual reports. In arguing for the abolition of the jury trial and the introduction of voluntary admission, White and the Board of Visitors were also making an argument for a reconceptualization of mental illness and psychiatry: mental illness should no longer be viewed as a disease different from any bodily disease. Even though dynamic psychiatrists had worked hard to de-emphasize the somatic basis of insanity—through an emphasis on maladjustment, the unconscious, and intrapsychic conflict, for instance—they still understood mental illness and their role in curing it within the same biomedical and public health framework that underpinned physicians' approach to disease more broadly. In other words, psychiatrists needed to engage in preventive measures, but they also needed to make interventions when an individual was in the early, incipient, or acute stage of mental illness in order to prevent it from becoming chronic and incurable. As White pointed out in the hospital's 1919 annual report, in which he reinforced the need for a reform of the District's commitment law, a policy of voluntary admission would allow someone experiencing mental stress to seek "treatment in the same manner that any sick person could go to a dispensary of a municipal hospital when he is in need of treatment."[13]

Although neither the secretary of the interior nor Congress responded affirmatively to requests to change Washington's lunacy laws, District officials did endorse an alternative clinical approach to mental illness that was consistent with dynamic psychiatry's emphasis on early intervention. In the first decade of the century, psychiatrists began to advocate for the development of separate clinical facilities in which individuals with acute symptoms of mental distress could be kept for a short period of time. Psychopathic hospitals or psychopathic wards in general hospitals would allow for the treatment of these individuals without having to sequester them in the large, prison-like structures that were state institutions. By 1920 there were only a handful of these clinical environments throughout the country: the Department of Mental Diseases at New York's Albany Hospital, the University of Michigan–affiliated Michigan Psychopathic Hospital, the Johns Hopkins–affiliated Henry Phipps Psychiatric Clinic, and the Boston Psychopathic Hospital.[14] In 1922 Washington, DC, opened its own when it established psychopathic wards at Gallinger Municipal Hospital.

Although Gallinger's main building, located in Southeast DC near the Anacostia River, was not completed until 1926, the four psychopathic wards were opened in 1922. The two-story building had two wings that allowed for the effective separation of patients by gender and race, in keeping with the standards of the psychiatric profession and, in the case of race, the segregationist policies and practices in the District, which were proliferating in the 1920s.[15] In 1923 alone, Gallinger admitted 2,401 individuals to its psychopathic wards. The psychopathic building, initially designed to accommodate 180 patients for a period of up to sixty days, ended up having space for 200 by 1930. The average daily census of the wards in that year, estimated the director of public welfare, exceeded 100.[16]

That same year Congress began to seriously consider amending the District's lunacy law. Even by the late 1920s Washington's commitment law was still woefully out of step with the rest of the nation. Forty-four of the forty-eight states provided for commitment through procedures that did not require a jury trial and at least half allowed for voluntary admission.[17] Senate Bill 5486 was introduced in December 1930, and a similar bill was introduced in the House two weeks later. The bill kept much of the 1904 law intact, including the circumstances under which the Metropolitan Police Department and the Board of Commissioners were authorized to temporarily detain and commit someone alleged to be insane, and the thirty-day maximum for temporary commitment. It provided protection to people who had been temporarily committed by requiring the superintendent of the hospital to show cause to the justice of the Supreme Court of the District of Columbia for why they should remain committed within three days after they, or someone on their behalf, requested their release in writing. Absent from the bill was the compulsory jury trial. Officials wishing to detain someone beyond the thirty days needed to prove to the court that he or she posed a danger to self or others; however, that proceeding would take place in front of a judge, not laypeople. The only condition under which a jury trial would be employed to determine one's mental condition was if the person whose sanity was being questioned—or a friend or family member—requested it.

White felt that this feature of the bill removed the criminal taint from what should largely be a medical process; he also thought that it would make the commitment procedure more egalitarian. Under the existing law, a person who had been committed had to initiate a habeas corpus proceeding in order to be discharged. This was a grave disadvantage to those whose family or friends did not have the resources to hire an attorney. Under the proposed law, the burden of proof fell on the hospital, making it easier for patients to challenge their detention and commitment. In addition to doing away with a mandatory jury trial, the bill authorized voluntary admission of any person "desirous of submitting himself or herself to treatment for mental disease." The hospital would be required to discharge persons voluntarily admitted within three days of written notification of their wish to leave.[18]

Despite the support of Saint Elizabeths' officials and the District's corporation counsel, the bill died in the House Committee on the District of Columbia in early 1932. A disappointed White and Board of Visitors continued to argue for the need to amend the city's lunacy law but made the decision to step back and encourage District authorities to take the lead.[19] They did so two years later. In the fall of 1934, E. Barrett Prettyman, the corporation counsel, submitted to the Board of Commissioners a proposed bill that would replace commitment by jury trial with a streamlined process that would be conducted by a three- to five-person lunacy commission. Such a change was supported by Richard Sylvester, a veteran of the Metropolitan Police Department, and Dr. Percy Hickling, the District's alienist, the municipal officer who signed off on all commitments of civilian residents and nonresidents. In much the same way that the presence of cranks in the federal city had prompted local authorities to lobby for an insane asylum in the nineteenth century, it was the increased number of disgruntled and dispossessed Americans coming to the nation's capital in the early years of the Depression that motivated District officials to press Congress for a more progressive lunacy law. Implementing a procedure that revolved around a small group of medical and legal experts would strip commitment of its criminal connotations and expedite the process by removing it from the sclerotic equity court, thereby making it easier to commit individuals suspected of being mentally ill before they had actually committed a crime or breached the peace.[20]

By the winter of 1935 the board's proposed bill had gained the support of the Medical Society of the District of Columbia and the Federation of Citizens' Associations. The federation, organized in 1910, was a network of neighborhood associations, some of which dated their founding back to the 1870s and 1880s. Given the inability to participate in the electoral process at either the municipal or federal levels, the federation provided one important avenue by which white Washingtonians could affect public policy. Beginning in 1925 the federation provided input to the Board of Commissioners and the congressional committees on the District of Columbia through the Citizens' Advisory Council, which consisted of the group's president and six delegates selected by the constituent associations. Although they had formed their own neighborhood associations, African Americans were excluded from the federation, which prompted black Washingtonians to establish a Federation of Civic Associations in the 1910s. In the case of the proposed lunacy law, there is no evidence that the Board of Commissioners consulted either the black federation or the African American medical professional association, the Medico-Chirurgical Society.[21] It would be approximately a year before the board's bill began wending its way through Congress with a substantial amount of support. But supporters of reform would have to wait an interminable two more years before the bill was passed, first by the Senate and later by the House. In June 1938 President Franklin Delano Roosevelt signed the bill into law. He handed his pen to Roger Cohen, an eminent psychiatrist and member of the Medical Society of the District of Columbia. Roosevelt might have handed the pen to William White had the bill passed a year and a half earlier, but White had died in March 1937.[22]

In late June 1938 the Commission on Mental Health began hearing its first cases. Drawn from a larger group of nine District residents who were appointed by the Supreme Court of the District of Columbia, the commission consisted of a lawyer and two physicians who served two- to three-month terms. The procedure for initiating a commitment proceeding—an affidavit from responsible residents, certifications from two physicians, and so forth—was largely the same one that had existed since the turn of the century. In a departure from the compulsory jury trial, the commission was empowered to conduct lunacy hearings where the allegedly insane person already was, be it Gallinger, Saint Elizabeths, or even a private residence. As in the proposed 1930 law, the option of a jury trial was available to the individual suspected of being mentally ill. The commission was charged with rendering a professional judgment as to the person's mental condition, resident status, and the ability of relatives to contribute to the person's upkeep should he or she be institutionalized. The commission only made a recommendation to the court, which ultimately issued a judgment as to whether a person was insane and warranted commitment. The commission's recommendation had to be unanimous; otherwise, another hearing would take place before a jury or the presiding justice.[23]

One aspect of lunacy legislation reform that was missing from the 1938 law—and a slight modification of the law in 1939—was voluntary admission. Although technically someone could self-commit by initiating the lunacy proceeding through the commission, the process required hiring a lawyer and waiting for ten days before being allowed to enter the hospital (or transfer from Gallinger to Saint Elizabeths). The bureaucratic red tape dissuaded some "borderline cases" from seeking treatment, according to one of the members of the commission. "Many become eager to avail themselves of needed treatment," Albert Marland alleged, "and chafe at the ten days' period of waiting imposed by law after the hearing."[24] There were several reasons why the Board of Commissioners and Congress may have opposed voluntary admission. The ambiguity around the question of whether someone who was of unsound mind could voluntarily enter into an agreement gave rise to concerns about individuals being coerced or manipulated into self-commitment. They may have also been concerned that a commitment policy with greater latitude would lead to increased admissions, putting more pressure on the resources of Saint Elizabeths. White had sought to allay this fear during the consideration of Senate Bill 5486 by pointing out that even as voluntary commitment might increase the number of admissions, earlier intervention would actually reduce the length of time individuals needed to stay in the hospital.[25] Still, overcrowding continued to remain a significant concern for Saint Elizabeths officials, leading them to embrace mental hygiene even more firmly.

The Racial Boundaries of Mental Hygiene

As much as psychiatrists and Progressive reformers wanted to make commitment a less cumbersome and traumatic process for those in need of medical treatment, they were equally desirous of improving the conditions within mental institutions. Early in White's tenure as superintendent, overcrowding was attributed to increased admissions from the District's civilian population. That situation prompted a three-man committee appointed by the Board of Commissioners to investigate the conditions of Saint Elizabeths to recommend that the District construct another mental hospital for the indigent insane and reserve Saint Elizabeths for "the insane of the army and navy and other classes coming under the care of the Federal government."[26] There is no indication that Congress ever considered appropriating funds for the building of an institution for the District's indigent insane. And to the extent that such a hospital would have potentially become a custodial institution for the chronic insane, it would have encountered opposition from the medical profession, mental hygiene advocates, and Progressive reformers.

District officials had no incentive to support a separate institution if there was a possibility that funding for the day-to-day care of its patients would come mainly from the District's congressional appropriations. Housing the city's mentally ill civilian residents with those who had been committed by some arm of the federal government allowed the municipal government to pass some of its fiscal responsibility off onto the feds. Although the city was obligated to provide financial support for civilian patients who were determined to be indigent, a typical practice, according to White, was for the District's Board of Charities to identify a relative or a friend and get him or her to promise to contribute to the patient's upkeep. That person was then committed as a pay patient. Once the relative or friend stopped contributing to the patient's support, the Board of Charities was not particularly aggressive about going after him or her. Nor would it change the designation of the patient to indigent. As a result, the District regularly owed the hospital exceedingly large sums of money.[27]

Efforts in the early twentieth century to move patients out of the institution, then, were in many ways financially motivated. Nonetheless they fit nicely with the larger Progressive goals of mental hygiene. One of the earliest iterations of mental hygiene was the practice of boarding out—placing "improved" patients in the homes of local families that were willing to care for and monitor them. It began in the 1890s largely in response to the fiscal strains that the maintenance of large asylums placed on state and county governments. By the second decade of the twentieth century, this move toward aftercare was framed within an explicit mental hygiene paradigm.[28]

It does not appear that boarding out was a widely implemented policy at Saint Elizabeths, although there were certainly instances in which patients were given parole with the expectation that they would stay with a family, blood-related or not. Fifty-two-year-old Ada R., diagnosed in 1919 as suffering from "constitutional inferiority, mental defective, with excitement," was one of those patients whose mental disorder did not warrant permanent institutionalization. When a former nurse who knew Ada offered to sponsor her parole, the clinical staff warily agreed. "Of course it is possible that this patient will not like it and if she does not she will return to the hospital," Dr. James Hassall informed his colleagues. "She may on the other hand make a good adjustment and so we feel she might be given a trial." Ada was on parole for several months, although she did not adjust to the outside world in the way that the psychiatrists had hoped. She worked for the former nurse, Irene Chappelear, and her husband for a few weeks before becoming "displeased" and leaving. Chappelear was probably relieved, as Ada was a more troublesome employee than she bargained for. "She has simply nearly worried me to death," Chappelear complained to Mary O'Malley. "I could not trust her for nothing, and [she] was such a terrible liar until she liked to have driven me mad telling me lies about the Hospital etc (and everybody). She is right much disturbed, and really she is a very dangerous negro to be at [large]." One thing that frustrated Chappelear was Ada's repeated attempts to patronize the exclusively white theater, "and when they refused to sell her tickets she would walk up and down in front of the theater and fuss for an hour or so."[29]

Apparently Ada had been absent from Chappelear's house for several weeks before Chappelear notified Saint Elizabeths. By then Ada had secured work as a domestic in the home of a storekeeper, Simon Tennyson. O'Malley assented to Tennyson's request that Ada remain in his employ. She worked for the Tennysons for several weeks while staying at her sister's home. However, Ada's new employers soon began to complain of similar behavior—"that patient's hours were irregular and that she became irritable when reprimanded." Eventually Ada ended up back in Saint Elizabeths, but only for a few months, before being paroled into the custody of her sister. Ada remained with her sister for about a month, her sister initially being grateful for the help she provided around the house. As with the case of the Chappelears and Tennysons, however, Ada's sister gradually became irritated by her behavior, including her "passion for 'sight-seeing'—exploring on foot various sections of the city." Compounded by the fact that her husband and Ada argued a lot, Ada's sister requested that the staff return her to the hospital.[30]

As assessments of Ada's behavior suggest, members of the community who took in paroled patients constantly weighed their own personal costs for providing care against the benefits—either financial or emotional—that they received. For Chappelear and Tennyson, Ada's unwillingness to be a model employee made their own status as temporary guardian less appealing. Moreover Ada's apparent unruliness extended to her behavior in public space, much to the chagrin of Irene Chappelear. It was, arguably, Ada's refusal to abide by the segregationist policies of private businesses in the District that made her a "dangerous negro" in Chappelear's estimation. And surely she was seen as such by white proprietors, white patrons, and law enforcement, an uncontrollable woman who refused to stay in her place.[31]

But, as Ada's sister's complaints also reveal, family ties could be tested in the guardian-parolee relationship, requiring the hospital to constantly reevaluate the environment in which they temporarily released their patients. Even though "working paroles," as staff members called these arrangements, might help to alleviate some of the overcrowding and fiscal pressure on the hospital, Saint

Elizabeths' psychiatrists were loath to release patients if they did not feel that the patients had a reasonable chance of readjustment or if they felt that the patients posed a threat to the community. And when they did release patients, White instructed his staff to make sure that the receiving family or friends were aware of the patient's condition and were willing to take responsibility for him or her. "We should not permit our patients to inflict themselves upon others by not knowing these facts," White declared in a directive shortly after he assumed leadership of the hospital.[32]

Parole need not always entail the relocation of a patient from the hospital to a local residence. Patients were often given ground parole, meaning that they could leave their wards and move around the hospital property with minimal supervision. At least in one case, the staff extended a modified working parole to a patient. Although not considered improved enough to be discharged, Washington B. was given a fair degree of autonomy within the hospital. The middle-aged man, an inmate of the institution since his early thirties, worked on the grounds for a "small remuneration" every month. The hospital administration possessed enough confidence in Washington's equanimity that they allowed him to stay in "a small house in the woods which he built himself, and where he keeps and raises rabbits, chickens, and other fowls, looking after them before and after working hours."

Even though a staff psychiatrist had asserted in 1905 that Washington "seems perfectly satisfied with his environment and never asks to leave," by 1906 he was requesting to be discharged. He continued to do so through 1909, with the support of his mother and sister and an attorney. White eventually signed off on the clinical staff's recommendation to release him into the custody of his mother for a two-month trial period. The original terms of the parole were never met. According to a conference report conducted three months after he was released, Washington "went to his home, but after [his mother and sister] learned that he didn't have his money with him, they thought they couldn't keep him as they could rent the room, so he was obliged to go out and earn his living." Apparently Washington found employment and lodging and managed to keep his follow-up appointments at Saint Elizabeths, which were scheduled every ten to fourteen days. In January 1910, despite the fact that the clinical staff thought there was "a certain amount of damage done" by his dementia praecox psychosis, they agreed to discharge Washington as a "very good social recovery."[33] As Washington's experience suggests, although parole and aftercare necessitated cooperation between the hospital, the patient, and the patient's social network, the shape that those interrelated forms of extra-institutional care took and the lines of cooperation needed to sustain them were not always predictable and clear.

Eventually aftercare would evolve into more professionally based therapeutic and intervention strategies. Hospitals would extend themselves into the community through the outpatient clinic, which provided the opportunity for psychiatrists to follow up on patients who had been discharged as well as the opportunity for mentally distressed people to seek treatment before their condition warranted institutionalization. Hospitals also increasingly employed or worked with psychiatric social workers, who evaluated the social environment that noninstitutionalized mentally ill individuals inhabited and coordinated with their friends, family members, and employers to facilitate their readjustment to that social environment.[34] But there were limits to the extent to which these forms of mental hygiene penetrated Washington's African American community—limits that were produced and maintained by a number of dynamics, including the segregationist culture of the District as well as the agency of patients and the members of their social networks.

The idea that Saint Elizabeths should more proactively project its psychiatric authority out into the community materialized within a few years of White's arrival as superintendent. In November 1909 he enthusiastically reported to the Board of Visitors that the new training school at the hospital was attracting a significant number of attendants who were interested in receiving a diploma in nursing. Earlier that year the training school had graduated a class of twelve, ten women and two men. Increasing the hospital's nursing staff was important to White not just because the patient population warranted it. He was also fielding more requests "to furnish to the community . . . employes trained as mental nurses in order that their services may be made use of in private work." He hoped, in fact, that as soon as the hospital had a large enough staff to provide sufficient care for those within the institution, Saint Elizabeths would "be in a position to furnish the physicians in the city with mental nurses so that cases of transitory mental disease can have the care of experienced and trained nurses in their own homes." The turn to mental hygiene—underpinned by a psychodynamic approach to insanity—was prompted, in part, by the community itself (or at least by noninstitutional psychiatrists and physicians).[35]

While White hoped that these nurses would function as a prophylactic measure to reduce the number of people who needed to be institutionalized, he also expected them to be instrumental in the aftercare of discharged patients. Yet by 1911 he expressed dissatisfaction with the hospital's lack of progress in this area. "The effort to extend the influence of the institution outside of the hospital reservation and into the community by the organization of an after care society has not been successful as yet," he informed the Board of Visitors. In the same report, he proposed a plan to improve the hospital's aftercare efforts. He had recently employed a fieldworker who had been trained by Charles B. Davenport at the Eugenics Record Office in Cold Spring Harbor, New York. Funded by the Carnegie Foundation, the fieldworker, a Miss Ross, was engaged in a large study of heredity and mental abnormality for the Eugenics Record Office and had requested access to Saint Elizabeths' records in order to survey local families. In granting her access to the records, White expected that whatever report was generated would be shared with the hospital. He also decided to enlist Ross's research skills for the purpose of investigating the home life of the families of patients who were being considered for discharge. If productive, this effort could be broadened by hiring more fieldworkers who, in addition to gathering information about patients' families, would also conduct follow-up visits once patients were released in order to prevent "another breakdown or recommitment."[36]

The fieldworker figure in aftercare was, in effect, a precursor to the more professionalized psychiatric social worker. Unfortunately we do not have much information on who these fieldworkers were or the extent to which they were used. In 1912 White reported merely that there were a "number of visits to families of patients." He pointed out with satisfaction that "friends and relatives of patients receive a field worker kindly when they know their mission," and he was confident that the information these researchers were obtaining was allowing the hospital to make important decisions about the patients who were being considered for discharge.

We do know that this method of gathering information for aftercare extended to African American patients. In the first semiannual report he made to the Board of Visitors after employing Miss Ross, White illustrated the utility of this new practice. "We had a tubercular negro woman patient whose friends were anxious for her discharge," he informed the board. "The field worker visited their home, found that it was crowded, and that there were several small children in the house. In view of these considerations it was believed by the hospital unwise to discharge the patient to these surroundings and thereby necessarily endanger the lives of these children, and the patient was retained in the hospital."[37] White gave no specifics as to where in the city this tubercular woman's friends lived, so we have no way of knowing for certain if the home that the fieldworker visited was a ramshackle shanty in one of the District's numerous alleys—which were almost exclusively inhabited by African Americans by the turn of the century— or a more spacious row house on one of the streets that formed the city's famous grid. While overcrowding and high rates of morbidity and mortality were still characteristic of alley life in Progressive-era Washington, housing conditions for most African Americans throughout the rest of the city were hardly better.[38] In any event, considering the assessment of the fieldworker, White and his clinical staff decided that the discharge of the woman would be imprudent. The crowded house would make it difficult for her to readjust to her social environment and her tuberculosis posed a threat to the health of those around her. In this sense White's vision of mental hygiene clearly incorporated the city's black population.

Saint Elizabeths' aftercare efforts evolved even more fully into mental hygiene when it opened an outpatient clinic in 1920. The clinic's purpose was to serve as the intermediary between the hospital and the discharged or paroled patient. Prior to its establishment, if former inmates' behavior or actions raised concerns among their family or neighbors, they primarily resorted to asking hospital staff to come and retrieve them. This was often inconvenient given Saint Elizabeths' distance from many neighborhoods in the District. With a centrally located clinic staffed by a psychiatrist and a social worker, the hospital could respond more rapidly when discharged or paroled patients had relapses. But the clinic also allowed the hospital to better monitor those patients by making it easier for them to report for checkups and more convenient for social workers to visit their homes. The clinic was opened in Trinity Community House, a nonsectarian community service organization affiliated with Trinity Church and located on Indiana Avenue, NW, just a few blocks from the Capitol. Trinity Community House made perfect sense. Run by Rev. and Mrs. David R. Covell, the newly established organization took particular interest in working with institutionalized populations, including those at the District's almshouse and Saint Elizabeths. Dr. Loren Johnson, senior assistant physician at Saint Elizabeths, ran the clinic, where he made himself available from 2:00 to 5:00 P.M. three days a week. He was initially assisted by a psychiatric social worker.[39]

As the 1920 annual report made clear, the outpatient clinic had dual objectives: "First, to assist the patient leaving the institution to an adjustment of maximum success; second, to aid other individuals at the onset of their difficulty to adapt to the community." Ironically it was this broad mandate that made Saint Elizabeths' outpatient clinic a short-lived endeavor—at least in the way it was originally conceptualized operating at Trinity Community House. The small staff was overwhelmed by the number of people they had to assist and the number of visits they had to make. The hospital's annual reports document the sheer number of hours put in by the social worker in the first two years of the clinic's operation and suggest the skewed division of labor between the male psychiatrist and the female social worker. In the first seven months after the clinic was opened, Johnson received 97 visits from 33 patients, an average of three visits per person every other month. In that same time span, the social worker made 557 visits to the homes of paroled and discharged patients as well as those who were being considered for parole. Over the following year, the social worker made 1,295 visits, an average of 3.5 per day, while the psychiatrist received 150 visits from 97 patients. By the summer of 1922, Johnson was receiving three times as many visits as the previous year. These were still a fraction of the number of visits being made by the social worker, but she was joined by another social worker in March of that year. On top of this, Johnson and the social workers received at the clinic or made visits to the homes of people who were referred by private physicians, social service organizations like the Associated Charities, or municipal agencies such as the Board of Children's Guardians or the Juvenile Protectorate. The number of these interactions increased from 308 in 1920 to 569 by 1922.⁴⁰ Even with two social workers, Saint Elizabeths could not handle the volume of Washingtonians seeking mental hygiene services and maintain the necessary work of assisting paroled and discharged patients in readjusting to their social environment. In May 1925 they ceased operations at Trinity Community House.⁴¹

The hospital administration hoped that the closure would be temporary, a hiatus until the fall, during which time it would beef up its resources. The actual clinic at Trinity Community House remained closed, but a year later Saint Elizabeths initiated a new, more robust social service department, one that would concentrate its energies on helping patients reintegrate into society. The social service department employed more social workers to do the kind of investigation necessary to determine the suitability of the environment into which paroled and discharged patients would be released. "This sort of preliminary contact," hospital officials pointed out, "paves the way for a more friendly relation which carries over into home visits."⁴² In addition to investigating the home life of the family member or friend into whose custody a patient was to be released and conducting follow-up visits, the social worker also collaborated with hospital staff in identifying employment and residential opportunities for improved or recovered patients who did not have close relations outside of the institution. During the latter half of the 1920s, Saint Elizabeths' social service department significantly expanded. Between 1928 and 1929 alone, the average number of outpatients on the monthly rolls increased by 25 percent, and the total number of visits went from 2,028 to 2,512.⁴³

One of the many patients handled by the social service department was Pearl B., an African American orphan who was admitted to Saint Elizabeths in 1925 at the age of nineteen. It is unclear when or how Pearl's parents died, but the five-year-old became a ward of the Board of Children's Guardians in 1911. Despite being placed in various boarding houses over the next ten years, Pearl managed to do well in school. It was not until she was fifteen and sent to Virginia for employment—presumably as a domestic—that she began to exhibit a "marked personality change." In 1921, after an examination at a psychopathic clinic, doctors concluded that Pearl was mentally defective. It became more difficult for her guardians to control her behavior. She began having trouble in school and not coming home in the evening. In December 1923 Pearl ended up in the District's Columbia Hospital for Women, where she underwent an "induced miscarriage." She was then sent to a home for "incorrigible girls." Five months later she ran away. Her whereabouts were unknown until December 1924, when a pregnant Pearl was "found working in the city" and taken to Gallinger for a mental examination. She remained in Gallinger for five months—during which time she gave birth to her child—before being committed to Saint Elizabeths.⁴⁴

According to her case file, Pearl appears to have been a rather typical patient. At times she was pleasant and tractable, at others obstinate and combative. Early in her confinement, Dr. Lois Hubbard described her as getting along "surprisingly well," even though she made "frequent requests to go home." Two months later she appeared to be in a foul mood and fought with other patients and nurses before being restrained with a cold pack. "This morning she is sullen, resentful, threatening," observed Hubbard, "complains that she was choked, beaten and otherwise abused, asserts her intention of writing to the authorities to report the ill-treatment received by her as an innocent victim." Nearly two and a half years after she was committed, Saint Elizabeths' staff considered releasing Pearl because she showed no signs of psychosis. They convened a conference to examine and discuss the patient in November 1927.

A review of the examinations conducted when she was admitted reveals the racist assumptions that undergirded the staff's medical opinion. "Orientation was correct and memory was good for one of her race and ability," the examining physician recorded. The staff psychologist, Winifred Richmond, concluded that Pearl was "sub-average but not feeble-minded for her race." The mental obtuseness of this young black woman, from the staff's perspective, was perfectly concordant with the natural intellectual aptitude that they considered people of African descent to possess. That this "normal abnormality" was as much a cultural product as a biological certainty was acknowledged by Richmond in the November 1927 conference. "The girl is not actually defective," she stated to her colleagues. "We must remember that we are examining these patients by tests developed for the use of white children and they cannot be expected to show up as well as a white person would. She has intelligence enough to make a go of it if her other qualities won't prevent [it]." The rest of the staff members agreed. Settling on a diagnosis of psychopathic personality without psychosis, Dr. Arthur P. Noyes, one of the hospital's senior medical officers, contacted the Board of Public Welfare to inquire about releasing Pearl back into the custody of the Board of Children's Guardians. When the assistant director responded that she was of majority age and no longer considered a ward, the hospital administration had to come up with an alternative plan.[45]

Pearl stayed in the hospital for several months after the conference, during which she was a regular in the occupational therapy classes while the social service department attempted to identify a suitable home for her. The hospital had been approached by Pearl's brother and sister-in-law, who requested that she be allowed to stay with them for short visits. But they disappeared before the social service department could investigate their home, a situation that did not inspire confidence. When Pearl's sister-in-law reappeared in March 1928, she was no longer with Pearl's brother and had remarried. Dorothy Sproul, the psychiatric social worker, was not impressed with Pearl's sister-in-law. Sproul found her to be "resistive about giving information about herself" and, although she acknowledged that the home was fairly clean, she reported that it was "a poorly kept brick house in a mediocre, mixed colored and white neighborhood. . . . This home apparently would have nothing socially constructive to offer the patient," Sproul concluded, "and visits might only serve to break down the good habits she has established in the hospital." In the meantime Pearl was becoming impatient. Ten days after Sproul filed her report, Dr. Agnes Conrad indicated that while she was, in the main, cooperative, Pearl "has so nursed her grievance of being kept in the hospital after other[s] less well behaved have been permitted to leave that she is likely to assume a worse rather than better attitude if her privileges are not soon increased."[46]

Sproul was clearly aware that keeping Pearl in Saint Elizabeths was not good for her or the hospital, and she intensified her efforts to find a suitable placement. She enlisted the assistance of Mary Stewart, the industrial secretary for the Phyllis Wheatley Young Women's Christian Association, the District's African American branch of the segregated social service organization. Stewart felt that many respectable African American women in the city who were capable of providing the necessary support and guidance for a "problem girl" such as Pearl were "for the most part, busy in their own professions and would have little time to care for anyone in the home." But Stewart held open the possibility of Pearl's staying at the Phyllis Wheatley house. Sproul took that opening and pressed Stewart. "Although it is quite possible that she will not make an adjustment, we think that she ought to have a chance to try life outside," the social worker remarked in a letter to Stewart in late March. On April 4 Sproul took Pearl to meet Stewart at the Phyllis Wheatley house. They took to each other immediately. From Sproul's perspective, placing Pearl in the home was the ideal scenario. She reported to the outpatient physician that Stewart was "a well educated, intelligent, sympathetic, superior, young colored woman, who gives the impression of being thoroughly capable and competent" and was already referring to Pearl as her "adopted little sister." Pearl moved into the Phyllis Wheatley house six days later.[47]

The first few months at the house were good for Pearl, and her case file reveals both the challenges of the outpatient experience and the extent to which the social service department went in facilitating her adjustment to her noninstitutional environment. Within a week of moving out of Saint Elizabeths, Pearl had secured work at the National Pants Factory, where she was reported to be a competent employee. Unfortunately her weekly salary was not sufficient to rent a single room in the house, and she had to room with another young woman; nor was Pearl making enough money to pay for all of her meals, a problem that Stewart rectified by allowing Pearl to eat dinners at her home. Pearl also had difficulties socializing with the other women in the house, which Sproul attributed to a "combination of her inferior financial status and her long residence in the hospital." By this, Sproul meant that Pearl had grown unaccustomed to interacting with "normal girls." Yet Pearl's reticence to engage may have been influenced by shame at having been institutionalized. Her guardedness may have been a desire to keep her seven years in Saint Elizabeths a secret. Indeed the women she spent the most time with—attending church and going to the movies—were two other outpatients, Rosina B. and Irene T., neither of whom appears to have lived at the Phyllis Wheatley house.[48]

Interestingly, outpatients not only served as a support network for one another; they also functioned as surveillance for the social service department. During Pearl's first few months out of the hospital, Sproul regularly called the Phyllis Wheatley house or Stewart to check up on her. Pearl was also expected to report to the outpatient office at Saint Elizabeths. The first time she did so she was accompanied by Irene. In addition to counting on Rosina and Irene to make sure that Pearl kept her appointments and remained responsible, Sproul relied on them to provide information that she could not necessarily obtain in her interviews with Pearl. "From Irene [T.] . . . it was today learned that Pearl has been visiting her brother's home in the vicinity of H and 9th Streets, N.W. to meet her gentleman friend, Frank," Sproul recorded in July. "She also introduced Irene to a man visiting at this house and according to Irene's report it is suspected that Pearl has been having at least occasional sexual relations with Frank." Three months later Sproul entered the following note in Pearl's file: "Reports from other out-patients regarding Pearl's activities recently have indicated that she was making a less satisfactory outside adjustment than when she first went out and Miss Stewart also reports various unfavorable points in her behavior." Once she lost Stewart's support, it was probably only a matter of time before Pearl ended up back in Saint Elizabeths. The last social service report was filed on October 10, 1928; by mid-November she had been readmitted.[49]

Not surprisingly, Pearl became a more difficult patient once she was back behind the institution's walls. Staff members consistently remarked about how uncooperative she was, especially when it came to work. She was also apparently a puckish figure on the ward. Pearl is "always more or less of a problem," Hubbard noted in April 1929. "She goes to all amusements and is ringleader in any mischief that crops up." Pearl yearned to be an outpatient again. She frequently asked to leave the hospital to go find work and became "very disappointed" when staff refused. In an examination in April 1931, Dr. Anita Harper characterized Pearl as "rather longely [sic] and anxious to get out and make her living and to be among her relatives." Although we do not know if she was able to achieve these goals, Pearl did finally get out of the hospital. One month after Harper's examination, while on an excursion with other patients to see the circus, Pearl and another patient managed to evade the nurse and escape into the District streets. After alerting the police and attempting to track her down through her brother and former sister-in-law, Saint Elizabeths' staff gave up their search for Pearl. In June 1932, a year after she disappeared, they convened a conference to consider discharging her. Even though the last observation made by a psychiatrist indicated that Pearl was lucid, "heard no voices [and] had no delusions," the staff agreed to change her original diagnosis of psychopathic personality without psychosis to psychosis with psychopathic personality before dropping her name from the rolls.[50]

Despite the racist-tinged language that characterized the clinical staff's diagnostic and evaluative assessments of Pearl, the hospital's social service department certainly worked on her behalf in facilitating her transition from an institutionalized to a noninstitutionalized environment. In doing so, it employed multiple resources, including psychiatric social workers, community-based reformers, and even other outpatients. In the end, however, the efforts to utilize a mental hygiene approach ran into Pearl's determination to challenge the medical authority that Saint Elizabeths' staff presumed they had over her.

The social service department certainly had cases they considered less troublesome than Pearl's. Twenty-four-year-old Adeline J. was admitted to Saint Elizabeths from the psychopathic ward at Gallinger Hospital in June 1930. She had been taken to Gallinger in early May from the District Workhouse in Occoquan, Virginia, where she had been serving a sentence for solicitation, although she denied this charge to the hospital staff. Even though Gallinger records indicated that Adeline was "extremely demented," the admitting physician at Saint Elizabeths, Dr. Elizabeth Vann, did not make an initial diagnosis. Her delirium may have been a symptom of malaria, for which she was treated at Saint Elizabeths. Adeline was also syphilitic, according to the physician at the workhouse. That fall, while undergoing treatment for syphilis, Adeline was diagnosed with general paresis and began malaria fever inoculation therapy. She also began making short visits to her mother's house. In January 1931 Adeline became an outpatient.[51]

Unlike Pearl's, Adeline's support network included family and neighbors, although this did not necessarily make for an easier transition to noninstitutional life—at least from the social service department's perspective. Whereas the problematic transition for Pearl was, in part, the result of her rebelliousness, for Adeline it was her social network itself. The psychiatric social worker K. F. Silber felt that Adeline was "getting along satisfactorily." The biggest problem was getting her to return to the hospital for her treatments for syphilis and general paresis. Her mother's Northwest home was far from the hospital's campus in Southeast, and neither her mother nor her cousin, also an outpatient who lived at the house, had enough disposable income to pay for taxi fare. Indeed Silber's constant reminders of the importance of treatment and Adeline's mother's assertions of "shortage of funds" are a running theme in Adeline's case file. With Adeline unable to work and her mother going through periods of unemployment—no doubt intensified by the Depression—it was too difficult to make the trek to Saint Elizabeths.

The family's lack of money even made it challenging to comply with the alternative arrangements proposed by Silber: having Adeline stay temporarily in the hospital for her treatment or having her receive her treatments at a Northwest clinic operated by Dr. Theodore Fong, a serologist on Saint Elizabeths' staff. "[Her mother] says that patient becomes so lonely and unhappy that it is necessary to visit her every week and this takes almost as much car fare as weekly trips to Dr. Fong's clinic," Silber documented in March 1933. Although one must be careful about presuming their physical ability, given that the clinic was approximately one mile from her home, it is possible that Adeline's mother may have pleaded poverty as a way of severing the connection between her daughter and Saint Elizabeths. Even though Adeline acknowledged that she liked the hospital, according to Silber, Adeline's mother managed to get her discharged. "[Her mother] agreed to bring the girl to the hospital in order that the doctors might decide as to her present condition," Silber noted, "her own feeling being that 'improved' better describes her than 'recovered.'" Silber recommended to the clinical staff that, since Adeline had completed a course of the malarial fever inoculation therapy, she should be discharged as improved even though she still needed treatment for syphilis. Six days later the clinical staff convened a conference and agreed to discharge Adeline as improved.[52]

It is impossible to know if Adeline's mother's assessment of her daughter as improved rather than recovered influenced Silber's professional judgment. The case file is clear that her mother played an active part in managing Adeline's outpatient therapeutic experience and did not cede her own authority as a parent to that of the doctors. Although Adeline's mother had agreed to take her to Fong's clinic as a condition of her release, once the staff dropped Adeline from the rolls, the hospital had no legal recourse to ensure that her mother complied. As Adeline's case suggests, the ability of Saint Elizabeths to extend its presence into the community could be dependent on the willingness of the patients and members of their social networks to cooperate.

Gilbert W.'s mother had a decidedly different collaboration with Saint Elizabeths' social service department. The thirty-year-old African American had been a soldier in the US Army for ten years. While attached to the Engineers' School Detachment at Fort Humphreys in southeastern Fairfax County, Virginia (now Fort Belvoir), he occasionally visited his mother and stepfather, who lived in Arlington County, sandwiched between Fairfax and southwestern DC. In February 1930 Gilbert was admitted to Fort Humphrey's station hospital. According to his stepfather, who filed a complaint with his commanding officer, Gilbert had shown up at his mother's house and threatened to kill his mother and stepfather if "they did not give him a Chrysler car to repay him for all the money they had gotten from him." Upon being diagnosed with dementia praecox, paranoid type, Gilbert was transferred to Walter Reed Hospital in the District. Army doctors also discovered that Gilbert had syphilis and began treating him with salvarsan and mercury. He would stay at Walter Reed for five and a half months before being admitted to Saint Elizabeths. At the admitting conference, the clinical staff, after examining Gilbert, found "no active symptoms of a psychosis." Although they concurred with the initial diagnosis of dementia praecox, they also agreed that he was on the road to recovery, noting that "he seems to be able and willing to go to work."[53]

Over the next few months Gilbert continued to improve, to the point that his mother, who had begun visiting him, requested that he be released into her custody. In an April 1931 conference, Dr. John E. Lind reiterated the initial diagnosis of dementia praecox but recommended that Gilbert be allowed to make short visits to his mother's home. "She seems reliable and I feel sure she would take care of him," Lind told his colleagues. Although the psychiatric social worker did not have an opportunity to assess the home of Gilbert's mother before his first visit, the social service department did conduct an investigation in June. One of the physicians on staff, perhaps Lind, gave a special charge to the social worker, S. F. Schroeder, to "learn whether patient's mother is afraid of him because of the threats he made before coming to the hospital." After interviewing Gilbert's mother, Schroeder reported that "she has seen nothing threatening in his attitude since out and they seem willing to have him there." However, Schroeder added, "she does not wish him discharged . . . as she wants to see how he gets on." Unfortunately he did not get on very well for long. By the beginning of the following year, Gilbert began acting in an erratic manner, preoccupied by the thought that his mother was withholding money from him. "His mother says that the patient insisted that she had his money, so on the 16th of January he would not eat because he said he did not want any food but wanted money," Gilbert's case record states. "The mother became rather alarmed and had him sent back." Gilbert would not return to his mother's house, despite the fact that the clinical staff felt that the paranoid psychosis associated with his dementia praecox had abated during his readmission to Saint Elizabeths. In May 1932, after receiving assurances from his Pennsylvania-based uncle that he could provide a home and employment for Gilbert, the clinical staff agreed to discharge him as improved.[54]

As Gilbert W.'s case suggests, it was possible for the hospital's clinical staff, social service department, the patient, and members of the patient's social network to collaborate in a set of relationships that would ultimately result in a favorable outcome for all parties involved. Gilbert, whose mother had always suspected he would take off for points north where employment opportunities were better, managed to end up with his uncle in Pennsylvania. Despite her troubles with him, the knowledge that he was in the home of a relative (but not hers) instead of an overcrowded and segregated facility must have comforted her. The clinical staff was probably also satisfied that it managed to provide sufficient care and treatment for a mentally ill individual to the point that he no longer needed to be confined in an institution.

Yet Gilbert's final conference report betrayed a great deal of skepticism on the staff's part. After Dr. Francis Tartaglino recommended that Gilbert be discharged as a social recovery, other physicians at the conference weighed in. Although Dr. Manson Pettit agreed to discharge, he balked at the designation of social recovery. "I doubt if he can make a social adaptation for any length of time," Pettit suggested. Dr. Roscoe Hall, the clinical director, also concurred but expressed a similar suspicion as to Gilbert's ability to reintegrate into society. "I think he is the type of patient that makes a better adjustment in hospital than outside," Hall admitted to his colleagues. "He may be able to get along for months, or perhaps even for years, but I should be inclined to doubt it." O'Malley supported Hall's estimation, although she confessed that she did not "know much about his condition." But O'Malley did examine Gilbert at the beginning of the conference and found him to be "fairly intelligent for a colored man who has been suffering from a regressive mechanism."[55] O'Malley's qualification of Gilbert's mental condition, along with other physicians' occasional references to the thirty-one-year-old as "boy," reminds us that these clinical encounters between white psychiatrists and African American patients were hardly devoid of racist signification, if not intention.[56]

As much as these racist assumptions figured into the diagnostic and therapeutic assessments of their black patients, Saint Elizabeths' staff do not appear to have substantially withheld resources from them in either the outpatient clinics or psychiatric social work services that were in place to manage their postinstitutional lives. This was not the case, however, in other efforts in which Saint Elizabeths was involved in preserving the mental health of Washingtonians who had not been yet been committed to the hospital. Even though it would be unfair to blame White and his staff, the marginalization of African American residents of the District in two mental hygiene clinics connected to Saint Elizabeths illustrate the racial boundaries of this new psychiatric approach to mental illness that White himself so adamantly advocated.

Of all of Washington's private mental hygiene clinics, the Life Adjustment Center and the Child Guidance Clinic had the closest ties to Saint Elizabeths. Founded in December 1928 by Reverend Moses R. Lovell, the center was housed in the Mount Pleasant Congregational Church in Northwest Washington. An advocate of the "new psychology," Lovell opened his church every Monday evening for troubled adults to meet with a mostly volunteer staff. The center's staff was an eclectic one, consisting of psychiatrists, social workers, a spiritual adviser, a general counselor, and a director of religious education. There was a significant presence of Saint Elizabeths personnel on the center staff, including Roscoe Hall; Dr. Amy Stannard, one of the hospital's chiefs of service; Dorothy Sproul; and Dr. Lucille Dooley, a medical officer who had resigned from the hospital in 1926. By 1932 the center had expanded its staff considerably, increased the number of days and hours for seeing adult patients, and opened its services to children.[57]

Saint Elizabeths had an even more direct hand in the opening and early operation of the Child Guidance Clinic. White was the president of the clinic, and the hospital's psychologist, Dr. Winifred Richmond, was an officer, as was Loren B. T. Johnson, head of Saint Elizabeths' first outpatient clinic, who had left the hospital in 1925. In June 1930, five months before the clinic opened, White appointed its director, Dr. Paul J. Ewerhardt, a psychiatrist who had extensive experience in mental hygiene clinics in Rhode Island. The clinic, initially located in an elementary school in the Shaw-Logan Circle neighborhood, operated full time, with hours from 9:00 to 5:30 during the week and 9:00 to 1:00 on Saturdays. Its staff was somewhat smaller than at the Life Adjustment Center, with a psychiatrist, a psychologist, and two psychiatric social workers. Unlike the center, however, the clinic's staff was employed full time. By 1936 the center and clinic were sharing a large, formerly private residence just north of Meridian Hill Park in Northwest.[58]

The clientele at the Life Adjustment Center, according to its staff, was diverse, even though it was hardly representative of the District's population. Its founder envisioned it as a nonsectarian service; as such, there was a distinct denominational heterogeneity among those who utilized the center. Protestants and Catholics topped the list, but there were also Jews, Mormons, and the unchurched among the center's clients. More women than men sought assistance there, and most of the clients were between twenty and fifty years of age. Apparently, too, the majority of those availing themselves of the center's services were educated professionals and federal employees.[59] One does not run a great risk in surmising that the center's clientele was not racially diverse. None of the newspaper articles on the center supplied a racial breakdown of the clients, though they did detail religion and gender statistics. The absence of race in any press coverage of the center itself, in fact, suggests that the clients were exclusively white.

Due to the lack of concrete evidence, any discussion of the nonuse of the center by African Americans is necessarily speculative. Some of the potential structural and cultural explanations are rendered less convincing given that we are talking about black Washington. For instance, the idea that psychiatry was considered to be alien by a population that was, in the main, skeptical of Western biomedicine, resistant to a naturalist understanding of the psyche, and reliant on religion and folk medicine as coping mechanisms is belied by the fact that the District had a large African American professional and educated middle class. Many blacks, employed by the federal government and perhaps having some connection to one of the most elite institutions of black higher education, would have been exposed to some of the scholarly research by Howard University academics on the impact of racism and segregation on African Americans' psychological and emotional well-being. And while it might be easy to invoke the lack of disposable income as a barrier to seeking psychiatric help—a lack that was exacerbated by the Depression—this becomes a nonfactor because the center's staff did not charge for their consultations.[60] Rather, the absence of African Americans at the Life Adjustment Center was most likely a product of the segregationist culture of the District. Although it is unclear whether the center had an official policy of segregation, the staff was probably inclined to discourage any prospective black clients from attending out of fear of offending its white client base. Moreover, given the rigid segregation that attended the District's churches, African Americans were most likely reluctant to seek services at a white church, as liberal as that church's congregation and pastor may have been.

But the scarcity of African Americans at the center does not mean that blacks were unconcerned about mental hygiene—or that Saint Elizabeths' staff were similarly aloof. Howard University invited Winifred Richmond to speak about mental hygiene and "what the minister should know about it" at its convocation dinner in 1928. Local civic organizations sponsored lectures and symposia on mental hygiene throughout the 1930s, inviting, among others, Richmond; Ewerhardt; Dr. Benjamin Karpman, senior medical officer at Saint Elizabeths; and Dr. Ernest Y. Williams, a black graduate of Howard University's medical school who had done his clinical rotations at Saint Elizabeths under the direction of Karpman. Williams would go on to establish a psychiatric service at Freedmen's Hospital in 1939.[61]

Where Saint Elizabeths' staff was more likely to engage in noninstitutional intervention in the lives of black Washingtonians was in the Child Guidance Clinic. Yet here, as in the Life Adjustment Center, there were significant racial boundaries. Early on, however, White recognized the importance of extending mental hygiene efforts to the African American community. He appointed the dean of Howard University's medical school to the Child Guidance Clinic's inaugural advisory board, which also included the deans of the medical schools of George Washington University and Georgetown University, as well as the superintendent of the District's public schools. Two years later, Mordecai Johnson, Howard University's first African American president, was also serving on the clinic's advisory board.[62]

The clinic, and the child guidance movement more broadly, was aimed at assisting "normal" children who were having difficulty adjusting to their surroundings because of minor emotional or behavioral problems. The "problem child," in other words, did not include juvenile delinquents, children with subnormal intelligence, the feebleminded, or children with neurological or psychopathic disorders.[63] While it would have been keeping in line with the prevailing thought about race, intelligence, and culture to characterize African American youth, especially those in working-class neighborhoods, as subnormal or delinquent, child guidance experts did not completely abandon them.[64] The clinic, for instance, worked with officials in the Child Welfare Division to evaluate "a group of older colored girls requiring special care" who were being considered for adoption. In 1935 the clinic hired an African American native of Massachusetts, Gertrude Williams, as a reading specialist. Williams most likely worked with black children who were referred to the clinic. In fact by 1941 there was such a substantial presence of African American youths at the clinic that Ewerhardt's successor, Dr. Rex E. Buxton, identified a "Negro boy, 11, who could not adjust himself to school routine and who showed evidence of mental illness to come," as one of the three typical cases with which his staff dealt.[65] But these child guidance efforts were made on a segregated basis. This is no surprise given that playgrounds in Washington were segregated until the early 1950s and the District's schools would not begin the process of integration until 1955. Freedmen's Hospital opened a child guidance clinic in 1941, providing services to African American youths and their families in an environment that they could call their own; in the other clinics throughout the city, however, consultations with black children were limited to only a few hours a week.[66]

In the end, the racial boundaries of mental hygiene were both ideological and social. As much as Saint Elizabeths' staff sought to employ this approach to assist their African American patients in readjusting to their social environments once they were released, there is evidence that racist assumptions about the black psyche continued to compromise how they evaluated and worked with those patients and their families. Yet the racial boundaries that circumscribed the staff's intervention in the psychic lives of noninstitutionalized African Americans were as much the product of the District's social landscape as they were the manifestation of any racism or racial ambivalence on the part of psychiatrists, psychiatric social workers, or psychologists. The mental hygiene project that White and others envisioned implementing in Washington was constricted by the segregationist culture and politics of the nation's capital. By the 1950s these boundaries would begin to dissolve, as they would in Saint Elizabeths itself. In fact if the Negro boy whom Buxton described ended up being institutionalized in his mid-twenties, he would have entered a hospital with integrated wards and African American clinical staff members.

8

"An Example for the Rest of the Nation"

Challenging Racial Injustice at Saint Elizabeths, 1910–1955

Despite the efforts by William Alanson White and his professional colleagues to promote mental hygiene among Washingtonians, Saint Elizabeths remained a massive institution whose patient population continued to increase in the 1930s. The hospital was a gigantic operation by any measure. Its size contributed to, at best, overworked staff who neglected many patients and, at worst, willfully inattentive staff who took out their frustrations on patients. In the summer of 1936 a thirty-two-year-old African American patient, Howard Hawkins, was the unfortunate victim of maliciously motivated staff members. Shortly before his death in July, Hawkins reportedly accused two white attendants, John Ferguson and Robert Brunner, of having beaten him following an argument he had had with his wife when she visited in late May. The Metropolitan Police arrested the attendants, but the assistant district attorney refused to bring assault charges on the grounds that the cause of Hawkins's death had not been established. Even though Ferguson and Brunner were released, they remained suspended from the hospital.

At a coroner's inquest, the attendants claimed that Hawkins's injuries were the result of his accidentally falling against the bed as they were trying to get him to return to his room. The inquest ruled that Hawkins died of peritonitis, which would not have been caused by a beating two months earlier. Armed with this information, the grand jury refused to indict Ferguson and Brunner on homicide charges. Despite their exoneration, however, the attendants did not return to work. Citing their ultimate responsibility for protecting patients, Dr. Herbert C. Woolley, the first assistant physician, made it clear to the *Washington Afro-American* that they would no longer be employed by Saint Elizabeths.[1]

The press never cast Hawkins's death as a racial incident, and indeed the violent treatment of patients by attendants occurred across racial groups, as is evident in the deaths of two white sailors allegedly at the hands of attendants in the summer of 1945.[2] Rather, what the Hawkins episode threatened to do was to render Saint Elizabeths a model institution in an alternative sense, as an archetypical madhouse whose mission was more custodial than therapeutic. Despite Woolley's appropriate firing of Ferguson and Brunner, and the involvement of Saint Elizabeths' staff in mental hygiene efforts in the 1920s and 1930s, the hospital could not avoid becoming tainted by the image of the mental institution as warehouse, a popular perception of institutional psychiatry that intensified after World War II. By the 1940s and 1950s Americans viewed the public mental hospital in general as a chaotic, overcrowded space populated by the chronically ill, indifferent administrators, and incompetent staff. References to mental institutions as "snake pits" entered the national lexicon.[3]

In the postwar period, African American civil rights activists and medical professionals began challenging Saint Elizabeths' practice of racial segregation. The treatment of African American patients and the practical exclusion of African American medical students from access to psychiatric training occasionally provided the District's black community targets for criticism before World War II. But it was not until after the war that a sustained challenge to the hospital's segregationist policy resulted in the integration of the staff, including the appointment of the first African American doctor in 1955. Two developments in particular were critical to the success of the activists' frontal assault on segregation at Saint Elizabeths. The first was the changing demographics of the hospital. With the cessation of military admissions in 1946 and the military's growing reliance on psychiatric services in hospitals run by the Veterans Administration, Saint Elizabeths' patients were increasingly drawn from the District's civilian population. A greater civilian population eventually meant a patient population with more African Americans. Like other urban public hospitals that were forced to integrate their staffs because of the changing demographics of the communities they served, Saint Elizabeths found its segregationist policy unsustainable. Even if the hospital's administration had been unwavering opponents of integration, it would not have been able to withstand the second development: the evolution of a more progressive stance by the federal government in racial matters in the postwar period.

"A Degree of Segregation": Race, Space, and Place in the White Years

As much as the psychiatric profession recommended that Saint Elizabeths' patients be segregated on the basis of race—a policy the District's political elites and white citizens demanded—occasionally the staff had to compromise the segregationist policy in order to accommodate all of the hospital's inmates. There were periodic attempts to more rigidly segregate the patients, to, in effect, racially territorialize the hospital. In 1911, eleven years after the Board of Visitors considered sequestering all of the black patients on the eastern side of Nichols Avenue with the "more disturbed and untidy of the white males," a special committee convened by the Department of the Interior to evaluate the needs of the hospital revisited the prospect of achieving a more durable racial segregation.[4] The committee pointed out that, given the number of African American patients—approximately 650, most of whom were civilian residents of the District—the federal government could consider building a separate institution for them. However, it also acknowledged that to maintain the level of care they were receiving at Saint Elizabeths, the federal government would have to increase per capita spending if a new hospital was created. The committee suggested as a compromise a "special colony for the colored insane" that, while operated by Saint Elizabeths, would "preserve the advantages of the top cost distribution and still effect a desirable segregation."[5] The special colony was never established, and it appears that this was the last serious discussion of creating a separate institution for mentally ill African Americans in the District.

The inability to consistently maintain appropriate racial boundaries exposed Saint Elizabeths' administration to criticism from a variety of quarters. A Department of the Interior inspector noted in 1924 that black and white male patients in a temporary tubercular building were "only separated by an imaginery [sic] line," having their meals in the same room, albeit at separate tables. He also pointed out that black and white residents of Howard Hall shared the same recreational space, although he did not indicate whether they intermingled. One of the inspector's recommendations was that White needed to "be advised that there is no proper segregation of black and white patients and that, in order to prevent criticism, that this receive his attention."[6]

Concern that patients be racially segregated extended beyond the walls of the hospital. In fact the concern may have been even more intensely expressed by those not directly connected to the hospital. Shortly before Christmas in 1907, the superintendent sent a letter to G. Lloyd Magruder, the dean of Georgetown University Medical School and a member of the Board of Visitors, who had apparently inquired about an incident in which black and white patients were fraternizing off the hospital grounds. "I cannot find out that we have ever sent parties out driving containing both white and colored patients," White assured Magruder. "It is possible, however, that a mistake may have been made owing to the fact that we send white nurses with our colored patients. The nurses would have probably had coats or shawls on so that their uniforms were not visible and therefore their identity would not have been evident." In an effort to further placate Magruder, White concluded his letter with the following declaration: "We do not employ, as you know, colored attendants or nurses on the wards at all."[7] Whether Magruder had witnessed this interracial party or was merely relaying a concern expressed to him by a local resident is not known. Either way, Magruder's or the residents' pique would have certainly been enhanced if they witnessed what they thought to be a black male patient and a white female patient riding together in the same vehicle. That White had to take time to explain the racial dynamics of the hospital's therapeutic procedures while also reinforcing its racist employment policy is indicative of the segregationist expectations held by the lay public as well as government officials.

To be sure, the hospital administration managed to maintain a largely segregationist regime during the White years, the overall lack of space and the bureaucratic and lay admonishments notwithstanding. Aside from the nominal segregation that existed in the tubercular cottage and a juvenile ward, a committee inspecting the hospital under the auspices of the navy reported approvingly that Saint Elizabeths' patients were separated on the basis of race, gender, emotional state, and underlying psychosis. "Whites and blacks may occupy different wards in the same building, but they are not treated together in the same wards," the report clarified.[8] As in the Godding administration, the necessity of achieving racial separation contributed to the overcrowding of wards, particularly those occupied by African American patients. The 1932 annual report, for instance, admitted that the colored male wards in Howard Hall were "extremely overcrowded" and that the West Lodge's receiving ward did not have enough seating space for all of its patients.[9]

This, then, was the predominant racial climate of Saint Elizabeths during the White years. Although the administration could not maintain impermeable racial boundaries within the inmate population, a general segregationist stasis prevailed at the institution. For the most part, the racially biased nature of inmate management policies did not provoke a sharp response from Washington's black press or political class, despite the fact that Saint Elizabeths was a federal institution and black Washingtonians were certainly sensitive to discriminatory policies in federal employment. There were moments, however, when racial controversies flared up, commanding attention, even if somewhat muted, from some quarters of the African American community.

One of these controversies actually had little to do with African American patients themselves. In keeping with his mission of turning Saint Elizabeths into a preeminent teaching and research hospital, White began to offer clinics to local medical students in 1910. His initial vision of the clinics did not conform to the racist strictures of Jim Crow, as he extended invitations to students from all of the medical schools in the District, including Howard University's. In early January 1911 the white students from Georgetown and George Washington— but not the Army Medical School—boycotted one clinic because of the presence of students from Howard. Apparently the white students were not the only ones who were uncomfortable in mixed-race company; according to hospital officials, some of the white patients "objected to being used as subjects at lectures delivered for the benefit of colored students."[10] Rather than give separate lectures, White decided to temporarily postpone them. "Because of the recent unpleasantness in connection with my clinics in psychiatry, based upon the attendance of the negro students," he wrote to Edward A. Balloch, dean of Howard's medical department, "I have concluded to discontinue them, at least until some satisfactory understanding can be reached among the several medical colleges."[11]

The African American newspaper *Washington Bee* struck a strident chord in its coverage of the affair. Reminding its readers that Georgetown and George Washington were private universities, the *Bee* indignantly pointed out that Saint Elizabeths and Howard "are institutions maintained and controlled by the Government, and yet these students of the two former institutions had the audacity to demand that the Government discriminate against itself in favor of outside institutions." The *Bee* further questioned the character of the white students and challenged the rationality of white supremacy, using a satirical idiom that barely obscured the seriousness of the matter. "These white students who went to hear Dr. White's lecture on insanity must be in need of brain cure themselves," the paper quipped, "because no sane medical student would have made an ass of himself, as the 100 white men did when they walked out of the lecture room or refuse[d] to attend with Negro students."[12]

Black Washingtonians praised White for his refusal to provide separate lectures. The *Bee* characterized it as a "fair and just decision" that acknowledged and reaffirmed that "science knows no color." Dr. Lucy E. Moten, principal of the District's Miner Normal School, commended White on his refusal to "draw distinction . . . on the superficial basis of color." White also received an official recognition from Howard's Council of Upper Classmen for his "whole-souled, dignified, and manly stand."[13] Yet within two weeks of receiving these accolades, White was proposing that a color line be drawn at his clinics. This is not particularly surprising given that three days after William C. Borden, the dean of George Washington's medical school, wrote him a letter asking him to reconsider separating the students into different lectures, White responded that he thought "it will be possible to make some arrangement that will be satisfactory." The alternative arrangement consisted of one of his assistants providing the clinic to Howard students, using African American patients as the subjects. The black press was extremely disappointed at this turn of events, as was Wilbur P. Thirkield, Howard's president, although it is not clear whether he or Balloch allowed African American students to attend the segregated lectures. But the *Afro-American* left no doubt as to its distress that Jim Crow was insinuating itself into the federal government. "It is inconceivable that all this could happen in the nation's capital," the paper intoned, "where the civil rights law is supposed to be in full operation and where culture is so thick that it can be cut with a knife."[14]

By April, White had discontinued the clinic indefinitely. He indicated to Borden that it was because of exhaustion. Whether the exhaustion was the result of the turmoil surrounding the clinic or the overall responsibilities of the superintendency—or whether his claim that he was "pretty well tired out" was itself a feint—we do not know. It very well could have been an unwillingness to tolerate racism in the realm of medical education. White appears to have been committed to the psychiatric training of interested and capable students, regardless of racial background, and in fact Saint Elizabeths had reestablished an academic relationship with Howard's medical school by the early 1920s. Nonetheless his initial acquiescence to Borden and others in the immediate aftermath of the student boycott suggests that, even though he had moderate views regarding race, he was still very much a pragmatist.[15] More important, the black press's response to the taint of Jim Crow at Saint Elizabeths was the first since the *New National Era* had raised the issue of discriminatory treatment of African American patients some forty years earlier. Here, though, it is telling that the press's concern was with racism's effect on the prospects of educated black would-be professionals. At a time when African American federal government workers were increasingly being buffeted by the employment policies associated with lily-white Republicanism and a nationally ascendant Democratic Party, it is not surprising that the black press would have been preoccupied with threats to the social mobility of black Washingtonians.[16] In the mid-1920s, however, another racial incident would occur that shifted the target of African Americans' concerns about Saint Elizabeths.

In July 1924 the *Washington Tribune*, an African American newspaper, reported "one of the most brutal murders in the history of Washington." Four white attendants at Saint Elizabeths had beaten William Green, an African American patient, to death. Apparently two attendants, William McIntyre and Irwin R. Sweeney, had attempted to take Green to the hospital barber. Green objected and appealed to the assistant physician on his ward. Upset that he had gone to the physician, McIntyre and Sweeney later forcefully dragged Green to the barbershop. When they learned that the regular barber was not on duty, the attendants, now joined by two others, held Green down and cut his hair. He died shortly afterward. At a coroner's inquest, the deputy coroner determined that Green died from an abdominal contusion, a ruptured pancreas, and "shock from violent assault." McIntyre and Sweeney were arrested on charges of homicide.[17] It took nearly a year and a half, but a grand jury eventually returned an indictment against McIntyre and Sweeney for manslaughter.

As part of the grand jury process, jurors visited Saint Elizabeths and were reportedly appalled at what they observed. Howard Hall housed twice the number of patients for which it was originally designed and did not have sufficient recreational facilities, and there was the promiscuous intermingling of the "dangerously insane," individuals who had become insane while in prison, and apparently sane people who had been committed for "ulterior motives."[18] Multiple organizations latched onto the grand jury report to call for more widespread investigations of Saint Elizabeths.

One organization that took particular interest in Green's murder and the resultant grand jury investigation was the Barry Farm Citizens' Association. The association represented the residents of Barry Farm/Hillsdale, a predominantly African American neighborhood whose founding dated back to 1867. Just to the north of the Saint Elizabeths campus, Barry Farm/Hillsdale was a solidly black middle-class enclave, counting among its denizens entrepreneurs, professionals, and political activists such as Frederick Douglass and his descendants. Unlike the citizens' associations that represented white neighborhoods, black civic associations did not provide African American residents direct political input into municipal governance or federal policy concerning the District.[19] Nonetheless the Barry Farm Citizens' Association sought to keep local blacks abreast of the situation at Saint Elizabeths. "The grand jury findings should interest citizens in general in reference to the startling conditions noted by that body at Saint Elizabeth's Asylum, a government institution," the *Tribune* reported shortly after an association meeting. "Many insane colored patients are in this asylum." A month later the association informed Barry Farm residents and the press of the Veterans Bureau's recommendation that Congress investigate Saint Elizabeths, reminding them, "Many of our shell-shocked soldier boys of the World War are inmates of this institution."[20]

The association's invoking of the presence of black veterans—along with its consistent reference to the hospital as a government institution—elevated the concerns that local residents should have about Saint Elizabeths above that of the singular incident of William Green's death. African Americans should be interested in the treatment of black patients because it was one index, among many, of the black community's civil status in the nation's capital, a city that was in and of the Jim Crow South. By reminding local residents that a federal facility needed to be held accountable for its ill treatment of black patients, particularly those who served in the war, the association enacted and reaffirmed African Americans' citizenship. It was a reaffirmation that the *Tribune* extended to black Washington as a whole by covering the discussion in its neighborhood issues pages.

The association and the *Tribune* were not the only advocates for further investigation into conditions at Saint Elizabeths. In the spring of 1926 a local white resident, Myrtle de Montis, attempted to rally support for passage of a Senate resolution calling for a congressional investigation of the hospital. The resolution was introduced by Henrik Shipstead, a Farm-Labor senator from Minnesota, in December 1925. De Montis, who charged that attendants were responsible for the deaths of two other African American patients in addition to Green, urged the National Association for the Advancement of Colored People (NAACP) and "all colored citizens" to support Shipstead's resolution.[21] Although de Montis's relationship to the NAACP is unclear, she had a larger interest in the jurisprudential aspects of the commitment of mentally ill people.[22] We do not know if the letter-writing campaign that she proposed garnered a great deal of support within the African American community. Shipstead's resolution appeared to go nowhere in the Senate, despite receiving an endorsement from the local District chapter of the American Legion. However, a number of investigations materialized in the wake of the grand jury's report. In addition to the Veterans Bureau, other bodies that conducted investigations or inspections of Saint Elizabeths throughout 1926 were three House committees—a subcommittee of the Committee on the District of Columbia, the Judiciary Committee, and the Committee of the House on World War Veterans—the Navy Department's Bureau of Medicine and Surgery, and the General Accounting Office.[23]

The fact that Saint Elizabeths was the primary treatment facility for service members and veterans suffering from neuropathological damage was clearly the overriding concern of those who pressed for investigations of the hospital. The demands that the war had placed on the hospital were immense. There was nearly a doubling of admissions between the 1918 and 1919 fiscal years. Between June 30, 1917, and June 30, 1918—itself a record year—Saint Elizabeths admitted 1,054 people, 886 of them men. During the following fiscal year, 1,549 men were committed, constituting 85 percent of the 1,802 admissions.[24] The increase in admissions, combined with a shortage of employees at the institution due to the conscription and voluntary enlistment of men into the armed forces, contributed to a horrendous patient-staff ratio. This imbalance did not begin to improve until 1920, a year after the US Army's decision to temporarily stop sending soldiers to Saint Elizabeths because of its overcrowded conditions and Congress's authorization of higher salaries and reduced hours for employees in order to recruit and retain more staff. In addition to achieving a better balance between patients and staff, Saint Elizabeths' resources were enhanced through a $1 million appropriation from Congress in 1920. This and subsequent funding led to per patient spending of $511 by 1923, more than double the amount spent prior to the war.[25]

Despite the progress made in the treatment of military personnel at Saint Elizabeths, some elected officials attempted to exploit lingering concerns in order to go after White and those who were perceived to be his allies. In December 1925, just two months after the grand jury issued its findings on the conditions at Saint Elizabeths, Thomas Blanton, a Democratic representative from Texas, brought impeachment charges against Frederick Fenning, one of the District's commissioners. Among the thirty-four charges leveled against Fenning, Blanton accused him of conspiring with White to commit and keep detained veterans who showed no signs of mental illness, merely to benefit financially from the management of their estates. In a remarkably scurrilous indictment that was clearly aimed at tapping into some sense of racial paranoia, Blanton claimed that White sold the bodies of deceased white veterans to Howard University so that they could be dissected by black medical students. The sensationalist deployment of imagery of white bodies being violated by African Americans was meant to amplify the corruptness of the deeds of White and Fenning—as they were imagined by Blanton—even as it inverted the very real history of the routine unauthorized autopsies of African Americans by white medical students in the nineteenth and early twentieth centuries. Representatives, however, were not persuaded by Blanton's fearmongering; after Fenning testified before a subcommittee of the House Committee on the District of Columbia and the House Veterans Committee, the Judiciary Committee decided not to impeach the commissioner.[26]

Congress did end up authorizing a fuller investigation of Saint Elizabeths by the General Accounting Office in the summer of 1926, which resulted in a comptroller general's report that was critical of both the hospital's physical plant and its administration.[27] Despite the report, White was never in danger of losing his job. But following the investigation, Secretary of the Interior Hubert Work appointed a committee of five "special medical advisers," all of whom were either psychiatric hospital superintendents or academics, to evaluate Saint Elizabeths and to develop a broad set of recommendations aimed at optimizing its administration. Many of the committee's conclusions and recommendations reiterated the comptroller general's findings, including the importance of expanding the number of beds in order to alleviate overcrowding. Importantly, the special medical advisers pointed to the diverse patient population as one factor that contributed to the housing problems at the hospital. "There is probably no hospital in the whole country which receives so many different groups of cases when admitted as St. Elizabeths," the report stated. The variety of civil status, gender, race, and diagnosis made it unfeasible to effect the necessary separation of patients. "These groups alone present a problem in housing, because a degree of segregation is demanded and expected," the advisers warned, "and when there is added the classification of mental conditions after admission, necessary to the best treatment and care, the problem, as here, becomes large and complex, and, in fact, impossible with the existing housing limitations."[28] This had been precisely White's point when the congressional committee questioned him about the lack of absolute segregation in 1906.

At least one inspection of the hospital concurred with the special medical advisers' assessment and did so in a way that highlighted the discriminatory impact of the institution's housing strategy on African American patients. The Navy Department's Bureau of Medicine and Surgery conducted an inspection of Saint Elizabeths in the fall of 1926 and described the receiving wards (the initial wards that newly admitted patients occupied before being reassigned) in the following language: "The reception service for colored males is a part of the Howard Hall Service which service embraces the male criminal insane and all colored males. Colored males are now, however, housed with or treated as criminals. This grouping is for administrative convenience only and is made because the wards used for colored patients are located near Howard Hall, the building in which the criminal insane are housed."[29] The special medical advisers also pointed out that the overcrowded wards were in older buildings that housed African

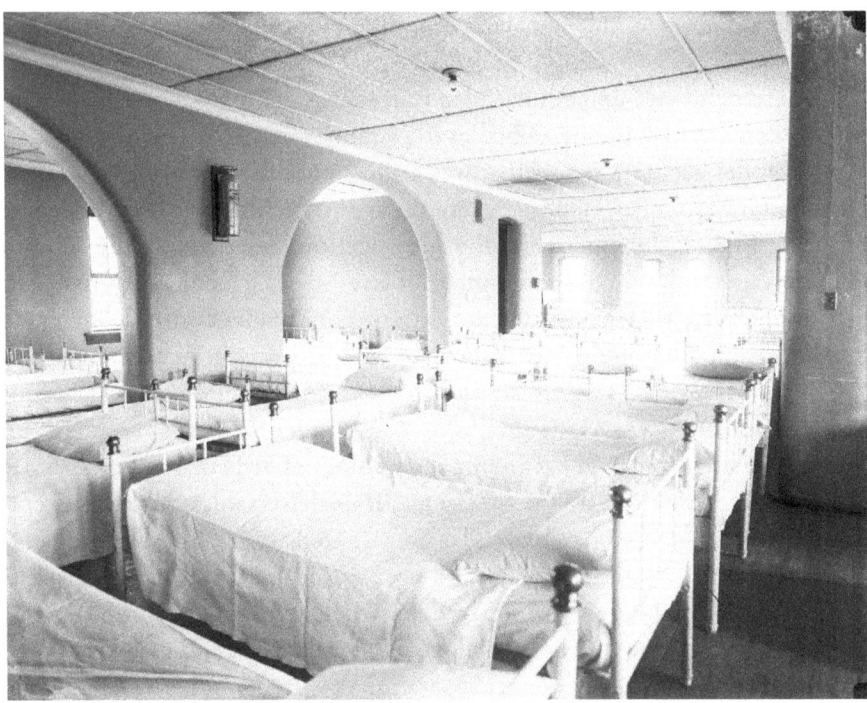

Tightly packed rows of neatly made, empty beds line a ward for colored patients in 1925. As the number of admissions increased between the world wars, overcrowding disproportionately characterized the conditions on the wards that were inhabited by black female and male patients. *National Archives, photo 418-G-344.*

American male and female patients as well as the "infirm, untidy . . . epileptic and feebleminded white women." They took special note of the dining room of Oaks B, a building for African American women, which they described as "dark and greatly crowded" and in such poor condition that it should be abandoned.[30] The administration continued to struggle with overcrowding in the wake of the special medical adviser's report. Five years later, for instance, it disclosed that the space in Howard Hall—especially the colored male wards—remained insufficient for the number of patients housed there.[31]

The problems of unequal treatment of African Americans at Saint Elizabeths fell off the radar of the black press and civic associations the further the death of William Green receded into the past. And the death of Howard Hawkins warranted no more than the *Baltimore Afro-American*'s listing his name in the week's fatalities as reported by the District of Columbia's health department.[32] Moreover it was not civilian African American patients at Saint Elizabeths who were the primary concern of those who judged the hospital to be deficient in the 1920s and 1930s; rather, it was primarily white male service members and veterans. As this category of patients grew in the 1940s with another world war, the federal government would move more assertively to redress the myriad problems at Saint Elizabeths.

World War II and Its Aftermath

It has perhaps become a cliché to say that World War II was a watershed moment in American history, but that does not make it any less true. Just as the global conflagration is credited with unleashing all kinds of economic and social changes—from southern industrialization and the rise of the Sun Belt to the civil rights movement and second-wave feminism—it also led to transformations in American psychiatry. The war contributed to changes in the numbers of physicians entering the psychiatric specialty and their intellectual orientation toward mental illness, ideas regarding the etiology of mental disorders, and the federal footprint in mental health policy. The psychological turmoil accompanying combat service in an especially brutal war made the soldier and veteran a target of psychiatric intervention. Unlike in the aftermath of the First World War, however, psychiatrists were more apt to approach the mental and nervous disorders of service people within a framework of dynamic psychiatry than one of neurology. And to the extent that dynamic psychiatry had posited the role of the social environment in the development of mental illness, postwar psychiatrists became increasingly open to the idea that broader structural forces, such as discrimination and poverty, might be important causal factors.

This emergence of social psychiatry encouraged a public policy approach to prevention that would accompany existing strategies associated with the earlier mental hygiene movement. A professional commitment to the prevention of mental illness and a New Deal liberal consensus on the importance of a robust federal state in tackling deadly diseases such as cancer facilitated the passage of the National Mental Health Act of 1946. That act, which created the National Mental Health Advisory Committee and the National Institute of Mental Health, inserted the federal government into a policy realm that had previously been largely reserved for the states. The legislation provided, through the new agencies, funding for research into cure, treatment, and prevention at both the national and state levels.[33]

The responsibility for managing Saint Elizabeths during this period of change fell to White's successor, Winfred Overholser, who took over the superintendency after White's death in 1937. A native of Worcester, Massachusetts, Overholser received his AB from Harvard and his MD from Boston University. His employment at several Massachusetts public hospitals—interrupted in 1918 by his overseas service in the Neuropsychiatric Section of the US Army Medical Corps—prepared him for his appointment as the state's commissioner of the Department of Mental Diseases, a position he held until December 1936.[34]

Overholser was a dynamic psychiatrist through and through. In a February 1938 speech before a joint meeting of the American Medical Association's Section on Neurology and Psychiatry and the Medical Society of the District of Columbia, he articulated a view of the mentally ill individual within an "organism as a whole" paradigm. "It is being recognized more and more that the distinction between mind and body is largely academic," he stated, "that the patient represents not a diseased liver or heart, or just a case of dementia praecox, but that he is a human being, a social animal, with certain assets and certain liabilities, who is attempting in his own peculiar way and conditioned by his own disabilities to adjust himself to the demands of his environment."

The responsibility of the modern mental hospital was to treat the mentally ill individual in his or her totality. This demanded that mental institutions have the characteristics of a general hospital, with the technology, facilities, and personnel that were capable of treating acute diseases. It also required more informal commitment procedures, including voluntary admission, as well as outpatient clinics to provide counseling for mentally distressed people in order to preempt institutionalization. Operating as a modern mental hospital meant employing a team approach to mental illness, in which psychiatrists, psychiatric nurses, psychologists, psychiatric social workers, and occupational therapists worked together to provide an effective and holistic therapeutic regimen for patients. Finally, in keeping with White's vision, Overholser stressed the importance of continuing psychiatric research to grasp a better comprehension of etiology and to develop more efficacious therapies.[35]

Overholser's ambitious designs for Saint Elizabeths, like those of his predecessors, were tempered by the institutional realities, especially the overcrowding and staff shortages that were repercussions of the war. In the latter years of the war, Saint Elizabeths saw the greatest growth in its annual admissions over its entire ninety-year history. The hospital admitted 2,599 people in the 1944 fiscal year, approximately 60 percent of whom were military personnel. The number of admissions was even larger the following year, totaling close to 3,000. Moreover, the military personnel admitted that year included 163 servicewomen. One positive development was that, even as the number of admissions increased, the rate of discharges also rose. Overholser attributed this to the high proportion of servicemen and women in the hospital. "Service people stand a better chance for recovery since the cause [of their illness] is usually some phase of military life," he told a local reporter, "and removal from the service, even though only temporary, often enables the patient to regain his equilibrium very quickly."[36]

Although the newspaper feature's positive image of the hospital—which emphasized its recreational facilities, massive laundry, extensive farmland, shoe and mattress factories, postgraduate training courses, and new therapies such as psychodrama—was predictable for a piece of wartime journalism, others were not hesitant to expose the many problems that plagued Saint Elizabeths. Republican representative Frank Keefe from Wisconsin, for instance, read into the record a description of a visit that he and fellow representatives made to the hospital in May 1945. While acknowledging that much of the hospital was modern and praising the hospital staff for their competent efforts in the face of dwindling government resources, the portrait he painted of Saint Elizabeths lingered on the parts of the hospital that "reek[ed] back to the Dark Ages." "There are places over there that would compare with the prison holds of the prison ships of old," he alerted his House colleagues. "The darkest, dankest, dirtiest, foulest, and most evil place I was ever in is the laundry over there, and they are compelled to ask people to work in it." Keefe's reference to a facility that was predominantly populated by African American patients as exemplary of the substandard state of much of Saint Elizabeths did not explicitly invoke race. Yet a comment later in his remarks on the House floor reveals his sensitivity to the fact that it was largely black faces that he witnessed in the laundry. "Therefore, when we went out there and saw the situation [at Saint Elizabeths as a whole]," Keefe intoned, "we came back just as amazed as were DEWEY SHORT and EWING THOMASON and the other Members who went to Europe and saw the horrors of the concentration camps."[37] As public mental hospitals were increasingly being characterized as snake pits, Keefe brought a particular racial valence to his

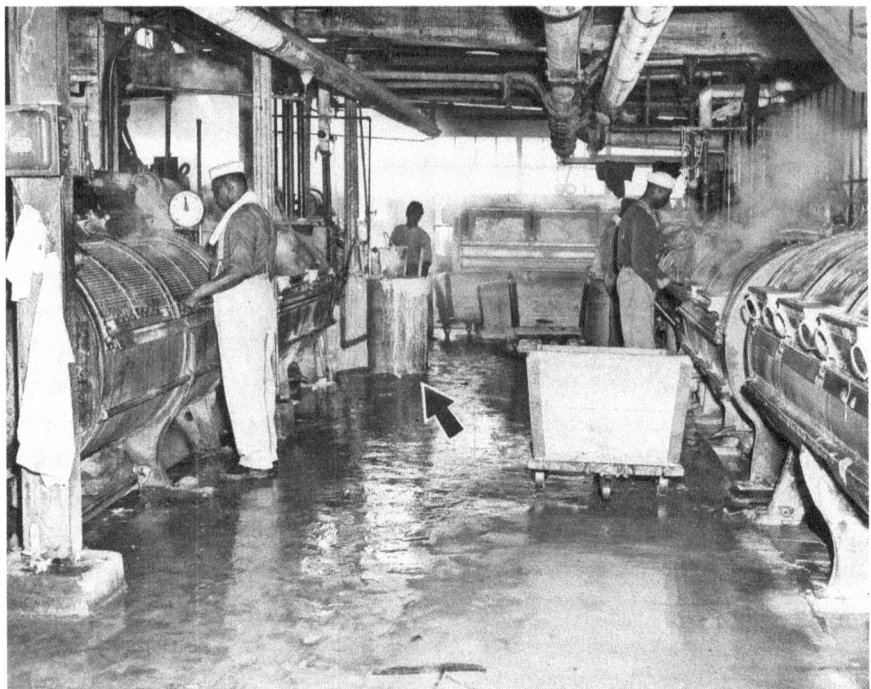

Black male patients stand on water-soaked floors and work outdated steam washing machines in a dimly lit section of the hospital laundry. An "old-fashioned soap bucket" sits nearby. Unlike workers in more modern laundries that existed by the 1940s, these patients still had to transport wet clothes in carts instead of overhead conveyers. *Washington Star Collection, Washingtoniana Division, DC Public Library. Reprinted with permission of the DC Public Library, Star Collection © Washington Post.*

criticism of Saint Elizabeths by implicitly associating it with the bowels of a slave trading ship and the sites of Jewish genocide.[38]

Several months later Saint Elizabeths came under criticism from another representative of the federal government, this time the Public Buildings Administration. Paul V. McNutt, the head of the Federal Security Agency (FSA), which took over control of Saint Elizabeths from the Department of the Interior in 1940, commissioned the Public Buildings Administration to conduct a study of the state of the hospital's infrastructure. The overall conclusion of the study was that the institution housed too many people in dilapidated buildings. Two of the most egregious examples of overcrowding were the West Lodge Service, which housed 979 African American men in a space that was meant to accommodate only 741, and Q Service, whose recommended occupancy was 491 but held 861 African American female patients.[39]

In part, the overcrowding of Saint Elizabeths could be attributed to the fact that it was practically the only mental institution in the District. Several studies

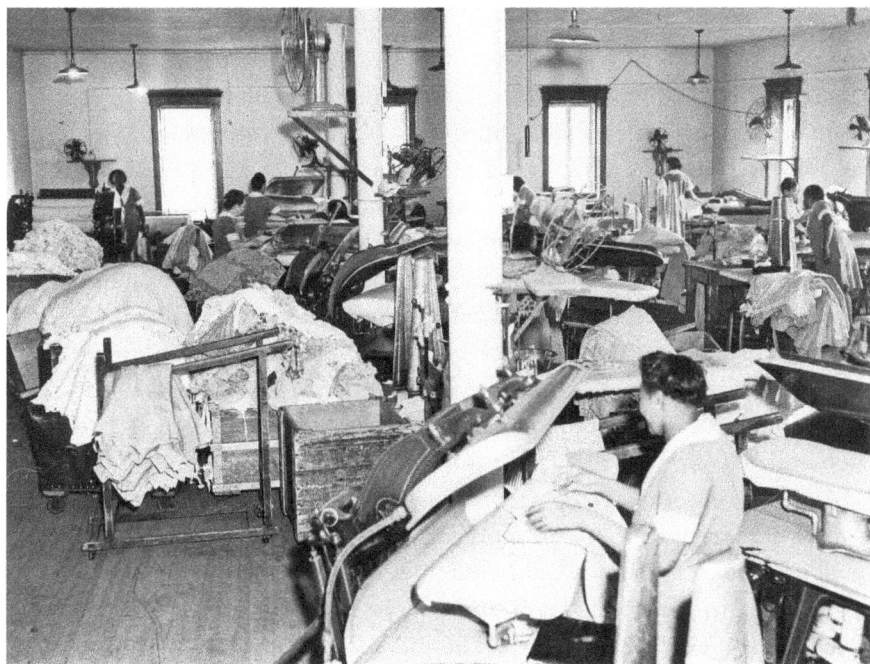

A well-lit and airy section of the hospital laundry, in which female patients in neat uniforms use mechanical wringers and steam presses to complete the laundering process. Although this space was cleaner, cooler, and better ventilated than that occupied by the black male patients who worked with chemical-filled vats, it was still filled primarily by black women. *Washington Star Collection, Washingtoniana Division, DC Public Library. Reprinted with permission of the DC Public Library, Star Collection © Washington Post.*

during the World War II era concluded that approximately 97 percent of all of the District's beds for psychiatric patients were in Saint Elizabeths. As the numbers of service people requiring institutionalization increased, there was no way of siphoning off the civilian population who similarly needed commitment to a mental hospital. And notwithstanding the fact that Saint Elizabeths surpassed professional standards and proved superior to most other state hospitals—if only in terms of per capita expenditure and staff-to-patient ratio—the outdated and inferior quality of many of its buildings remained a persistent problem and the subject of public censure. A survey of the health infrastructure of the District of Columbia and surrounding areas conducted by the Washington Metropolitan Health Council in 1946 recommended the expansion of the hospital campus and renovation of many of the existing buildings.[40]

The overcrowding of Saint Elizabeths led to a change in military policy with respect to commitment of service members with mental disorders. In the spring of 1945 President Harry S. Truman issued a directive to reorganize the hospital. In addition to changing the administration structure by abolishing its Board of Visitors, the proposed plan would end the practice of sending active-duty service members to the hospital. The White House denied that Truman was motivated by the deaths of two sailors at the hands of attendants, but he was clear, according to the *Star*, that the inability of Saint Elizabeths to accommodate all of its patients was a central factor in his decision. At approximately the same time, the administrator of veterans' affairs began the process of transferring veterans from Saint Elizabeths to Veterans Administration hospitals close to their families. The mental health resources within the VA hospital system had matured by the eve of World War II. There were twenty-seven VA mental hospitals throughout the nation and forty-six general VA hospitals with psychopathic wards. By 1938 the VA system was handling twenty-six thousand veterans with mental disorders.[41]

Along with some members of Congress and some military physicians, Overholser was opposed to the reorganization plan. To the superintendent, the main problem was that it would create deficiencies within the hospital's therapeutic regime. He credited a diverse patient population with creating an efficacious therapeutic environment. The presence of both military and civilian patients contributed to a discharge rate of almost 80 percent the previous year, a rate "so high we could hardly believe our eyes," Overholser claimed.[42] Despite opposition from various quarters, the Senate Judiciary Committee ultimately approved the president's proposals. With Reorganization Plan No. 3, the US Army and Navy ceased admitting their active-duty service members to St. Elizabeths in 1946 and began sending them exclusively to VA mental hospitals. The percentage of military admissions dropped precipitously. In fiscal year 1946 the hospital estimated that only 41 percent of admissions were service members, down from a high of 60 percent just two years earlier. Only 2 of the 1,339 individuals admitted in fiscal year 1947 were active-duty members—both from the navy. The cessation of the long-term relationship that Saint Elizabeths had had with the military warranted a melancholy remark in the hospital's 1947 annual report: "The loss of this contact with the armed forces is a source of keen disappointment to the hospital personnel." Although there were still patients with military and federal status at Saint Elizabeths—including soldiers and sailors who had been admitted prior to 1946—the hospital was well on its way to becoming a primarily civilian institution.[43]

Within a year of the change Overholser found himself having to combat moves within other branches of government that threatened to strip Saint Elizabeths of its status as a federal institution. In February 1947 the District's budget officer, Walter L. Fowler, floated a proposal before the Board of Commissioners that would have given the city policy and budgetary control over Saint Elizabeths. Fowler's rationale was that since the District's fiscal burden was becoming greater as the civilian patient population increased, the city might as well take administrative control of the hospital. By the mid-1940s the amount of money that the District spent on the upkeep of civilian residents at Saint Elizabeths consumed a third of its congressional appropriation for public welfare, and yet the city's Board of Public Welfare had no input into how the institution was run or what the daily per capita expenditure should be.[44] Overholser was unequivocally opposed to the proposal, arguing that the loss of federal status and the funds that went with it would lead to a diminution of Saint Elizabeths' prominence in the field of mental disease research.

Fowler's recommendation to combine the care and treatment of the elderly, the feebleminded, juvenile delinquents, and the mentally ill into a municipally controlled Saint Elizabeths prompted opposition from other powerful entities. Fowler's proposal was met with "unqualified condemnation" by the Coordinating Board of the Washington Metropolitan Health Council, and the American Board of Psychiatry and Neurology sent a veiled threat to the Board of Commissioners that Saint Elizabeths risked losing its accreditation if the plan was adopted. Even some of Saint Elizabeths' patients weighed in on Fowler's proposal. "Some time ago some of the downtown politicos conceived what they thought to be the 'bright idea' that St. Elizabeth's should be taken over by the district," an editorial in the patient-run *Elizabethan* remarked. "We hope that in the final analysis the 'idea' will remain paralyzed permanently into a state of 'just talk.' Common sense alone dictates that St. Elizabeth's identity as a top-ranking mental institution and research center in nervous disorders, unburdened by weakening incumbrances [sic] of any plan designed to confuse the cardinal aim of treating mental illnesses. Making St. Elizabeth's an Old People's Home, a House of Correction and a haven for juvenile delinquents as well as a mental institution would not advance this aim."[45] The board elected not to pursue Fowler's plan, but four months later Congress revisited the question of whether it was best for the federal government to manage the hospital.

The political establishment's wartime propaganda about the United States as democracy's champion contributed to a congressional reevaluation of the District's relationship to the nation. Encouraged by prominent black and white Washingtonians who formed the Washington Home Rule Committee in 1947 to lobby for the right of District residents to elect their municipal officials, Congress formed a joint House and Senate subcommittee to explore the prospects of reorganizing the District's government. For more than three weeks in July, the subcommittee heard testimony from stakeholders on the question of reorganization and home rule. One of the areas that interested the subcommittee was the health care infrastructure of the District, including the feasibility of transferring control of the city's public hospitals from the federal government to a reorganized municipal government.[46]

Even though District residents constituted approximately three-quarters of the patient population by the time Congress began its hearings, Overholser thought it was not in the best interests of either the city or the federal government to change the status quo. And it was certainly not in the best interests of the patients. Part of his argument played to the fiscal conservatism of some of the subcommittee members. If the District took over Saint Elizabeths and transformed it into what amounted to a state hospital for the city's residents, the federal government would have to figure out what to do with the remaining patients who had federal status. Though the veterans could be moved to VA hospitals, it was not at all clear where the other federal patients—including American Indians, residents of the Canal Zone and US Virgin Islands, and military prisoners—would go. The other alternative was to keep these federal patients in Saint Elizabeths and build a new mental institution for the District's residents. Yet in order to achieve a high standard of care, something that the families of these patients would expect, the District would need to spend between $40 million and $50 million to build a modern hospital with appropriate facilities. Overholser also reprised a version of the argument that he had made against Truman's reorganization plan, claiming that it was the "great variety of patients . . . that gives St. Elizabeths the national atmosphere it has enjoyed through the 92 years of its existence." He sought to capitalize on the recent commitment made by the federal government to combat mental illness. Obliquely referencing the freshly passed National Mental Health Act, Overholser pointed out that "it would be taken in many quarters as a decidedly backward step for the Federal Government to give up St. Elizabeths Hospital."[47]

But no matter how resistant Overholser was to the prospect that Saint Elizabeths would become "just another municipal hospital," he could not stem the demographic sea change that was under way. The change in military admission policy not only altered the military-civilian patient distribution; it also led to a "graying" of the patient population. Overholser had predicted before the end of the war that the nation as a whole would see higher rates of mental illness as the life expectancy of Americans increased. But the cessation of military admissions and the transfer of veterans created an inverse dynamic at Saint Elizabeths, in which the siphoning off of younger patients led to an institutional population that skewed toward an older demographic.[48] Moreover, in Overholser's estimation, Saint Elizabeths was increasingly seen by families as a potential dumping ground for their elderly and senile members, an option that was all the more appealing in difficult economic times. He attributed a sharp increase in admissions in 1947, for instance, to an acute housing shortage in the District. The economic pressures placed on families in the postwar period, he believed, even motivated some to attempt to institutionalize the eccentric or doddering elderly member who might be difficult to care for in his or her old age but who was hardly insane. In the end, whether justified or not, the elimination of military commitments and the surge in admissions of elderly civilians—"whose prognoses on the whole are less favorable than those of younger persons"—dampened the therapeutic optimism that characterized the psychiatric profession as a whole.[49]

The disappointment in the changing demographics of the hospital could not even be tempered by a development that Saint Elizabeths' staff and the District's psychiatric profession had long argued for: a change in the city's lunacy law in 1948 that allowed for voluntary admission.[50] In the first four months after that change, twenty District residents committed themselves. The gender breakdown was more or less equal, eight men and twelve women, and their ages ran the spectrum from the mid-twenties to seventy-five. Apparently there was only one African American, a forty-year-old woman. Over the next eight months more than sixty people sought admission to the hospital. While there was a growing gender imbalance—with female admissions double those of male—the proportion of African Americans remained much lower than in their total population in the District. Of the eighty-three Washingtonians who committed themselves in the first year after the legislation passed, only three were African American. Dr. Addison Duval, Saint Elizabeths' first assistant physician, speculated that the paucity of self-committing African Americans was due to the fact "that the Negro population is not as aware as the white population that one can obtain the services of St. Elizabeths without going through the process of legal commitment." By 1950 the proportion of voluntary admissions had increased, accounting for 15 percent of the approximately 1,500 admissions; it is unclear if the presence of African Americans within this particular treatment-seeking population increased as well.[51]

As the general patient population was increasingly drawn from the ranks of the District's civilian residents in the postwar period, the proportion of admissions to Saint Elizabeths who were African American similarly grew. This was particularly the case beginning in the 1950s, as more and more white Washingtonians—and people moving to the metropolitan area to work in an expanding federal government and its auxiliary services—moved to the existing suburbs and to new, planned communities in Maryland and Virginia.[52] The sheer demographic shift in the city's and the hospital's population alone would have made the exclusion of African Americans as employees an unsustainable practice by the 1950s. But Saint Elizabeths was a federal facility in the capital of a nation that sought to project a self-image as a beacon of freedom and equality. As such, its personnel policies were susceptible to being changed by New Deal liberalism, the exigencies of World War II and the cold war, and the percolating civil rights activism of the postwar period.

The Uneven Process of Integrating Saint Elizabeths' Staff

There is no single moment when the staff at Saint Elizabeths became integrated. The institution was a massive operation with many moving parts, making the elimination of discriminatory employment policies a process that played out over years and even decades. The first sectors of the workforce that saw the racial barrier fall were the nursing and attendant staff, which began hiring African Americans in the 1930s and 1940s. In the immediate postwar period, the hospital started to open up positions in psychiatric social work to blacks. But it was not until the mid-1950s, a period during which the wards were also integrated, that Saint Elizabeths began hiring black physicians.

African Americans had worked at Saint Elizabeths as menial laborers on the grounds of the hospital going back to the nineteenth century, but it was not until the latter part of White's administration, during the presidency of Franklin Delano Roosevelt, that the hospital started to employ African Americans in positions on the wards. The decision to do so was most likely influenced, in part, by White's personal views about the capacity of blacks to become good psychiatrists and to perform caregiving duties. Charles Prudhomme, a black medical student at Howard, recalled that White encouraged him to apply for an internship at Saint Elizabeths in 1936 and again in 1937, after his first application did not successfully pass the civil service evaluation process. Prudhomme did not explicitly attribute the failure of his application to the racial attitudes of the civil service examiners, but the young doctor from Kansas appealed directly to First Lady Eleanor Roosevelt, his senator, Harry S. Truman, and Secretary of the Interior Harold Ickes. Although his appeals were unsuccessful, his attempt to elicit the assistance of Ickes was politically astute. Saint Elizabeths was still under the authority of the Department of the Interior and Ickes was progressive on matters of race. He was the first secretary to appoint a special adviser on race relations; he ordered the cafeterias in the new Interior building to operate on a nonsegregated basis; and he implemented a "policy of fair employment" in the agency's hiring and contracting.[53]

This policy of fair employment also contributed to the hiring of African Americans on the hospital's wards. The first staff position in which African Americans were hired in significant numbers was that of nurse. Even though *Opportunity*, the journal of the National Urban League, reported rampant discrimination in "nursing services operated by the federal government" in the late 1930s, Saint Elizabeths had black ward nurses and black supervisors. In December 1938, for instance, the hospital promoted Myrtle Coy, a registered nurse and graduate of the Freedmen's Hospital and Howard University School of Nursing, to ward instructor. Coy's responsibility was to supervise Freedmen's nursing students who were receiving their "affiliation in psychiatry" at Saint Elizabeths.[54] These nurses would have worked primarily—if not exclusively—on the wards that housed African American patients.

By World War II black nurses were tending to white patients as well, although it is unclear how closely black and white nurses worked with each other. Two sources provide different pictures. As a professor of psychiatry at Howard University's School of Nursing during the war, Prudhomme coordinated the clinical rotations of nursing students at Saint Elizabeths. The African American nursing students "were kept completely separate during work and mealtimes from the White student nurses from various schools on the East Coast that had 'official' affiliate relations with St. Elizabeths," he recalled. On the other hand, toward the end of the war, someone connected to the hospital wrote a letter to the editor of the *Washington Post* suggesting the existence of a different racial climate. The letter writer praised Saint Elizabeths' progressive stance on hiring and argued that it should serve as a model for some of the other federal nursing services—especially the Army Nurse Corps and Navy Nurse Corps—that continued to discriminate against African American nurses even as they experienced severe personnel shortages. Pointing out that black practical nurses and attendants made up close to half of Saint Elizabeths' workforce, the writer represented an idyllic racial environment. "There have been absolutely no race incidents," a "South Carolinian" enthusiastically remarked. "There is, indeed, the finest imaginable spirit and cooperative relationship between the white and colored employes."[55]

The overall shortage of nurses during the war also affected Saint Elizabeths. Indeed there were so few registered nurses available that the hospital began enlisting "some of the older and more reliable attendants" to perform their duties.[56] American nationalism in a period of national crisis might have fostered a harmonious racial environment at Saint Elizabeths, but it is more likely that it contributed to the South Carolinian's romanticizing the interaction between black and white staff and patients. To be sure, the presence of African American employees primarily as practical nurses and attendants was probably tolerated by physicians and white patients because of their lack of medical and institutional authority, an image that particularly resonated in a culture that associated black women and servitude. As a report on the integration of the nursing profession several years after the war suggested, the predictable conflation of nursing and domesticity in the minds of nonnurses allowed white physicians and patients to more easily accept African American women in that position. "This is perhaps to be explained in part on the basis of a persisting tendency to view the nurse as a servitor rather than as a professional practitioner," the National Association of Intergroup Relations Officials surmised in 1952. "In the South, furthermore, there is a tradition of Negro nursing in white households. Many southern white children grow up in the care of Negro nursemaids. A somewhat paradoxical effect of this is even more general patient acceptance of Negro nurses in the South than in other parts of the country."[57]

Many white nurses at Saint Elizabeths undoubtedly bristled at having to work with African Americans, especially black registered nurses, whom white nurses largely considered to be less competent and professional than themselves. Just two years before the nation entered World War II, two white nurses resigned from the staff of the District's tuberculosis hospital when it hired African American nurses. Moreover, the District affiliate of the American Nurses Association did not begin admitting black women until three years after the national body ended its racial exclusion policy.[58] There was, in other words, surely racial tension as Saint Elizabeths began the process of integrating its staff. We only need to look at the case of the employment of African American attendants to better place the South Carolinian's assessment of race relations at the hospital in perspective.

Saint Elizabeths probably began hiring African Americans as attendants in the 1930s. But it was the manpower shortage created by the war that accelerated the employment of African Americans in those positions. Conscription or better employment opportunities in war-related industries led to a high turnover rate among the attendant population, particularly white males. From January to November 1942 more than 50 percent of the attendants left their jobs, only 5 percent because of enlistment. Hospital officials expressed concern about the quality of the attendants they were hiring, especially the African American attendants, whom they labeled a "special problem." "Before the war, the Hospital used to be able to hire [Negro] male attendants of a very high quality," officials reported, "but few Negro men are now available." Although the officials estimated that the overall number of blacks was increasing, they still constituted only 10 percent of the attendants in 1942. By the summer of 1943, however, they made up a majority of those hired as attendants. Interestingly, a report on black attendants conducted that summer concluded that African American employees were more likely than white attendants to have completed grammar and high school, illustrating the discriminatory hiring practices that existed in other sectors of the economy.[59]

The hiring of African American attendants was also the product of federal policy. In June 1941, feeling pressure from black labor activist A. Philip Randolph and the March on Washington Movement, Roosevelt issued Executive Order 8802, which prohibited racial discrimination in hiring practices in government agencies and defense industries and created the Fair Employment Practices Committee. In October the director of personnel of the FSA directed the heads of the FSA's subagencies to remove all questions regarding race from their applications. In a June 1943 letter to the director of the National CIO Committee to Abolish Racial Discrimination, Arthur McLean conceded that the integration of the staffs of FSA subagencies had not come without difficulty, but he added, "None of the constituent agencies have reported any indications of racial tension following the employment of Negroes."[60] Ironically McLean's letter was attached to a report on the work conditions of African American attendants at Saint Elizabeths that was written up two months later, a report that evinced a great deal of racial tension on the hospital wards.

Even though one of the report's findings was that "a slightly greater proportion of Negroes than whites felt that the hospital is a friendly place in which to work," the anecdotal evidence from interviews with African American attendants indicates otherwise. The black attendants had many of the same complaints as the white attendants—such as low wages and more work due to staffing shortages—but they also reported dissatisfaction with the racism they experienced. Despite the fact that employee cafeterias in federal facilities were supposed to be open to all regardless of race, an informal segregation, and even exclusion, still existed in Saint Elizabeths. Some black employees bemoaned their exclusion from the hospital cafeteria and attendants' club, for instance, a grievance that also appeared in a separate study on the attendant turnover problem. "A colored attendant complained because there is no cafeteria to serve colored attendants so that they are unable to get their hot dinners on the evening shift," the report revealed. "They have not actually been forbidden to eat at the hospital cafeteria, but . . . they feel that the attitude of white attendants is too markedly hostile for them to try to eat in the cafeteria." Segregation extended to the bathrooms and the dressing rooms. A female attendant on Q Service, the African American women's department, stated in her interview that "the women are dissatisfied because their dressing room is in another building, the equivalent of a couple of blocks away."[61]

Relations among supervisors, staff, and patients similarly became grounds for grievances by black attendants. Although one study found that African American attendants were slightly less likely than their white counterparts to complain about unfair treatment by their supervisors, another report highlighted the belief of a substantial proportion of employees that favoritism permeated the way supervisors ran their units. One female attendant suggested in her interview that race-based favoritism was rampant: "The colored girls are never given an opportunity to prove what they can do. They are always supervised by a white attendant regardless of how old they are on the job and how new the white girl is."[62]

African American attendants had their own form of favoritism, further indicating the existence of racial tension on the wards. One male attendant disclosed that his colleagues "treat the colored patients better." Others voiced the opinion that African American patients preferred black attendants because "they are kinder and more sympathetic." Even though there was no uniform racial solidarity between black staff and patients, many of the African American attendants who were interviewed attributed their preference for working on the colored wards to the negative interactions they had with white patients. "Some dislike of working with white patients was expressed by Negro attendants," hospital officials remarked, "because they said white patients, particularly officers, treat Negro attendants with less respect than they treat whites."[63] It is clear from these wartime reports on the working conditions at Saint Elizabeths that African American employees were not confined to the colored wards. However, even as the exigencies of war and a somewhat progressive federal employment policy dismantled the racial barrier, the relations between black and white staff and patients were shaped by everything from cultural preconceptions born of a lack of familiarity with another group to deep-seated racist hostility.

White attendants who were interviewed expressed a range of opinions about working alongside African Americans. In general, according to the study on the employment of black attendants, white staff members developed a "grudging acceptance" of their new colleagues, and "general disapproval and prejudice" weakened as they increasingly came into contact with "competent colored employees." Nonetheless racist attitudes were clearly evident in the 1943 survey of white attendants. Most who answered the questionnaire, for instance, expressed a desire to maintain "strict social segregation" even as they worked with African Americans on the wards. Some wanted even more extensive segregation, confining black attendants to the colored wards. Others believed they should be paid more than their black counterparts, and a few harbored a fear—rooted in ignorance and a generations-old mythology about black sexuality—that they would catch syphilis by working with them.[64]

One response by a female attendant from Virginia, however, illustrates the conflicted emotions some white employees had as they attempted to cope with their new work environment:

> I think there are more of them [black attendants] who are irresponsible because they are afraid. Sometimes if there is trouble on the ward, the colored girl just stays out of it until it's all over. Of course after they get used to the work they are just as good as the whites, I think. But one reason we object to them, if they have been here only a few days longer than a white girl they try to run right over her. Most of the girls complain about it. It just seems that being colored they are determined to be boss and the strange thing is that it's not the lighter skinned ones who are like this, it's the darker skinned ones.[65]

Putting aside the erroneous association she made between complexion and assertiveness or sense of entitlement, the attendant's estimation of black women on the ward reveals a number of interesting things. On the one hand, her unquestioning acceptance of the "bossy" nature of African American women ignored the pervasiveness of employment discrimination that conditioned their existence in the labor market, a reality that was expressed by the African American female attendant who spoke of supervisors ignoring seniority when it came to their black subordinates. Having to constantly assert themselves was a necessary strategy for African American women in the workforce, but it was incorrectly interpreted by whites as a character flaw of the entire black race. On the other hand, any racist assumptions about black women's ability that the white attendant may have had dissolved once she began to work with them. Working on the wards together could produce racial antagonism and racial misunderstandings, yet it also had the potential to produce racial enlightenment.

White attendants also confirmed the existence of racial tensions between African American attendants and white patients. A female attendant, who indicated in her interview that the black and white employees on her ward eventually developed a good working relationship, suggested that this was not the case with the white patients. "The patients resented it at first and some still don't accept it," she remarked. One white male attendant originally from North Carolina reinforced some of his colleagues' unwillingness to work with African Americans by emphasizing white patients' dismay at the integrated staff. "Most of the patients won't get along with them either," he told his interviewer. The attendant put a fine point on his assessment of patient attitudes by channeling an older argument—reminiscent of that made by John M. Galt in the mid-nineteenth century—about the only suitable conditions under which black attendants should tend to white patients: "It's alright on a degenerate ward where the men are so far gone they don't know what they are doing." As these remarks make clear, there was a great deal of racial friction at Saint Elizabeths that could not be contained by the single-mindedness of the national war effort.[66]

Even though the study on black attendants concluded that they had an overall positive impression of Saint Elizabeths and their work experience, it indirectly attributed those positive attitudes to the development of a critical mass of black staff during the war. "Some of the Negro attendants," the report acknowledged, "said that it had been hard for them when they first came, and there were few Negro attendants, but that the situation had changed now."[67] The labor demands caused by the war amplified the racial progressivism of New Deal liberals in federal agencies—particularly Ickes in Interior and McNutt in FSA—and accelerated the emergence of this critical mass.[68] But this phase of integration occurred only within the nursing and attendant staff. The dismantling of the racial barrier among the psychiatric social workers and physicians would take another ten years.

African American physicians and medical students had been affiliated with Saint Elizabeths as early as the 1920s, when White reestablished an academic relationship between the hospital and Howard University after the unfortunate events of 1911. Largely responsible for this resuscitation was Benjamin Karpman, a clinical psychiatrist who joined the staff shortly after World War I. A native of Russia, educated in North Dakota and Minnesota, Karpman took an early interest in the education of African American medical students, teaching courses in dynamic psychiatry at Howard University in the early 1920s and convincing White to resume his lectures. Through their relationship with Karpman, Howard students evaluated African American patients at Saint Elizabeths and undertook more elaborate research studies. One of his students was Ernest Y. Williams, who went on to establish the psychiatric service at Freedmen's Hospital in 1939. Other African American physicians had relationships with Saint Elizabeths, including John S. Perry, a clinical assistant in neuropsychiatry at Freedmen's Hospital in the 1930s, who did research with John E. Lind.[69] Saint Elizabeths continued to offer educational opportunities for Howard students throughout the 1940s. Medical students from Howard had access to the hospital's clinical facilities and received psychiatric instruction along with students at the District's other medical schools, although it is not clear whether the classes, lectures, and clinics were segregated. By 1947 Saint Elizabeths' staff were training social work students from Howard and Catholic University in psychiatric social work.[70] But as much as the hospital extended its teaching resources to African Americans interested in psychiatry and psychiatric social work, it did not employ any on its permanent staff in the years following World War II.

In a sense, the demographic changes that Washington, DC, and Saint Elizabeths experienced in the decade after World War II would have made continuing exclusion of African Americans from these positions untenable. In 1957 Washington became the first major American city in which African Americans made up a majority; by 1960, 71 percent of the District's population was black. Blacks also constituted more than 40 percent of the patients treated in Saint Elizabeths in 1957. As the hospital increasingly served a civilian and African American population, it would have inevitably hired African American physicians, in much the same way as New York's Harlem, Chicago's Cook County, Detroit Receiving, Boston City, and other public hospitals did in the 1920s and 1930s. But these hospitals did not integrate their staffs without political pressure from civil rights and black professional organizations. This was also the case with Saint Elizabeths.[71]

Those agitating for the integration of Saint Elizabeths, and District hospitals more generally, had a rich tradition of civil rights activism to draw on. In 1933 black Washingtonians formed a cross-class group called the New Negro Alliance to pressure white-owned businesses along U Street in Northwest—the District's

Harlem—to hire more African Americans. The alliance's "Don't buy where you can't work" boycott managed to generate jobs for blacks, but its concomitant goal of desegregating the lunch counter at Peoples Drug Store was less successful. A decade and a half later, members of sixty-one progressive black and white religious, civic, labor, and social service organizations founded the Coordinating Committee for the Enforcement of the DC Anti-Discrimination Laws. The committee sought to pressure the municipal and federal governments to enforce antidiscrimination laws that Congress had passed in the 1870s but that had vanished from the District's municipal code in 1901. Through a campaign of sit-in strikes in the early 1950s, led by the prominent black educator, reformer, and activist, Mary Church Terrell, the group forced several downtown businesses to open their lunch counters to all customers regardless of race. The sit-in protest at one particular restaurant prompted a legal challenge to segregation in public accommodations, resulting in the US Supreme Court's 1953 decision in *District of Columbia v. John R. Thompson Co.*, which affirmed the District's "lost laws" and guaranteed equal access to services.[72]

Fully integrating a federal mental hospital, however, required different tactics. Spearheading the campaign were the NAACP and the National Medical Association (NMA), the principal professional organization for black physicians. Although these organizations relied on the work and support of many, the efforts of both organizations seemingly converged in one individual: W. Montague Cobb. A physician and professor of anatomy at Howard, Cobb was also chair of the NAACP's National Health Committee and a contributing editor to the *Journal of the National Medical Association*. Shortly after the war, Cobb, in his capacity as president of the Medico-Chirurgical Society—the District's African American physicians' association—challenged the District's Board of Commissioners, which was considering a policy that would grant black doctors admitting privileges to Gallinger Municipal Hospital but also require that they use separate facilities and quarters. Cobb and others were outraged that such a policy would be implemented in a hospital that had a shortage of admitting physicians and whose patient population was 70 percent black. Cobb's letter to one of the commissioners was reprinted in the *Journal of the National Medical Association*, with the endorsement of its editor-in-chief, John A. Kenney, a longtime leader within the NMA.[73]

Another prominent figure who supported Cobb's challenges to the exclusion of black physicians and medical students from Gallinger was President Truman's federal security administrator, Oscar Ewing. As head of the agency that oversaw, among other constituent agencies, Freedmen's Hospital, Howard, and Saint Elizabeths, Ewing expressed grave concern over the dearth of African American physicians in the country. He attributed this shortage to the fact that most black physicians received their training at Howard and at Meharry Medical College in Nashville, Tennessee. Freedmen's Hospital, which was smaller than all of the other teaching hospitals in Washington, was the only facility that allowed black physicians, residents, and interns to practice, placing an artificial cap on the number of African Americans who could successfully complete their medical training. The insufficient numbers of African American doctors compounded the existing health deficit within Washington's black community as a whole, a product of segregation that received a great deal of attention in the immediate postwar period. The Council of Social Agencies of the District of Columbia and Vicinity published a report on race relations in 1946 that listed lower life expectancy and higher tuberculosis and maternal mortality rates among blacks as direct effects of racism. A year later Truman's Committee on Civil Rights issued a report that contained a section on racial discrimination in the District, characterizing the health care disparities between blacks and whites as among the nation's "greatest inequalities."[74]

In addition to the very practical argument that allowing African American physicians and medical students to practice at Gallinger would alleviate the pressure on white physicians and improve the overall health of the District's black community, those who were opposed to the continued exclusion framed their arguments within the more lofty language of democratic idealism. Employing the kind of rhetoric that was used by civil rights activists during the cold war to expose the hypocrisy of the country's stated commitment to spreading democracy across the globe, they pointed to the particular indignity of Gallinger's policy existing in the capital of the free world. Kenney's admonishment that "of all places in the United States, our Nation's Capital should be the last in which such a discriminatory measure is contemplated" resonated quite well with the Committee on Civil Rights report's statement that the "District of Columbia should symbolize to our own citizens and to the people of all countries our great tradition of civil liberty." With the "tacit approval" of Truman and his committee, Ewing began discussions with the Board of Commissioners about integrating the physician staff of Gallinger. Ewing's proposal enjoyed the support of the DC League of Women Voters and, most likely, the Federation of Civic Associations, the alliance of black neighborhood associations that had been agitating for African American employment at Gallinger since the late 1930s. In February 1948, facing federal and public opposition, the board relented and ordered Gallinger to allow black physicians and medical students to practice medicine there.[75]

An unidentified newspaper article suggests that Ewing also wanted to leverage the policy change at Gallinger to effect a similar change at Saint Elizabeths.[76] This may very well have been the case, but Ewing was unsuccessful in convincing Overholser, despite the superintendent's welcoming of Howard medical students for classroom and clinical instruction. When the NAACP, the NMA, and the black press made a more frontal assault on segregation in the District's hospitals in the early 1950s, they included Saint Elizabeths in their sights. In 1951 the NAACP, with Cobb as the chair of its National Medical Committee, passed a set of resolutions at its annual convention in Atlanta that addressed what it considered to be the pressing health concerns for African Americans. The organization praised the federal government's infusion of funds to build a robust mental health infrastructure for Americans, but it castigated the government for allowing the perpetuation of segregation in public and private hospitals—a reality that was facilitated by the "separate but equal" provision in the landmark Hospital and Survey Construction Act of 1946—and the VA system.[77]

Two years later Cobb, the president of the local chapter of the NAACP, Eugene Davidson, and the president of the Medico-Chirurgical Society, Edward Mazique, collaborated in an effort to eliminate segregation in District hospitals. The *Baltimore Afro-American*, pointing out that African American physicians were still excluded from Saint Elizabeths, pondered whether the new president, Dwight D. Eisenhower, could use his executive power to abolish segregation in the District. A few months later Cobb, Davidson, and Mazique sent a letter to eighteen hospitals—private and public, municipal and federal—demanding that "racial discrimination or segregation of any form" be eliminated. As with those who had begun the campaign immediately after the war, the three urged "the hospitals' full cooperation" in "making the city of Washington an example for the rest of the nation."[78]

Despite the preoccupation of Overholser and his predecessors with maintaining Saint Elizabeths' status as a symbol of enlightened medicine for an enlightened nation, he was not particularly responsive to civil rights activists' rhetoric. Overholser was a racial moderate. He and his wife, Dorothy, were Unitarians, and he was proud of having descended from a long line of New England antislavery activists. Dorothy was active in civic affairs, leading a fight by a Unitarian women's association to remove some of the barriers against African Americans, including the employment of black physicians at Gallinger and the prohibition of segregation at District restaurants.[79] While a medical student at Boston University and a resident at Westborough State Hospital for the Insane, Overholser himself had studied under Solomon Carter Fuller, a Liberian-born psychiatrist who did his own postgraduate work with the psychiatric luminaries Emil Kraepelin and Alois Alzheimer. So he was likely respectful of black people's capacity to be medical professionals.[80] Yet Overholser was skeptical of what he considered extremism on either the right or the left. Charles Prudhomme, recalling his first encounter with Overholser in the late 1930s, said that the superintendent expressed his disagreement with the existence of segregation at Saint Elizabeths but pleaded his lack of power to do anything about it.[81]

It was only a matter of time, however, before the racial barrier within the physician ranks at Saint Elizabeths fell. Within six years of the integration of Gallinger's staff, African American physicians were appointed to the staffs of the Georgetown University, Providence, and George Washington University hospitals—all private—and the District's public tuberculosis sanatorium in suburban Maryland. In 1952 African American physicians were admitted to the Medical Society of the District of Columbia, which subsequently exited the all-white Federation of Citizens Associations because it opposed the integration of the professional association.[82] By the middle of the decade Saint Elizabeths had its first African American clinician. Dr. Luther D. Robinson was a Meharry graduate who worked at Lakin State Hospital, West Virginia's colored asylum, from 1947 to 1949. After serving a tour overseas as an army physician, Robinson pursued postgraduate education in psychiatry at both Freedmen's Hospital and Saint Elizabeths. He became the first African American to complete a residency at Saint Elizabeths, becoming a permanent member of the physician staff in 1955.[83] Within the year the staff included two more general medical officers who had done their internships at Freedmen's Hospital, and by 1957 Robinson was the physician in charge of the West Lodge Service.[84] By the time these African American physicians were walking the halls of Saint Elizabeths, moreover, they were interacting with black and white patients who were occupying integrated wards. As the hospital began the process of integrating its wards in the mid-1950s, African American and white staff and patients would all have to adjust to some new realities.

9

Whither the Negro Psyche

Integration and Its Aftermath, 1945–1970

The year 1955 marked a significant milestone for Saint Elizabeths, as the hospital reached its hundred-year mark. The administration thought there was much to celebrate. Announcing the formation of a commission to organize the centennial, a press release trumpeted the fact that military psychiatry was developed there, that the hospital had trained hundreds of psychiatrists and psychiatric nurses working with military personnel, and that its staff members were pioneers in "the use of the arts, including psychodrama, music and the dance, as therapeutic tools." The commission had big plans for the centennial. It organized a two-day conference in which distinguished American and foreign psychiatrists presented papers on, among other things, the history and scientific contributions of Saint Elizabeths, forensic psychiatry, psychiatric nursing and social work, psychopharmacology, and the psychiatric profession in an international perspective. The conference proceedings were published the following year. In addition, patients who were in psychodrama therapy classes wrote, produced, and acted in a play, *Cry of Humanity*, dramatizing the life and work of Dorothea Dix.[1]

The same year, the National Broadcasting Company televised a half-hour program examining the state of care of the nation's mentally ill population. "We, the Mentally Ill . . . ," the second episode in *The March of Medicine* series, was set in the Washington hospital and consisted of interviews with the staff, footage of the wards, and scenes from *Cry of Humanity*. Although it highlighted the most important challenges confronting hospital superintendents across the country—including "lack of facilities, lack of supervisory and medical personnel, lack of funds for modern medical care"—the program introduced an optimistic note into its coverage: the future of mental health care looked bright because of the recent development of effective pharmaceutical agents—especially chlorpromazine. One staff member lauded new drug treatments as "the greatest opportunity of this age to rid the heavy burden of mental illness upon all." It is not surprising that the benefits of psychopharmacology were a main topic of the documentary, given that the program's sponsors were the American Medical Association and Smith, Kline and French Laboratories, the American-based marketer of chlorpromazine under the brand name Thorazine.[2]

Developed in the early 1950s by the French pharmaceutical giant, Rhône-Poulenc, chlorpromazine and a set of other alkaloid compounds such as reserpine promised to transform the treatment of patients in mental institutions. Their powerful sedative effects obviated the need for the use of hydrotherapy and other more controversial treatment modalities such as insulin/metrazol shock therapy and electroconvulsive therapy. The psychopharmacological revolution, moreover, came at a time of heady optimism that science was triumphing against some of the most intractable medical problems of the day—from polio to venereal disease.[3] Even though the typical institutionalized patient still resided in a large public hospital, where clinical staff had little time and few resources to conduct psychotherapy on a massive scale, the psychiatric profession maintained a degree of optimism that the psychotropic drugs offered new routes to recovery, not just easier patient management.

The psychopharmacological revolution also came on the heels of two related, but distinct, postwar developments that influenced a subtle shift in the way the psychiatric profession approached mental illness among African Americans. The 1940s and 1950s were decades in which the belief in race as a biologically determined and deterministic category of human difference began to decline

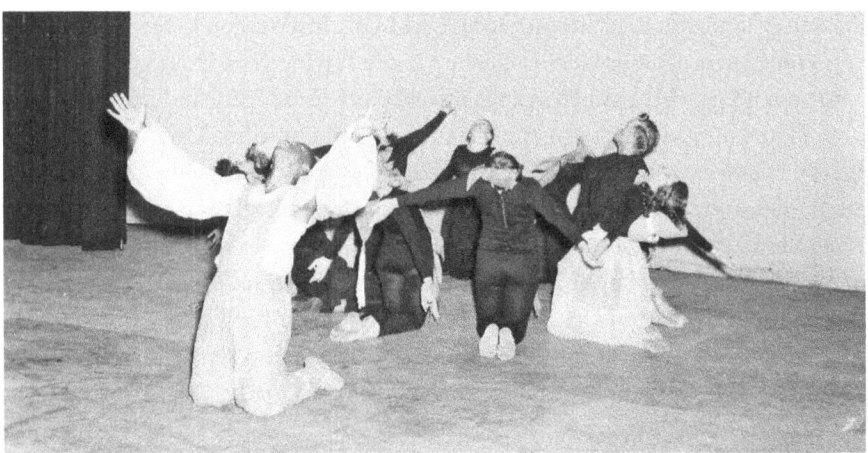

A black male patient, on his knees with his arms stretched upward, along with white female patients, acts out a scene from a play dedicated to the life and work of reformer Dorothea Dix. By the mid-1950s Saint Elizabeths, which was a pioneer in psychodrama therapy, had begun to integrate its wards, therapeutic practices, and recreational spaces. *Scene from Cry of Humanity, 1955. National Archives, photo 418-P-441-445.*

within academic and public policy circles. The horrific revelations of Nazi racism contributed to the delegitimizing of the field of eugenics, whose central principle of better life through better breeding was premised, in part, on the incompatibility of distinct races. In the United States the biological justifications for racial segregation began to crumble as natural scientists and medical experts increasingly rejected the idea that black and white blood was fundamentally different. And although United Nations officials were not completely prepared to accept some scholars' claims that race had absolutely no biological basis and therefore was an invalid measure of human variation, in its second statement on race, in 1950, a UNESCO panel did categorically repudiate the use of biological difference to promote and justify racial purity and racial discrimination. To be sure, the belief in race as a type of human difference persisted in the emerging fields of population studies and genetics. And for both liberal and conservative academics, politicians, and public policymakers, culture would increasingly serve as a proxy for biological difference when it came to debating black-white relations or the status of black America in the 1950s and 1960s.[4] When psychotropic drugs became available to physicians in mental hospitals, however, they used them on their patients regardless of those patients' racial backgrounds, indicating that they understood blacks and whites to have the same physiological responses to medication.

As the concept of the irreducible biological difference between blacks and whites was increasingly regarded as a shibboleth within the scientific and medical communities, the psychiatric profession was undergoing an important transformation. Psychodynamic psychiatry, which certainly had many American practitioners prior to World War II—including William White and Winfred Overholser—became even more dominant in the postwar era, especially among institutional psychiatrists. The ideas that everyone fell on a spectrum with mental illness and mental health at opposite poles, and that mental illness was essentially an individual's failure to adapt to his or her environment and the people within it, gained even more currency in the wake of the nation's war experience. Psychiatric screening of draftees suggested that a significant proportion of young American men had inadequately developed personalities. The prolonged stress of combat, moreover, further damaged the already fragile psyches of many servicemen.

Following the war, a younger cohort of psychiatrists brought many of their observations and experiences with military patients into their work with civilian populations and sought to infuse the profession with a more socially responsible vision. For instance, they recognized that prolonged stress did not come only from the immersion in a physically dangerous environment; it was also the product of the harsh everyday environment of living in poverty or being the target of discrimination. This new generation was also appalled at the state of the nation's mental hospitals, which were all too often overcrowded and understaffed. The responsibility of psychiatry, they argued, was not only to ameliorate the conditions for patients within these institutions but to also make meaningful interventions in the lives of those people whose mental health was jeopardized by society's structural inequalities and the daily indignities associated with being unemployed, homeless, or occupying the position of social outcast. This new iteration of the discipline, social psychiatry, would take seriously the role of racism in producing mental illness. As such, psychiatry's growing interest in the psyche and emotional interiority of African Americans neatly dovetailed with postwar social science's preoccupation with the psychological damage of racism and segregation.[5]

In some respects, psychopharmacology and social psychiatry naturally led to, respectively, race-neutral and racially liberal approaches to mental illness among African Americans.[6] They were not incidental forces in the integration of the wards at Saint Elizabeths, a process that began in earnest in 1954 and was more or less complete by 1956. But acknowledging that black and white bodies responded similarly to drugs did not inevitably translate into race-neutral ways of thinking about the etiology and pathology of mental illness among African Americans and whites. And for all the progressive intent behind social psychiatry's embrace of racial liberalism and patient autonomy, African American patients and employees at Saint Elizabeths still had to deal with both institutionalized and run-of-the-mill racism in the postintegration era.

The Strange Career of Race in Postwar Psychiatric Thought

Although psychiatrists and mental health experts were not prepared to completely abandon the salience of race as a factor in the causation and manifestations of mental illness, ideas about the black psyche that had animated late nineteenth- and early twentieth-century physicians' understanding of insanity were clearly on their way out by the eve of World War II. The civilized/primitive binary had less currency when it came to framing questions about the prevalence of mental illness or the prospects for mental health among African Americans. The explicit project of developing a comparative psychology that presupposed distinctive black and white psyches commanded less interest among medical and psychiatric journal editors and their readers. Lamarckism and recapitulation theory, underlying ideas about evolution that informed the thought of many of those who pursued comparative psychology research, were rejected by most of the psychiatric profession by the 1930s. Racial differences were still considered important in many quarters of the psychiatric profession, but those differences were increasingly attributed to environment rather than biology.[7]

Still, the belief in biological difference between the races persisted in psychiatric circles. Based on the clinical research that he conducted in Panama in the early 1940s, Dr. Siegfried Fischer of the University of California Medical School in San Francisco published findings on the incidence of manic-depressive psychosis among whites, mestizos, Indians, and blacks. His conclusions echoed the comparative psychology research of the early part of the century. Patients who were more "negroid" exhibited more "outspoken" and "intense" symptoms of mania than patients of white, Indian, or mestizo backgrounds. On the other hand, the naturally stoic nature of Indians was responsible for the "mildest symptoms" of mania among the mestizo population. In the end, for Fischer, it was biology more than culture that influenced the development of mental illness, with the "distribution of the manic-depressive psychosis among various peoples" shaped by "the differences in the constitution, the structure of the body of the various races."[8]

Unlike Fischer, the chief psychiatrist of New York's Bellevue Hospital, Dr. Lauretta Bender, was more amenable to considering the role of culture and environment in producing mental differences between blacks and whites. She invoked the earlier work of comparative psychologists—particularly the work that situated African Americans within a primitive typology—but as a point of departure rather than as gospel. Yet Bender advanced some of the same ideas, even if they were couched in more muted language. Some of the behavioral disorders that she observed in African American children were rooted in blacks' "capacity for so-called laziness" and their "special ability to dance." While the average African American child was not necessarily more promiscuous than the average white child, black children were more open than white children when it came to discussing sex. Ultimately Bender was cognizant of the potential for culture, experience, and environment to produce feelings of inferiority in African American youths. However, she refused to let go of biology, suggesting that there was something peculiar about black people's cellular development—and especially the mesoderm, the middle layer of cells in an embryo that evolve into bones, muscles, connective tissue, and so forth—that interacted with their vascular system, thereby creating the possibility for "special deviations in organic brain condition."[9]

Increasingly physicians and psychiatrists who remained wedded to biologically reductionist and determinist explanations of the causes and evolution of mental illness in individuals would become outliers. Even those who insisted on thinking about mental disease and race within a civilizationist framework were more likely to invoke primitive culture than the primitive body as the controlling factor. Moreover, they abandoned simplistic explanatory models that posited the mentally healthy primitive in contrast to the civilized races that were more prone to mental illness.

On the basis of fieldwork off the coast of Papua New Guinea, for instance, Géza Róheim, an anthropologist and staff psychoanalyst at Worcester State Hospital, expressed a relativist understanding of insanity, acknowledging that what constituted normality and what constituted psychosis were often contingent on the cultural context. Róheim was also part of a generation of psychiatrists, many working in colonial settings, that was beginning to take seriously the fact that the mental illness experienced by people from what were considered to be primitive societies could develop independently of any interaction with Western civilization as easily as it could be the product of social disorganization as a result of contact with colonizers. Reflecting the growing unease with Nazi propaganda about Aryan superiority, he expressed discomfort with race as a biological fact. "There is no such thing as a German race or a Jewish race and therefore statistics about disease or behavior variations in these groups do not prove anything," Róheim insisted. "On the whole, it can be stated that if race exercises any influence on the choice of certain types of psychical reactions, this influence is exercised through the type of culture evolved or assimilated by that race."[10] Róheim could not square the circle of rejecting the existence of the German and Jewish races and taking as a given that there were still races that could develop or assimilate cultures. When it came to the question of the influence of biology or culture on the development of neuroses and psychoses, however, he came down firmly on the side of culture.

Róheim's carefully considered conclusions about race and mental illness were informed as much by his background in anthropology as by his psychiatric clinical experience.[11] The fact that his article was published in *Psychiatry: Journal of the Biology and the Pathology of Interpersonal Relations* is particularly significant in this regard. Begun by the William Alanson White Psychiatric Foundation in 1938, *Psychiatry* became a venue for "all serious students of human living in any of its aspects, and to those who must meet pressing social needs with current remedial attempts." Its coeditor was Dr. Harry Stack Sullivan, a protégé of White, who had worked at Saint Elizabeths as a liaison to the US Veterans Bureau in the early 1920s. Sullivan was also the first president of the foundation. An ecumenical thinker, he promoted interdisciplinary conversation between psychiatrists and social scientists, and he rejected the idea that humans were the "unalterable product of heredity and constitution"; rather, he believed, they were the "most remarkably complex representation[s] of . . . culture and experience." Sullivan's interest in interpersonal relations led to his involvement in the postwar period in UNESCO and the World Federation of Mental Health.[12]

Sullivan's opposition to biological determinism and his insistence that the social context of mental illness and health needed to be addressed as much as the individual personality certainly account for the amount of space given to race and racism in *Psychiatry*. Arguably one of the most influential figures in the intellectual assault on biological determinism, the anthropologist Ashley Montagu, published no fewer than nine articles in the journal between 1940 and 1946. In his first article for *Psychiatry*, Montagu took aim at the vulgar biologism associated with early twentieth-century thought, calling race no more than a myth of the same class as "pixies, ghosts, satyrs, [and] Aryans." He did not categorically deny that some physical differences existed between human populations that had settled in distinct areas of the globe over the course of generations. But the leap that was required to go from this point to the conclusion that these groups were irreconcilably different and inevitably unequal ignored the fact they had never existed in isolation. Indeed these human populations were not static but had histories that were marked by movement and interaction.

The leap also required believers in racial difference to ignore the fact that there was greater variety in the physical features and mental functions within groups defined as races than there was across groups defined as races. As such, Montagu concluded, there was no validity to the claim that different races had distinctive psychical reactions to stimuli. Montagu's article was an early version of the first statement on race by UNESCO, of which he was the lead author, which called race not a biological fact but a social myth. "Race is not a biological problem at all," he wrote in *Psychiatry*, "and furthermore, does not even present any biological problems which society needs in the least to consider. Race is a term for a problem which is created by social factors, and by social factors alone; it is, therefore, entirely a social problem."[13] It would be easy to dismiss *Psychiatry* and Montagu's interrogation of the biological reality of race as the obsession of a few progressive psychiatrists and social scientists and not representative of the profession as a whole. But their viewpoint about race—and its relationship to mental illness—was clearly ascendant by the 1940s. Even though it published a review that was critical of Montagu's 1945 book, *Man's Greatest Myth: The Fallacy of Race*, the editors of the *American Journal of Psychiatry* still had to confront the questions that he and a growing number of psychiatrists were raising.[14]

One of the last articles that Montagu wrote for *Psychiatry* had the provocative title "Racism and Social Action." The article was a manifesto of sorts, offering a theoretical explication of racism and advocating for forceful political strategies and public policies to combat it. Montagu also elaborated on earlier work in which he attributed race hatred to an underdeveloped personality. Rooted in the interpersonal interactions that structured an individual's early childhood, race hatred was a manifestation of the repressed feelings of anger and fear that one developed as a result of being deprived by one's caregiver. These repressed emotions were released through safety valves in one's youth and adulthood, largely through the processes of displacement and projection. "The insecurities incident to life in highly industrialized societies are continually productive of frustrations," he argued, "and race prejudices constitutes [sic] a socially sanctioned outlet for the resulting accumulated aggressiveness, which at once serves to explain the person's failure to himself and at the same time enables him to revenge himself upon the imagined cause of it."

But for Montagu, racism was not just a personality deficiency that would be remedied through intensive therapy or an intergroup phenomenon that could be solved by greater education. It had become embedded in the very soul of the nation and could only be torn out by radically transforming the country's educational, legal, and economic institutions. To that end, Montagu advocated for the implementation of antidiscrimination laws at state and local levels. He also pressed for greater federal involvement, particularly the permanent establishment of President Roosevelt's Fair Employment Practices Committee.[15] For Montagu, there were no barriers to be erected between the psychiatrist's concern for healing the minds of individuals, the larger public-oriented project of preserving mental hygiene, and the pressing social issues confronting the nation. Rather, it was incumbent on the psychiatric profession to address the interrelated nature of these problems and opportunities.

Montagu's ideas about the social capacity of psychiatry reflected a zeitgeist. In the same year that he published "Racism and Social Action," a small group of members of the American Psychiatric Association (APA), led by William C. Menninger, a brigadier general and head of the neuropsychiatry division of the US Army Medical Corps, formed the Group for the Advancement of Psychiatry (GAP). Menninger and his like-minded colleagues believed that the profession as a whole had allowed the mental health infrastructure of the nation to deteriorate and that it was too detached from some of the major moral problems of the day. GAP developed and maintained its membership through invitation only, the main criterion being one's willingness to delve into social problems through intensive group study. The organization consisted of groups that investigated and produced reports on various aspects of the care and treatment of mentally ill people—including shock therapy, the state of public mental hospitals, and commitment policies and procedures. It also expanded its purview beyond the institutionalized patient. One of the first study groups formed was devoted to "racial and economic problems," indicating the social activist orientation of GAP's members. Throughout the mid-1950s the organization produced a report on school desegregation, and its members were among the experts who consulted with educators and government officials.[16]

Thus an increasing number of psychodynamic psychiatrists were directing their attention toward the environmental stressors that had the potential to elicit abnormal psychical reactions. As Overholser remarked in the waning years of the war, mental illness was a threat to everyone. "Nobody's immune," he told a reporter from the *Washington Star*. "It's partly a question of the resilience of the individual and equally as important is the amount, the duration and the intensity of the stress to which he is exposed. In other words, everybody has a breaking point." For some, that breaking point was the intensely congested environment of the "apartment civilization" that characterized America's cities.[17] For others, it was racial discrimination.

The psychological effects of racism became the subject of numerous studies in the decade and a half following World War II. Within a year of the war's conclusion, Dr. Rutherford B. Stevens presented findings on the impact of racial discrimination on the emotional well-being of African American soldiers at the annual meeting of the APA. An African American army doctor himself, Stevens compiled observational data from his work with various black troops over the course of five years. He found that in the case of African Americans, the "chronic emotional tension" that soldiers would have experienced under normal wartime conditions was exacerbated by the racial segregation that existed on bases, the racism of local communities, the tendency for them to be assigned to quartermaster or service engineer units, the paucity of black officers, and the "fascist" attitudes of many of their white commanding officers.

Importantly, Stevens began his presentation by suggesting that his findings had broader applicability than the military. Psychiatrists would do well, he told his audience, to recognize the extent to which racism could have adverse effects on the entire black population. "Unquestionably, in post-war America," Stevens warned, "large numbers of Negroes need psychiatric care and will go in search of it to civil and industrial hospitals and clinics as well as to the hospitals of the Veterans Administration." He concluded his talk by revisiting this point and stating it in even more forceful language that must have spoken to the more socially activist members of the organization. "And this is far more than a military problem in wartime," he reminded his audience. "It should be obvious that psychiatrists, not to mention all the others who deal with the health problems of American citizens, of whatever color, have a duty to society and to themselves to study, understand, and aid in the prevention of these problems by furthering the practice of the principles of real democracy."[18] Over the next ten to fifteen years, psychiatrists, psychologists, social scientists, and educators would echo Stevens in producing a massive body of knowledge about racism's damaging psychological effects on African Americans and the most efficacious public policy remedies.[19]

Much of this work was done by psychologists and social scientists, although psychiatrists with a more interdisciplinary bent—like many of those involved in GAP—welcomed the opportunity to collaborate. Some who were interested in the psychological damage wrought by racism explored this dynamic within a clinical setting. Two of those psychiatrists were Henry J. Myers and Leon Yochelson, both medical officers at Saint Elizabeths. In a clinical study conducted among black male patients in West Lodge Service in 1948, Myers and Yochelson concluded that the disconnect between the American creed and the reality of black subordination produced a state of chronic and intense anxiety among African Americans, leading to "one or more of a number of possible reactions from marked servility to pronounced aggression; from invalidism to frank psychosis." Although they suggested that the postwar environment was contributing to a newfound "racial consciousness and racial pride" within the black community, African Americans still attached a great deal of shame and embarrassment to their color.

But what was perhaps most telling about Myers and Yochelson's study was their blatant rejection of the earlier comparative psychology theories that had been advanced by previous Saint Elizabeths' staff. Specifically, they pointed to the studies by Mary O'Malley and W. M. Bevis in the World War I era and characterized their conclusions that African Americans possessed a psyche that was different from and inferior to whites as nothing more than base stereotypes. "Naturally," they authoritatively stated, "little contribution to the understanding of the Negro and his problems can be expected from such sources."[20] Here was a clear repudiation of the psychiatric thought that had dominated the profession's approach to black mental illness from the post-Reconstruction period to the interwar era. It was also reflective of a more universalist understanding of the mind, in which African Americans' mental capacities and psychological reactions to external stimuli were not assumed to be different from those of whites.[21]

Although it is not certain if Myers and Yochelson identified themselves as social psychiatrists, their thinking about racism and mental illness clearly aligned with the liberal politics of GAP and other like-minded psychiatrists and psychologists. As more clinicians like Myers and Yochelson who rejected assumptions about the existence of a distinctive black psyche joined Saint Elizabeths' staff, there was bound to be growing acceptance of, if not internal pressure for, the dismantlement of the institution's segregationist policy. But a lofty and noble antiracist turn in postwar psychiatry was only partly responsible for the eventual integration of the hospital's wards. Logistical realities—in terms of the stresses placed on the hospital's infrastructure through overpopulation and underresourcing—and external pressure from the federal government and activist organizations all contributed to the complete removal of the racial barriers that had largely separated black and white patients for a century.

"Not as a Crusade": Integrating the Wards

The same year that Myers and Yochelson published their study on black male patients in West Lodge Service, Overholser participated in a two-day conference to discuss the prospects of desegregating hospitals operated by the Veterans Administration. The conference was at the behest of black physicians and activists who had approached General Omar Bradley, the recently appointed head of the VA. Bradley instructed the VA medical director, General Paul R. Hawley, to invite experts on both sides of the issue to debate the merits and challenges of integrating the hospital system. Even though his views may have been in accordance with social psychiatry, Overholser, who was now the president of the APA, was one of the most vocal opponents of integration. According to Charles Prudhomme, a black psychiatrist who was at the meeting and who himself had known Overholser since he was a medical student, the Saint Elizabeths superintendent argued "that such integration was not in the best interest of the patients, that psychiatric care could be best delivered in a segregated setting."[22] Four years later Overholser expressed a similar sentiment in an article in the *Times Herald*, in which he explained that racial separation of patients was for their own good, for "mentally ill persons have more acute prejudices than normal ones."[23]

As had been the case for decades, there were limited occasions and certain circumstances under which white and black patients intermingled in the postwar period. As early as 1947 black and white male patients in Howard Hall's maximum security ward were taking occupational therapy classes together, even though they continued to live in separate quarters. Their numbers were roughly equal and, according to the occupational therapist who ran the sessions, for the most part the "shop atmosphere has been one of a 'good group spirit.'" But the therapist also reported racial tension. Some of the white patients, for instance, objected to the display of the crafts made by the African American patients in a talent show, as they "thought that they were receiving too much recognition."[24] Overholser's continued support for the segregation of patients was probably influenced by this anecdotal evidence more than it was conditioned by the inheritance of a legacy of psychiatric research that posited an innate, unbridgeable difference between the psyches of whites and African Americans. These ideas and their influence on how racial groups were managed in hospitals were certainly changing over the course of the decade, but the superintendent did not have the luxury of determining the pace at which these changes would occur at Saint Elizabeths. Beginning in 1953 President Dwight D. Eisenhower began to aggressively extend civil rights into areas that were under federal jurisdiction.

During his 1952 presidential campaign, General Eisenhower spoke frequently and forthrightly of wanting to eliminate "every vestige" of segregation in the District of Columbia and the federal government more broadly. Within two weeks of his election, civil rights organizations, meeting in Washington under the auspices of the National Association of Intergroup Relations Officials, expressed their expectations that he fulfill his campaign promise. Initially the new president hoped to extinguish Jim Crow in the capital by convincing Congress to extend home rule to the District, which would give the city's residents—a sizable proportion of whom were African American—direct input into municipal governance. When it became clear that segregationists in Congress would block such legislation, Eisenhower decided to work through the District commissioners, two of whom were appointed by the president. He managed to get the Senate to approve Samuel Spencer, a native Mississippian, Harvard graduate, and navy veteran who had worked on Eisenhower's presidential campaign. Spencer was instrumental in moving the president's desegregation agenda forward. In November 1953 the Board of Commissioners ordered twenty-three District agencies to prohibit racial discrimination in employment and services and to integrate their workforces. The order did exempt some agencies—including the Fire Department, the District Jail, and a few public welfare institutions—but this was largely for logistical reasons, with the understanding that these agencies would eventually comply. Two of the areas in which African Americans experienced segregation most acutely—recreational facilities and schools—were also exempt from the order because the board did not have jurisdiction over them. Eisenhower sought to flex his executive muscle elsewhere, creating committees to lobby private firms that had government contracts to implement nondiscriminatory employment policies and to resolve nonwhite federal employees' complaints of discrimination.[25]

Eisenhower was most effective in addressing segregation in the VA system. President Truman had issued an executive order in 1948 abolishing discrimination in the armed forces on the basis of race, color, religion, and national origin, but actual racial integration of the military occurred primarily during Eisenhower's administration. Along with the active-duty military force and schools on military bases, VA hospitals and facilities were priorities for the president, both because of the executive relationship that he had with them as commander-in-chief and because of the particular symbolism they held. How could government institutions that employed black men and women for the defense of the nation continue to discriminate against them and their families? Early in his first term, Eisenhower ordered the VA administrator, H. V. Higley, to move forward with integrating the system, a move that pleased civil rights activists. W. Montague Cobb, chair of the NAACP's National Health Committee, wrote to Higley in September 1953 that his organization appreciated that, "in keeping with the President's program, the Veterans Administration has already agreed to the principle of non-segregation in its hospitals." Maxwell Rabb, secretary to the president's cabinet and one of Eisenhower's closest advisers on race relations, reported in July 1954 that forty-three of the forty-seven VA hospitals were integrated. By September the entire system was.[26]

Where Saint Elizabeths fit in Eisenhower's maneuvering against segregation is not entirely clear. Although it was located in Washington and served the city's residents, it was not a District government agency, so it was not subject to the Board of Commissioners' order to desegregate. Nor was it in the VA system or a military installation, despite the large numbers of veterans who continued to be institutionalized there. Yet it did become completely integrated—but not until the middle of the decade.

The letter Cobb wrote to Higley offers a clue to the timing of the hospital's integration. The argument against integration offered by Overholser in 1948 still had some support in 1953. Higley had written to Clarence Mitchell, director of the NAACP's Washington Bureau, explaining why the VA was not moving more expeditiously to integrate its mental health facilities. "This is an area in which we may expect unpredictable and often violent reactions to prejudices and outside stimuli," the VA administrator wrote. "The safety of patients must always be our first consideration." Cobb dismissed Higley's and, by extension, Overholser's logic by pointing out that the argument that any integration of large populations would only exacerbate existing racism was also used by those opposed to the intermixing of the "mentally fit young men in the fighting forces." Integration of the armed forces—although not without its problems—had illustrated that argument's fallaciousness. He also employed his own psychiatric-based argument against the VA's policy of delay. Cobb acknowledged that "racial antipathy" was a form of hostility and that understanding the causes of hostility fell within the purview of the psychiatric profession. But he also reminded Higley that the causes and expressions of hostility—even those which manifested as racism—were specific to individuals. To reduce the sources and mechanisms of an individual's mental disorder to some notion of a group psyche was "unsound and unscientific." Cobb could draw only one conclusion: "Resistance to a policy of non-segregation is more a matter of the mental attitudes of administrators and possibly staffs than of the mental illness of patients." Cobb's assertion echoed that of the author of *The Snake Pit*, Mary Jane Ward, who, after investigating several public institutions in the late 1940s, found "little color bias among the insane themselves, but much among those who are supposed to cure the mentally unbalanced."[27]

Cobb pointed to the racially mixed group therapy sessions "being successfully operated" at Saint Elizabeths as evidence that VA mental health facilities could integrate without significant problems. What Cobb failed to notice or admit was that these sessions were taking place within the maximum security ward. As much as they might have been a progressive therapeutic development, the integrated group therapy sessions were also the residuum of the long-held belief that racial intermixing was tolerable as long as it was done among the most deviant subgroup of the patient population. It is hardly surprising, then, that it was groups of patients within Howard Hall, the Maximum Security Division, that were the first to experience sustained and deliberate racial integration.

Even with the limited success of the integrated group therapy sessions in the maximum security ward, it was a pragmatism born of the gap between expectation and capability that propelled integration of the wards. As it had for decades, the segregation of patients redounded to the detriment of African Americans. Although the hospital's bed-to-square-footage ratio fell well short of the APA's standards, there were certain wards that were "seriously overcrowded," according to hospital officials. West Lodge Service, the department for African

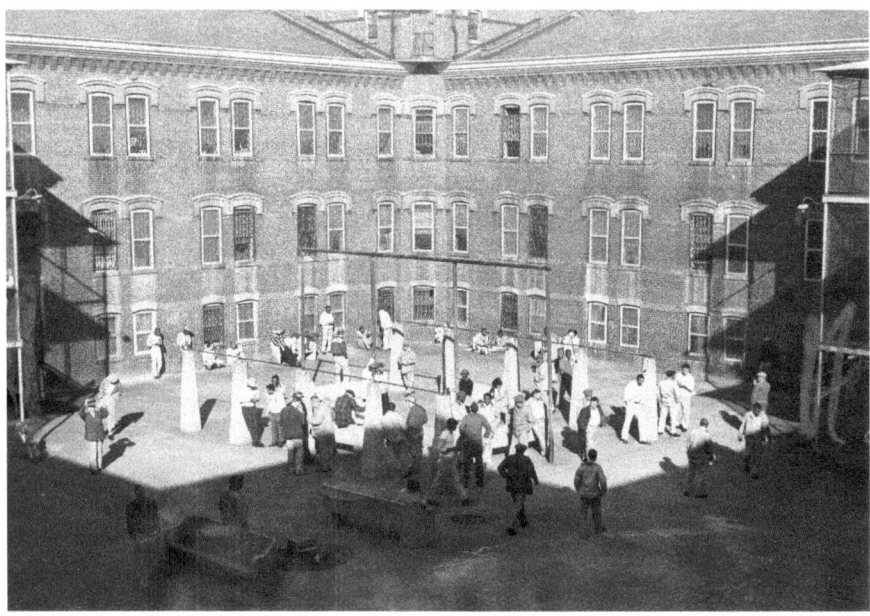

An interracial group of male patients mills about the inner courtyard of Howard Hall in 1956. It was among these "criminally insane" men that hospital staff began to experiment with racially integrated group therapy sessions, providing them, according to a local newspaper, a "new hope" that they could overcome their disease. *Washington Star Collection, Washingtoniana Division, DC Public Library. Reprinted with permission of the DC Public Library, Star Collection © Washington Post.*

American men, was 38 percent overcrowded, according to the 1950 annual report. The following year, both West Lodge and Q Service, the African American women's department, were reported to be 47 percent overcrowded. At the end of the 1951 fiscal year there were 1,076 African American male patients in a service that had a bed capacity of only 731.[28] Serious overcrowding in West Lodge Service meant that staff had few options to separate especially disturbed patients from the general population. It also forced the service to deny admission to individuals, particularly prisoners. In 1952 the inability to accommodate eight mentally ill African American men who were in the DC Jail prompted the intervention of the District courts, which made a survey of the hospital's facilities. Although Saint Elizabeths was held blameless, it was clear that the demands placed on the hospital—both in accepting patients and racially segregating them—were untenable. As early as 1950 the physician in charge of West Lodge Service suggested that his unit would need another receiving building or wards on other services would have to be opened up to African American men.[29]

West Lodge Service was not the first service to begin integrating its wards. That distinction fell to West Side Service, which included Howard Hall. Along with West Lodge and the Detached Service—a department consisting of primarily chronically ill patients—West Side Service made up Clinical Branch #3.[30] Beginning in early 1953, the director of the West Side Service and his staff began discussing the possibility of grouping the patients not by race but according to their behavior and the particular therapy they were undergoing. One of the problems with continuing to classify the patients by race was that it contributed to the inefficient use of space. The floor for African American patients, for instance, was often overcrowded, while the floor above them, for whites, was underutilized. Moreover the policy of racial segregation presented challenges for staff and newly admitted patients. The strict division of patients based on race meant that classes of patients who exhibited similar behaviors—such as being disturbed or assaultive—were distributed throughout Howard Hall rather than being concentrated on a few floors. This made it difficult for staff to interact with patients in ways that "most effectively utilized" their psychiatric expertise, and it potentially hindered therapeutic progress for the patients themselves. "Newly admitted patients who were quiet and cooperative were assigned willy-nilly to a ward with the most disturbed and uncooperative patients" merely to observe racial separation, the director noted, creating obstacles to their recovery. On June 30, after multiple meetings with nurses, attendants, and physicians, the eight wards of Howard Hall were racially integrated "without incident," and the director confidently reported that "both patients and personnel are highly gratified by the change."[31]

Within a year the entire West Side Service, which also included wards in the Center Building that housed patients who were considered troublesome and deviant—patients described as "mostly chronic," "senile," "untidy," "disturbed and semi-disturbed," "unpredictable," "assaultive," and "sexual psychopaths"— became racially integrated. Over the next year the director, Dr. William G. Cushard, reported to Overholser that the patients were functioning in this new environment "with very few problems and none of them serious."[32]

Integration proceeded apace throughout the rest of the hospital. Staff members were cautious in relocating patients. African American male patients were transferred from West Lodge Service to the Detached Service, thereby alleviating some of the crowding on African American male wards. Within the Detached Service, Dr. David W. Harris, the physician-in-charge, initially sought to introduce African Americans to white wards in a way that made all parties comfortable. Admitting black men in pairs would provide them with some emotional and psychological security and, at the same time, would not unduly alarm the white patients. In his report to Overholser in July 1954, however, Harris confessed that his careful approach had been unnecessary. He admitted that he may have been "too concerned" after a few occasions in which he had to move African American male patients in larger numbers produced little comment on the wards.[33]

This sentiment was, in fact, reflected in most of the reports summarizing the efforts to integrate the patient population. In the fall of 1954 the Women's Receiving Service and the female wards of the Geriatric Building began admitting African American women. By the summer of 1955 West Lodge Service and Detached Service had become, like West Side Service, thoroughly integrated, with Dr. F. N. Waldrop, West Lodge's physician-in-charge, proudly reporting that "no difficulties of significance" had accompanied the process. By the end of the 1955 fiscal year racial segregation, for all practical purposes, had ceased to exist. And integration had been achieved with little disruption to the staff or patients, according to Dr. Jay L. Hoffman, the first assistant physician. "No fanfare attended this move, and it would appear that the people concerned have been appropriately conditioned and oriented by the public press and similar means of mass information," Hoffman declared. "It was not considered necessary, therefore, and, in fact, it proved unnecessary to have any formal preliminary orientation or preparation of those concerned." Wards were not the only spaces being integrated. Administrators also began allowing racial intermixing in leisure settings, including dances. In December 1954 Hoffman characterized an annual party sponsored by an organization of navy mothers that was integrated for the first time as "an unqualified success."[34]

Yet these positive assessments by the staff were often leavened with sobering remarks about dissatisfaction with desegregration. Just as in the cases of the occupational therapy sessions and the nursing and attendant staffs, whenever the administration integrated hospital spaces, tension was inevitable. If the reports by staff are to be believed, the racial nature of this tension was negligible, yet it is more likely that this tension reflected a discontent in which race was a subtext even if not the centrally expressed concern. Dr. Evelyn B. Reichenbach, the clinical director of Clinical Branch #1, the division of female patients, pointed out that most of the difficulties encountered during the integration of the Women's Receiving Service were "due to the difference in the social level of the white and colored patients rather than to their color." Other staff members reported complaints coming from the relatives of patients rather than the patients themselves. The physician-in-charge of West Lodge Service indicated that there were complaints from "a number of the relatives of white patients" who were transferred to his service but that they were "not so much because of the mixing of the races as because of the relatively poor physical facilities of the wards."[35]

Given the sparseness of these reports, it is impossible to untangle what may have been racist motivations for opposing integration from genuine concerns over the new living conditions of one's relative or, as in the case of the Women's Receiving Service, of the prospects of sharing one's room or common area with someone of a different class level. Disentangling these becomes less important, however, when we consider that white employees, patients, and their families had long associated blackness with lower class, criminality, and uncleanliness. For white female patients to invoke class distinctions or for white relatives to complain about the substandard conditions of what had previously been African American male wards revealed these associations and exposed what had become their material manifestations.

Racial integration was fairly muted in the hospital's official publications, and, in internal communications, staff members emphasized that the shift in policy was done "not as a crusade" but for practical medical reasons. "In accordance with our practice to date," Hoffman wrote to Overholser, "such integration has been arranged to meet a definite need and not just for the sake of integration per se."[36] Hoffman may have been downplaying a widespread integrationist impulse among his staff to placate his racially moderate superintendent, but this is doubtful. There were a variety of opinions among the clinical staff, making any liberal consensus regarding integration unlikely. Hoffman's statements are nonetheless a reflection of the turn within the psychiatric profession toward a universalist understanding of the psyche. As racial distinctiveness became less of a fixed variable in the comprehension of mental illness, the clinical staff at Saint Elizabeths was able to emphasize symptoms, behaviors, and prognosis in their classification and treatment of patients. The universalist approach to mentally ill African Americans had progressive implications for their care and treatment. But these psychiatrists and the patients they sought to heal still had to contend with a long history of African American mistrust of the medical profession and a larger institutional, social, and political environment that was marked by skepticism, if not downright hostility, toward the idea of black equality.

Race-Neutral Psychiatry and the Persistence of Racism in Postintegration Saint Elizabeths

In 1948, a few years before the administration began integrating the hospital wards, a staff psychiatrist published an article on his therapeutic work with an African American patient that paralleled Myers and Yochelson's repudiation of the comparative psychology approach of an earlier generation of Saint Elizabeths' psychiatrists. Dr. William L. Granatir presented a paper at the tenth annual meeting of the Medical Society of St. Elizabeths Hospital in which he shared his insights into the challenges of working with a "disturbed psychotic patient" who happened to be black. In fact the difficulties in establishing an effective therapeutic relationship with the "29 year old, light-skinned, Negro, male patient" had more to do with the patient's individuated personality than his racial background, and Granatir's identification of his race in the beginning of the talk seemed more a perfunctory ritual of the clinical presentation than grounds for asserting some larger racial truth. The patient was especially troublesome, attempting suicide multiple times and engaging in other self-abusive behavior, assaulting attendants, and urinating and defecating in his room. Nonetheless the physician in charge of the patient's ward suggested to Granatir that he might be a suitable candidate for "intensive psychotherapy."

Granatir carefully and thoughtfully engaged the patient, changing the room that he interviewed him in, for instance, once he realized that the patient had received multiple electroshock therapy treatments there. But establishing an effective rapport with the patient was particularly challenging, and Granatir had only just reached that point when he presented the case to the medical society. Toward the end of the article, Granatir cursorily (and cryptically) referenced race, when he wrote, "More data is available to provide clues for further study about the operation of [the patient's] low self-esteem and closely related ideas about racial differences and the mechanisms he employed to avoid anxiety." This was, however, a far cry from the article that Philip Graven had published eighteen years earlier, in which he drew conclusions about the child-like nature of blacks based on his psychotherapy sessions with a young, middle-class, African American professional. By the postwar period, racial difference remained a clinical variable for Saint Elizabeths' psychiatrists, but it hardly occupied the same position that it had for the previous generation.[37]

One of the tactics that Granatir used to break through his patient's guardedness was the administration of the sedative sodium amytal. It was not successful, but Granatir attributed its failure to his own inexperience with interviewing someone on the medication. Within seven years Saint Elizabeths' psychiatrists would be utilizing two new drugs to assist them in their psychotherapeutic work with patients. Chlorpromazine and reserpine—marketed in the United States as Thorazine and Serpasil, respectively—were critical tools in the psychiatric armamentarium by the mid-1950s. They heralded a new age in patient management and therapy, and the psychiatric profession wasted little time in trumpeting their efficacy.

The new drugs were considered superior to the various shock therapies that were developed and deployed on the wards from the late 1930s through the 1950s. The use of insulin and metrazol to induce, respectively, temporary comas and convulsive seizures in patients were considered effective treatments for people suffering from dementia praecox (schizophrenia). After going through several treatments, patients' mental clarity tended to improve, and they became more amenable to the regimentation of hospital life, as well as to psychotherapeutic engagement. Saint Elizabeths' staff began employing insulin and metrazol shock therapies regularly in 1937, but their use was initially limited to white patients. By the winter of 1938 African American patients were undergoing both treatments, albeit on a segregated basis. The use of these therapies was short-lived, however. Minimal long-term recoveries, combined with the lack of staff needed to carry out the complex procedures, led to the determination that insulin treatment was ineffective. Metrazol shock therapy had its own problems, the least of which were the injuries that ensued from the seizures. Ruth C., a twenty-seven-year-old black Washingtonian who was being treated for schizophrenia in 1938, "dislocated her jaw on almost every treatment day," according to her medical record. Although insulin at lower doses would continue to be used through the mid-1960s, insulin coma and metrazol shock therapies were eventually displaced by electroconvulsive therapy.[38]

Electroconvulsive therapy was not developed until the late 1930s, but it was quickly in use in almost half of the mental hospitals in the United States by 1941. Although Saint Elizabeths' staff were cautious about using the therapy because of the possibility that it could lead to permanent brain damage or death, patients suffering from severe depression were routinely subjected to it. It was also used on patients who were particularly agitated, but less frequently. Electroconvulsive therapy was seen as an effective tool of patient management even as it was considered a treatment modality that would potentially facilitate the development of good psychotherapeutic relationships between patient and psychiatrist. However, it could hamper successful treatment by prompting patients to associate actions of the hospital staff with fear, pain, and loss of self, as Granatir recognized when he moved the location of his patient's psychotherapy sessions from the room in which he had received shock treatments.[39]

The new psychotropic drugs, Saint Elizabeths' officials believed, brought the same advantages as shock therapies without the risks of physical injury, brain damage, or death. They were especially effective with particularly disturbed and assaultive patients, but their advantage over other sedatives was that they did not impair the patient's consciousness. As Overholser reported on chlorpromazine in the journal of George Washington University Hospital, "This drug . . . calms the motor activity of an overactive or aggressive patient while at the same time his unconscious is not clouded; indeed, he is likely to become less confused, and to recognize the nature of his disability!" The introduction of these drugs was nothing short of a revolution. Overholser attributed a calmer, less tension-ridden environment at the hospital to the new medications. At the dedication of the new Dorothea Lynde Dix Pavilion in the spring of 1956, the superintendent told the attendees, "The climate at the hospital has changed remarkably." In fact a reporter covering the dedication pointed out, "A number of the patients watching the ceremony yesterday were beneficiaries of the new drugs."[40]

Psychiatrists argued that one of the advantages of the new drugs was that they obviated the need for staff to utilize more coercive practices of restraint and seclusion. But this was certainly open to interpretation. One Saint Elizabeths patient, interviewed in the late 1970s, recalled his introduction to the new tranquilizing drugs. Remarking on the discontinued use of tactics like wet packs and brute force to subdue patients, Lester reasoned, "That's because they don't need it. The medication's all they need. The first time I saw it, we had a guy in West Lodge, big bastard, made me look like a midget. Take eight attendants to get him into the room. One day he was standing off the whole goon squad when this little bit of a nurse comes up and zzzzzzzzip shot him full of thorazine. . . . They just stand back and wait for him to melt. Weak as a goddam baby."[41] No matter what one thought of the morality of this new form of chemical restraint, there was no doubting its efficacy. But the value of chlorpromazine and reserpine extended beyond patient management, psychiatrists argued, and into patient therapy. The drugs served as "valuable adjuncts" to other forms of therapy, including occupational therapy, recreational therapy, psychodrama, and psychotherapy. Because they did not just put individuals to sleep, the new drugs made "the patient much more accessible to psychotherapy," Overholser told the hosts of a local public affairs television program in 1963.[42]

From all indications, African American patients were as likely as whites to be given reserpine and chlorpromazine.[43] But we do not know if Saint Elizabeths' staff were more likely to administer the drugs to African American patients than to white patients. It is entirely possible that this new adjunctive therapy was disproportionately applied to African American patients given the historic tendency to characterize mentally ill blacks as combative, intractable, and downright "vicious." But by the mid-1950s the hospital was no longer providing a racial breakdown of administered treatments in its annual reports, so there is little way of assessing this. Moreover the inaccessibility of patient records places limitations on the archival evidence. Unfortunately, any racial differential in the use of chlorpromazine and reserpine must remain entirely speculative.

What is also necessarily speculative is the quality of the psychotherapeutic experiences of African American patients, including their relationship with staff psychiatrists. There was certainly a racial differential in the distribution of resources, even as the hospital was on the verge, or in the midst, of integrating its wards. In the summer of 1953, for instance, clinical director Francis Tartaglino reported that group therapy had to be suspended in the West Lodge Service because of a "lack of qualified personnel," and it did not resume until a year later. In the Geriatric Service, the recently reopened beauty salon did not employ a beautician "for our colored female patients," noted Dr. Theodore Fong in July 1958. The presence of beauty salons was considered a vital aspect of the therapeutic environment, something that William Alanson White was extremely proud of when he introduced them during his superintendency. By the late 1930s there was a beauty parlor for African American female patients. However, even though the salon in the Geriatric Service had become integrated by the late 1950s, as Fong indicated, he had trouble staffing it. It is not clear from his report whether this was the result of the racism of white volunteer beauticians who did not want to work on black women's hair, his own acquiescence to the racism of white female patients who did not want the same woman working on black women's hair and their own, the administration's lack of effort in recruiting black volunteer beauticians, or the reluctance of black beauticians to volunteer. It was most likely some combination of all of these. Nonetheless, during the period of integration there was still explicit discriminatory application of therapeutic principles, reflected in the establishment in the mid-1950s of a "charm class" for young white female patients, from which African American female patients were apparently excluded.[44]

Tartaglino's report notwithstanding, by the 1940s Saint Elizabeths' staff were conducting individual as well as group psychotherapy with African Americans. Dr. Joseph Abrahams reported on a group therapy program for African American male schizophrenics in Howard Hall, which began in October 1946. After several weeks of working together, Abrahams noted that an "atmosphere necessary for deep therapy was achieved when the group came to the conclusion that they wanted to listen to one another without showing disrespect in any of the infinite number of ways possible, that they wanted to try to understand the other fellow, and through that understanding try to help him achieve his goals."[45] The success of group therapy not only depended on the patients developing a sense of empathy and accountability toward one another; it also required that group members interact with each other in a way that validated the equal status of everyone. In this sense, these men on Howard Hall constituted a therapeutic community, a treatment model that utilized the corporate identity to address individual illness and that privileged democratic process over the older paternalistic clinician-patient relationship. This treatment model, known as milieu therapy, proliferated in mental institutions after the war.[46]

One of the principles of milieu therapy was that patients would become more amenable to psychotherapy and other treatment modalities if they were made to feel that they had a say in how their wards were run. Implementing milieu therapy first in Howard Hall, the hospital administration sought to "cultivate an atmosphere which is reasonably permissive" and that included patient self-government, social functions, guest speakers, and an orientation process for new patients that paired them with more settled patients.[47] Patient self-government took the form of patient administrative groups (PAGs). The maximum security building PAG met twice a month with the chief of the Howard Hall Service, and, according to the clinical director, the chapel in which the meetings were held was "usually filled to capacity." Other wards within the service also had PAGs. These groups functioned as deliberative bodies, making decisions about patients' responsibilities for chores, coming up with program schedules for the ward television, sanctioning patients for improper behavior, and selecting patients to receive "Man of the Month" awards. Each PAG appointed three of its members to serve as the ward's representatives on a service-wide Patients' Administrative Council, which met regularly with staff to discuss problems on the wards, including troublesome patients. The hospital administration provided a positive assessment of the new milieu model therapy. "An interesting therapeutic development was the organization of patient ward committees and an overall patients' congress which permitted greater participation in the operation of the hospital by patients than ever before," the 1957 annual report stated. "Patients received this change with great enthusiasm and cooperative understanding."[48]

By the late 1950s PAGs were extended to the hospital's other services. The clinical director of the West Side Service, Dr. William G. Cushard, reported to Overholser in 1958 that several of the wards' PAGs were up and running. He singled out the Cedar-Spruce Administrative Group, whose executive committee "has been a very positive force in the total treatment program in this area." Cushard was particularly laudatory of the PAG's role in enforcing discipline on the ward by reporting to staff patients who violated rules that the PAG itself had imposed. But ultimately, Cushard suggested, the PAGs were only as effective as the professional administration. Two years later, after the Cedar and Spruce wards were transferred from the West Side Service to the West Lodge Service, Cushard had a decidedly different assessment of the PAG. "Some difficulty was encountered during part of the year with the Spruce-Cedar Patients' Administrative Group in the West Lodge Service," he wrote in his annual report. "Because of some laxness in administrative control and a too easygoing or permissive attitude, the PAG became somewhat too active in the operation of the Service."[49] Clearly, for Cushard as well as others, there was a fine line between granting patients a certain degree of autonomy and allowing them to run the institution.

Even as the administration saw PAGs as conducive to the development of a therapeutic environment, they considered them helpful in assisting the attendants and clinical staff in policing the ward. PAGs were ward-based, and since the wards had been integrated by the mid-1950s, the patient democracy was theoretically a biracial one. There was ample opportunity, however, for racial antagonism to seep into the organizational and deliberative processes that occurred among the patients. There is no direct archival evidence that demonstrates this, but we do get a clue about the postintegration racial dynamics on the wards from the fieldwork of the sociologist Erving Goffman. Based on the observations he made at Saint Elizabeths from 1955 to 1956—which would form the empirical foundation for his classic study on total institutions—Goffman offered an assessment of race relations on the ward that suggested a generational transition was already having a positive effect. "I often heard old-line white attendants and old-line patients grumble about the occasional sight of a Negro male patient dating a white female," Goffman wrote. "Opposed to this old-line group, and separated from it by some kind of social epoch, were the hospital administration, which had desegregated the admissions and geriatric services and had begun desegregating the other services, and the leading cliques of patients, who were young and more concerned, apparently, to be 'hip' than to hold the color line."[50] Goffman's use of the term "often" suggests the existence of a great deal of racial friction, despite the countervailing administrative policy of integration and a somewhat more liberal attitude among the younger patients. This racial friction certainly would have negatively affected the patient autonomy and group sessions that were at the center of milieu therapy.[51]

But the patient administrative group could also be the vehicle for progressive change in race relations—or at least a mechanism for holding the hospital administration accountable to its claims of adopting more racially liberal policies. In the spring of 1957 members of one PAG in the William A. White Service wrote to Overholser requesting that he explain a decision to terminate racially mixed dancing at the hospital. Overholser and some staff had become uncomfortable with the interracial socializing—including sexual contact—that was becoming more and more common in the aftermath of desegregation. The members of this particular PAG expressed concern that the "abolishing of our dances is a segregation order" and made no effort to conceal their resentment. Overholser cryptically responded that the members take up the issue with the chief of their service, who "is familiar with my views in the matter." Despite some opposition to his policy among the staff itself, Overholser continued to ban interracial dancing through the rest of the decade. The exchange between Overholser and members of the PAG—and the fact that female patients on another service similarly complained about the decision—reveals the growing sense of empowerment among patients that was a hallmark of milieu therapy. It also confirms

Goffman's observation about a younger cohort of patients that, compared to its older counterpart, supported more racially liberal policies implemented by the administration, even if there was not complete agreement within the administration itself.[52]

Goffman also observed that the African American patients, along with former prisoners and homosexual patients, were one of the groups that "exploited the social possibilities" of confinement in Saint Elizabeths. "Some of these who so wished were able to *some degree* to cross the class and color line, cliquing with and dating white patients, and receiving from the psychiatric staff some of the middle-class professional conversation and treatment denied them outside the hospital," the sociologist concluded.[53] But Goffman's own qualified statement needs to be elaborated further, considering that both African American patients and white psychiatrists brought their own preconceived ideas and personal histories with them into the therapeutic encounter.[54]

Psychiatrists working with African American patients frequently remarked about the difficulty in establishing a rapport with them. Dr. Harvey R. St. Clair, a psychiatrist at the VA Hospital in Perry Point, Maryland, pointed to the tendency for his black male patients to be either suspicious of or submissive to him. The degree to which a history of mistrust shaped African Americans' perception of whites, he cautioned, should force white psychiatrists to reconsider utterances from their black patients that they might have initially attributed to paranoia. "From a dynamic point of view," St. Clair further offered, "it is felt this 'submissiveness' is probably a result of repression and suppression of intense resentment of the white man, that the Negro fears the threat of retaliation by the white man and wishes to protect himself by disguising his fear and hate behind a placating submissiveness." These fraught emotions, born not solely of interpersonal or intrapsychic conflict but of a collective sense of oppression, could hamper the ability of the patient and psychiatrist to develop an appropriate bond, according to Harold Rosen and Jerome D. Frank, professors of psychiatry at Johns Hopkins University School of Medicine. "The distrust which the Negro often brings to the white therapist," they noted, "may manifest itself in obscure ways which lead either therapist or patient to misinterpret what is going on."[55]

It was not just the fear and distrust that African Americans had of the medical profession and white society as a whole that threatened to undermine the therapeutic relationship. The erroneous ideas that white psychiatrists had about black culture also posed a problem. Even though St. Clair recognized that class differences made Negroes a diverse group, his generalizations about working-class blacks' "emotionalism, . . . greater affective demonstration, more alcoholic intake, [and] more exhibitionism," among other things, most likely shaped his approach to his black patient as much as mistrust or anger shaped the patient's response.[56] Culture had always been considered an etiological factor in mental illness, but it became a particularly prominent one as psychodynamic psychiatrists consolidated their dominance in the 1940s and 1950s. Postwar medical understandings of mental illness reflected a turn away from foregrounding the somatic, constitutional, and hereditarian origins of mental disease, a turn that had certainly begun in the early twentieth century. Many mental disorders were increasingly understood as an individual's failure to adapt to his or her social environment, which could be the result of emotionally traumatic early life experiences, inappropriate parenting, constant social stress, and more—all ultimately thwarting adequate development of the ego. The hegemony of psychodynamic psychiatry was solidified in 1952 with the publication of *Diagnostic and Statistical Manual: Mental Diseases*. The *DSM-I*, which would serve as the principal diagnostic guide for psychiatrists until it was revised in 1968, classified mental disorders into those with a somatic basis and those that were psychogenic. It included within the latter schizophrenia and manic-depressive disorder, in addition to the "milder" psychoneurotic disorders such as anxiety, phobia, and obsessive-compulsion.[57]

Psychiatrists allowed ample room for culture in the epidemiology of mental disease.[58] They thus kept the door open for persistent myths about the black psyche that had been present since the postemancipation period. Just as freedom had challenged the psychological and emotional capacities of the negro, some psychiatrists suggested that integration and the prospects of having to compete with whites on a level playing field threatened to undermine Negroes' already low self-regard. Being confined to a particular caste had afforded blacks— especially in the South—a certain psychological protection that was now being eroded by "enforced relationships with whites." African Americans' inability to cope with their new status as citizens unencumbered by caste restrictions was, in part, the product of a family structure characterized by an absent father and a domineering mother. One legacy of slavery, the matriarchal culture of African Americans, many psychologists and social scientists believed, prevented black children from becoming productive, normally functioning adults with adequate coping mechanisms to deal with disappointment, adversity, and failure.[59]

Some of the ways in which psychiatrists discussed mental illness among African Americans were clear reverberations from late nineteenth- and turn-of-the-twentieth-century ideas about black insanity. One was the assumption that blacks rarely experienced depression. This diagnostic fallacy turned on a century-old myth of the naturally jovial negro even as some postwar psychiatrists cloaked it in the psychodynamic rationale that blacks had less to lose than whites—including prestige and self-esteem—and therefore were less susceptible to depressive feelings.[60] A corollary idea that was, in fact, nothing more than a retread of the late nineteenth-century notion that blacks were more prone to mania, held that their psychoses were more likely to manifest as schizophrenia. In addition to the mental breakdowns that were accompanying the rapid change in race relations in the South, for instance, two psychiatrists working with data on state hospital admissions in Virginia claimed that African Americans were succumbing to "psychoses and aggressive crimes." In particular, they pointed to increased rates of schizophrenia as evidence that the political agitation over civil rights was harmful for a generation of African Americans that was accustomed to occupying a lower social caste. Equality with whites, to echo many nineteenth-century psychiatrists, was detrimental to the mental health of blacks.[61]

Much of the resuscitation of postemancipation mythologies of black insanity was done by psychiatrists working in the civil rights–era South and reflected a defense of Jim Crow. But an emergent portrait of the typical African American sufferer of mental disease was being produced by psychiatrists on both sides of the Mason-Dixon line. Three health care professionals working with mentally ill Philadelphians in the early 1950s, for instance, sustained a particular image of the atavistic insane negro in a study they conducted on the "mental breakdown patterns" of two groups: a high-status group that consisted of all whites and a low-status group that included all nonwhites. One of the hypotheses of the study was that "the pattern of mental disorder will show a greater prevalence of extreme aggressive behavior (paranoid schizophrenic reactions) or extreme withdrawal behavior (other schizophrenic reactions) for the low-status than for the high-status group." The authors attributed the preponderance of schizophrenic reactions among nonwhites to their "frustrated environments" rather than their biology and recommended that mental health care workers pay particular attention to their patients' social context. They also advocated "removing social barriers" as a critical tool for the prevention of mental disease. Even as the authors' prescriptions might be considered more progressive, however, the image of nonwhite mental illness that the study proffered was hardly a significant departure from what predominated before World War II.[62]

Characterizations of black insanity as especially deviant—and perhaps not amenable to conventional therapy—persisted well into the 1950s and 1960s. At Saint Elizabeths this characterization contributed to a veritable conflation of mentally ill blacks and the criminally insane, a throwback to the late nineteenth century. As Walter Barton, the medical director of the APA, testified before an ad hoc congressional committee holding a hearing on the federal institution, the typical criminal patient at the hospital was an uneducated, unskilled, single, African American male "with a history of anti-social acts." This development could not be laid solely at the feet of the psychiatric profession or Saint Elizabeths' staff; demographic changes and patterns of policing in the District certainly contributed to it. But despite a universalist turn with the emergence of social psychiatry and the elimination of official segregationist policies, there were clearly residual elements of late nineteenth- and early twentieth-century thought about mentally ill African Americans.[63]

An inherited legacy of racist constructions of the black psyche could combine with learned defense mechanisms to produce misdiagnoses and, subsequently, misguided therapeutic efforts. Rosen and Frank alerted their fellow psychiatrists to this potential problem in their 1962 *American Journal of Psychiatry* article. "Many Negroes, especially of lower class status, tend to defend themselves against unanticipated demands from the white by assuming an exaggerated air of indifference and stupidity," they pointed out. "The white psychiatrist may be misled by this into making an unwarranted diagnosis of mental deficiency or even of simple schizophrenia; yet the same patient may show normal responsiveness and intelligence when interviewed by a colored psychiatrist."[64] In suggesting that white psychiatrists were potentially led into misdiagnosis by a number of factors—including an unfamiliarity with black cultural cues and deliberate dissembling by black sufferers—Rosen and Frank stopped short of labeling the psychiatric profession racist. Yet they did implicitly point out the existing problem of the paucity of African American psychiatrists.

Perhaps the biggest difference between the postemancipation and postwar eras was that more people—both inside and outside of the profession—were willing to confront the psychiatric profession about the racist undercurrents that propelled the production of psychiatric knowledge and the actual treatment of mentally ill people of color. Some of this critique emerged in the antipsychiatry movement, a loose, organic collection of psychiatrists, humanists, and social scientists in the 1960s and 1970s, who criticized psychiatry for functioning as a form of social control and, in some cases, challenged the validity of mental disease as a real biological or psychological phenomenon.[65] Much of the criticism came from progressive white and African American psychiatrists and psychologists—many of whom were influenced by the radical politics of the Black Power movement and the anticolonial ideology of the Martinican psychiatrist Frantz Fanon—and characterized the predominantly white psychiatric profession as "an instrument in the service of the Establishment."[66]

Increasingly psychiatrists were taking up the issue of institutional racism, both as a problem in the profession and as a societal reality that could serve as a catalyst for mental disorder and an obstacle to proper treatment. Melvin Sabshin, Herman Diesenhaus, and Raymond Wilkerson, all professors in the University of Illinois Department of Psychiatry, delivered a paper at the annual meeting of the APA in 1970 in which they addressed the myriad ways that the psychiatric profession both underserved and did a disservice to the African American community. The absence of mental health clinics in black neighborhoods, income disparities that inhibited access to private treatment, and a legal system that was all too eager to criminalize the psychopathological behavior of African Americans were the principal manifestations of institutionalized racism in mental health care. Dominant cultural representations of blacks as naturally deviant continued to shape white psychiatrists' approach to mentally ill African Americans. "White American psychiatry has its equivalent racist stereotypes about the black psychiatric patient," they noted, "*hostile* and *not motivated for treatment, having primitive character structure, not psychologically minded,* and *impulse-ridden.*" In the end, the structural inequalities that existed in the nation and the unconscious (and conscious) prejudicial attitudes of white psychiatrists perpetuated a racist mental health care system as far as African Americans were concerned. As the professors succinctly stated, "White societal forces have created a network of institutions and gateways that regularly channel the disvalued black away from needed treatment by failing to provide accessible facilities, by defining certain behavior as criminal in blacks but as sickness in whites, and by defining blacks as untreatable."[67]

Challenges to the racial inequity in the mental health care system also came from patients. In 1966 a thirty-three-year-old African American resident of the District of Columbia, Maurice Millard, sued Saint Elizabeths over what he described as inadequate treatment. Millard had pled guilty to indecent exposure in 1962 and was committed to Saint Elizabeths under the District's sexual psychopath law. His ability to bring suit against the hospital was the result of a landmark legal decision the same year, *Rouse v. Cameron*, in which the US Court of Appeals ruled that patients at mental hospitals had a right to receive treatment and that treatment could be reviewed by trial judges. Millard claimed that during his five years at the institution, he had not received treatment. Instead he spent most of his time either watching television or mopping the floors. At the trial, Dr. David Dabney, an African American psychiatrist and former employee of the hospital who testified on Millard's behalf, attributed his inadequate treatment to his race and socioeconomic status. "Dabney said that as a practical matter the patients at St. Elizabeths least likely to get psychotherapy are low-income Negroes," related a *Washington Post* reporter covering the trial. When asked by Millard's lawyer why this was the case, Dabney chalked it up to "built-in bias." Judge William B. Jones of the US District Court ultimately held that Saint Elizabeths was providing Millard extensive treatment and that, based on the conditions of his commitment, he would remain at the hospital until the clinical staff determined he had recovered.[68]

But Millard's legal challenge had raised some thorny issues that went beyond determinations of the adequacy of treatment. One was the question of whether racial bias influenced the therapeutic regime at Saint Elizabeths. Another was the increasing criminalization of people with mental illness. Dr. Michael Miller, a private physician in the District and a former staff member at Saint Elizabeths, wrote a blistering letter to the editor castigating the "inhuman, outrageous and unjust" manner in which Millard's disorder had been treated in the first place. Characterizing him as a "sexually passive neurotic" but "relatively harmless," Miller argued that his disorder would be better treated through outpatient therapy than institutionalization. Locking up Millard, a husband and father of six children, would not only retard his own chances of recovery; it would also unnecessarily damage his family. "Is it in the public interest for the public to have to pay for the care of the family indefinitely," Miller asked, "while the father is not being given treatment so he can return to society to assume his responsibilities?"[69] Although the court's decision to Miller's rhetorical question was a maybe, the larger challenge to the idea that the best way to handle mentally ill people was to institutionalize them would only intensify.

Centennial Postscript

In the June 1955 issue of the patient-run journal *Elizabethan*, a patient commemorated the hospital's centennial by lauding the innovations that it had made in the field of psychiatry since its founding. One in particular resonated with the recent changes occurring at Saint Elizabeths. The writer noted that in constructing a separate lodge in 1855, Saint Elizabeths had become "the second hospital in the entire world to make provision for the colored insane."[70] The writer did not mention that the hospital was in the middle of abandoning its tradition of racially segregating patients so it is impossible to say whether he or she wanted to draw a connection between how race figured in the founders' vision of the asylum and the racial realities of mid-twentieth-century American society. In fact the writer might instead have pointed out that Saint Elizabeths was pioneering in another way. As a federal hospital in the South, it was among the vanguard of hospitals serving a primarily civilian population to begin desegregating its wards, a full decade before the Supreme Court's decision in *Simkins v. Moses Cone Memorial Hospital* in 1964 and the creation of Medicaid and Medicare in 1965 began the systematic dismantling of Jim Crow in the nation's healthcare system.[71]

The *Elizabethan* writer's decision to highlight the hundredth anniversary of the construction of the "colored lodge" is rich with irony. The endpoints of the centennial represented an inverse (and perverse) relationship between the demographics of the patient population and how it was managed, on the one hand, and the status of the hospital, on the other. Saint Elizabeths enjoyed a reputation as a leader in the field of asylum medicine and institutional psychiatry from the mid-nineteenth century to World War II, when the population it served was predominantly military and it practiced racial segregation. Following the war, as the army and navy stopped sending its active-duty service personnel to the hospital and veterans began transferring into the VA system, Saint Elizabeths' patient population became increasingly civilian and older. With the continued in-migration of African Americans and white flight in the 1950s and 1960s, the patient population also became blacker. Hospital officials still expressed a great deal of optimism and confidence in the wake of the centennial, and Saint Elizabeths remained an important component in the federal mental healthcare enterprise for some years to come. But by 1955 the institution's best days were behind it. Within a decade and a half, Saint Elizabeths, once touted as a model institution, would become synonymous with poor, elderly, criminal, and mentally ill black Washingtonians, and deinstitutionalization would turn it into a shell of its former self.

10

From Model to Emblem

Community Mental Health and Deinstitutionalization, 1963–1987

In 1961 a twenty-two-year-old white man, Charles H. Rouse, was committed to Saint Elizabeths as criminally insane after being arrested on illegal weapons charges. The reason for his arrest was that he had been found walking in a black neighborhood after dark with a gun and ammunition. Rouse was found not guilty by reason of insanity, diagnosed as a sociopath, and institutionalized. Rouse appealed his commitment, and in 1966 the case *Rouse v. Cameron* ended up in the US Court of Appeals, where it was heard by Judge David L. Bazelon. Bazelon was sympathetic to Rouse's Legal Aid lawyers' arguments that his commitment was unconstitutional. To acquit someone on the grounds of insanity, institutionalize him, and then fail to provide some form of therapy amounted to cruel and unusual treatment, the appellate judge ruled. Although Rouse was ultimately released because the court found that his insanity plea had been entered over his objection, Bazelon's ruling established the "right to treatment" legal principle that served as the basis of Maurice Millard's case the same year.[1]

The defendant in the *Rouse* case was Dale Cameron, who had become superintendent when Winfred Overholser retired in 1962. Cameron inherited the helm of an institution that was still plagued by many of the problems of his predecessors: overcrowding, underfunding, and a patient population that was increasingly suffering from chronic illnesses. By minimal space standards, Cameron wrote in 1963, Saint Elizabeths was 33 percent over capacity; if one applied optimal standards, the hospital's overcapacity was at 61 percent. Seventy-eight percent of admissions were residents of the District, continuing a trend that had begun in the mid-1940s. Of those District residents who were committed, nearly 50 percent were suffering from chronic functional mental illness, and 33 percent were geriatric patients who had organic neurological problems. Just over 11 percent were forensic patients—either individuals who had been committed after having been found not guilty by reason of insanity or who were undergoing court-ordered psychiatric evaluation to determine whether they were sufficiently competent to stand trial.[2]

The persistence of the problems associated with massive state mental hospitals triggered another lawsuit against Saint Elizabeths in 1974. In the case of *Dixon v. Weinberger*, however, the plaintiffs successfully sued for the right to receive treatment in the least restrictive setting. Both *Rouse* and *Dixon* were part of a larger patients' rights movement that emerged in the 1960s and 1970s.[3] This movement intersected with another movement driven less by patients and their lawyers and more by government officials and the psychiatric profession itself. The development of psychopharmacology and social psychiatry combined to usher in a new phase of care for people with mental illness. Concerned with the deteriorating conditions of the large public hospitals that existed in nearly every state, the profession as a whole began to advocate for a decentralization of the services provided to mentally ill people. Present since the early twentieth century, the desire to amplify psychiatric care beyond the walls of the hospital—for both those who became outpatients or former patients and those whose mental stress had not yet warranted commitment—coalesced into the comprehensive community mental health care movement by the 1960s. Unlike the earlier mental hygiene movement, this postwar community psychiatry envisioned giving patients and the communities from which they came more control over their care, and it would eventually lead to full-blown deinstitutionalization in the late 1960s and 1970s.

Certainly inspired by concern for the mentally ill and their families, the movement to decentralize mental health care delivery was a long and complex drama that introduced new problems even as it nobly confronted old ones. The results of deinstitutionalization—the relocation of chronically ill geriatric patients to nursing homes and the increase of the mentally ill homeless population in American cities—as well as the multitude of factors that hindered more successful outcomes, are well known by public policymakers, academics, and the general public.[4] In the nation's capital, community mental health care and deinstitutionalization were made all the more challenging by the larger political question over who would control Saint Elizabeths: the federal government or the District?

Even though the changes in policy approaches to mental illness in the District cannot be reduced to being "a superb example of mental health as pure politics," as drafters of a 1972 task force claimed, community mental health and deinstitutionalization were political and deeply politicized processes nonetheless.[5] Residents of the most marginalized neighborhoods in Southeast and Southwest Washington, DC, understood that these new policy approaches were riven with organizational and governmental politics and, in engaging with Saint Elizabeths around community mental health care, expressed a rights consciousness in the process. Black Washingtonians initiated some of the first lay-professional partnerships around community mental health care and sought a place at the table where decisions would be made over how best to deliver that care. Ordinary citizens considered themselves stakeholders in one of the preeminent mental hospitals in the country, and they were seen as such by many officials associated with the institution. In the end, as Saint Elizabeths became more "local" in character—serving a largely civilian population that was disproportionately black and poor—it, and the patients it served, became victims of federal neglect, despite the hopes of its staff and some government officials that the hospital would continue to serve as a model of humane and enlightened care.

The Politics of Community Mental Health Care

The growing concern about the decrepit conditions of state mental hospitals and the poor treatment of mentally ill people in the immediate postwar years evolved into a national reexamination of mental health care policy by the mid-1950s. Hospital superintendents took steps to ameliorate the problems that existed within their institutions, and Saint Elizabeths was no exception. In the early 1950s Overholser implemented a family care program in an attempt to alleviate some of the overcrowded wards in the hospital. The successful but small-scale effort to place improved patients in the homes of nonrelatives was aided, in part, by the calmative effects of chlorpromazine and reserpine. Family care also required stronger connections between the hospital and the surrounding community, which Overholser sought to foster by holding "open houses" so that local residents could visit and become familiar with how the institution operated. During one such open house, more than five hundred community members attended. These efforts to tap into community resources notwithstanding, the admissions at Saint Elizabeths continued to increase, which, combined with personnel shortages, led to an enhanced use of restraint and seclusion in some services.[6]

The success of the new medications created another set of challenges for Saint Elizabeths staff, however. On the one hand, they led to an increase in demand for services by Washingtonians seeking to take advantage of the voluntary admission law and obtain treatment for their mental disorders. On the other hand, according to the 1957 annual report, the drugs "produced a return to reality in many long-term care patients, without improvement to the point where they could be released from the hospital," which in turn put more pressure on staff to keep these previously withdrawn patients occupied. These developments put extra strain on the hospital personnel, which was already understaffed by the loss of psychiatrists to private practice.[7]

The conditions at Saint Elizabeths were representative of the nation's mental health care system as a whole. Confronted with an increasingly geriatric and chronically ill patient population in overcrowded and underresourced wards, leaders in the mental health care field began an intensive study of the systemic needs of the mentally ill population and the programs that served them: from prevention to postinstitutional care, from treatment in institutions to the provision of outpatient services. Initiated by the American Psychiatric Association and the American Medical Association and funded by the Mental Health Study Act of 1955, the Joint Commission on Mental Illness and Health (JCMIH) included representatives from the American Hospital Association, the VA, the Council of State Governments, and the National Institute of Mental Health (NIMH), as well as nursing, psychiatric social work, and clinical psychology organizations. Although Congress provided some funding for the commission, it was a nongovernmental body. Over the course of five years, the commission produced ten studies on various aspects of the problem of mental illness and the medical, social, and policy responses to it. The commission's final report, *Action for Mental Health*, released in 1961, made several far-reaching recommendations, including additional investment in research on mental disease, a more concerted campaign to recruit and train professional and lay mental health care workers, greater efforts to educate the public about mental illness, and a formidable increase in federal funding for mental health care services, including community-based clinics.[8]

Also in the JCMIH's final report was a recommendation that newly built public mental hospitals should contain no more than one thousand beds and that existing large state hospitals should be turned into centers for the long-term care of people with chronic diseases, including but not limited to mental illness. Although Overholser agreed with much of the commission's emphasis on the importance of integrating the inpatient services of existing hospitals with the prevention and postcare services offered by community facilities such as nursing homes, halfway houses, and outpatient clinics, he objected to the premise that a large institution was by definition antithetical to effective care and treatment. He certainly thought that overcrowding was a problem, but he cautioned against breaking up Saint Elizabeths into smaller hospitals without maintaining "control or coordination" of existing services. Overholser concluded his 1962 annual report—the last of his tenure as superintendent—by raising a concern about the JCMIH's recommendations for overhauling the nation's mental health care system, couching it in a language of exceptionalism: "It seems clear to all who are familiar with the history of the hospital, its international reputation, and the consistent support which has been given to it by Congress that the founders intended that there should be a national institution to set the pace for the various States in the lines of patient care, training, and research. Saint Elizabeths is in a unique position to do this, yet there are certain forces which appear to be interested in downgrading the institution to that of a District hospital."[9]

Despite Overholser's concern that there was a movement afoot to transform Saint Elizabeths into nothing more than a glorified nursing home, the joint commission did at least advocate for the preservation of the state mental hospital system. Evolving as a response to the joint commission's set of recommendations was an alternative approach, advanced primarily by NIMH officials, which was based on the shift of services from institutions to community-centered organizations. Both approaches had much to commend them and received varying levels of support from politicians, elected officials, and policymakers. The Democratic Party's platform in 1960 reflected support for both approaches, promising to increase federal funding in all phases of mental health care: basic research, training of mental health care workers, and community programs. Advocates for reform welcomed the election of John F. Kennedy, who, shaped by his own family's experiences of dealing with a mentally disabled child, was more than open to expanding federal authority in the care and treatment of the mentally ill and the promotion of mental health.

Robert H. Felix and Stanley Yolles, the director and deputy director of the NIMH, respectively, were staunch advocates for the community-oriented approach to mental health care. They also argued for an emphasis on prevention rather than institutional care. Felix and Yolles were instrumental in Kennedy's Interagency Task Force on Mental Health, which ultimately recommended that comprehensive community mental health care form the core of the president's policy. The task force proposed the creation of 500 community mental health centers by the end of the decade and an additional 1,500 by 1980, which would effectively eliminate the need for the large public mental hospital. And whereas the JCMIH emphasized federal funding of existing state hospitals, the task force suggested that the federal government should provide initial funding for demonstration projects and construction of centers but that states should eventually assume responsibility for operating costs and any future construction.[10]

Kennedy ended up endorsing the approach of the task force—and hence the NIMH and the Department of Health, Education, and Welfare (HEW)—and the comprehensive community mental health center (CMHC) became the basis for his administration's policy on mental illness. On February 5, 1963, the president submitted a message to Congress that laid out the new policy direction. Ten days later, in a letter to the secretary of HEW, Anthony Celebrezze, he stressed the importance of Washington as an ideal site for the development of the model CMHC. Like Saint Elizabeths' superintendents throughout the hospital's history, Kennedy invoked the unique nature of the nation's capital; however, he ignored the institution itself. "It is my desire that you provide every possible help to the [District's Board of] Commissioners in this important endeavor, so that in this significant area of human need the Capital of the United States may become ... a city of which the Nation may be proud—an example and a show place for the rest of the world," he wrote to Celebrezze.[11] Overholser was supportive of Kennedy's policy of federally funding state efforts to develop CMHCs, although he expressed skepticism that the training of mental health care workers would be able to keep pace with the centers' needs.[12]

In October 1963, eight months after Kennedy submitted his special message to Congress, both houses passed and the president signed the Mental Retardation and Community Mental Health Centers Act. The law authorized $150 million in federal grants for three years for the purpose of building CMHCs. Upon approval of construction applications submitted by states, the federal government would fund between one-third and two-thirds of the construction costs. The law also granted HEW authority to establish standards and regulate CMHCs. In 1964 HEW promulgated guidelines that required the centers to provide inpatient and outpatient services, partial hospitalization services, around-the-clock emergency services, and educational and training programs for community organizations and mental health care professionals.[13]

Shortly after the 1963 legislation passed, HEW formed an advisory group to assess how Saint Elizabeths would fit into the new model of comprehensive community mental health care, and particularly how it might straddle its relationships with, and responsibilities to, the federal government and the local community. Although the group was tasked with producing a forward-looking analysis, much of the report zeroed in on the institutional problems that had plagued Saint Elizabeths for years. The advisory group identified several deficiencies in the hospital's operation and its existing relationship with the District of Columbia. Many of them—such as overcrowding, personnel shortages, a deteriorating infrastructure, and a growing geriatric and chronically ill patient population—had been perennial problems and had certainly intensified over the previous two decades. Some, however, commanded much more attention, even if they were not particularly new developments.[14]

One of the problems that was gaining more consideration was the presence of two categories of patients—the elderly and the young—who would be better served in other facilities. The report indicated that there were approximately one hundred children and teenagers who were housed in adult wards, a problem that was the result of the lack of any residential treatment facilities for mentally disturbed youths in the District. Elderly, chronically ill patients were also ill-served at Saint Elizabeths. Ideally, the advisory group acknowledged, these patients should be in foster care facilities or nursing homes with psychiatric beds. However, the District's public nursing home, D. C. Village, had stopped accepting patients from Saint Elizabeths in 1962. Most of the elderly patients at Saint Elizabeths could not afford private nursing homes, and the District's public assistance payments could hardly cover the nursing homes' fees. The city's monthly public assistance benefits were roughly half of what nursing homes in the Washington area charged. The dearth of public eldercare facilities, the unaffordability of private homes, and the tendency of private home operators not to accept Saint Elizabeths patients contributed to a graying, chronically ill institutional population.[15]

The advisory group also identified the existence of prisoner patients as a problem that needed to be addressed. It was not so much the numbers, as only roughly 11 percent of the patients were of "prisoner status." Rather, it was the fact that their numbers exceeded the capacity of the maximum-security John Howard Pavilion, which had replaced Howard Hall in 1959. As a result, a number of patients escaped and then committed crimes, prompting criticism from both the press and public officials. The advisory group proposed the establishment of a separate facility for male prisoners, built around the Howard Pavilion and administered by both Saint Elizabeths and the US Public Health Service. Eventually, the group suggested, control of the facility could be transferred to the District, which would pay for the incarceration of DC prisoners and be reimbursed by Congress for the incarceration of federal prisoners. Superintendent Cameron supported the creation of a separate facility but opposed separating administration of the facility from the overall administration of Saint Elizabeths as well as the transfer of control to the municipal government. In the end, HEW did not act on this particular recommendation, and the maximum-security division remained part of the institution.[16]

The final report from the advisory group contained two overarching recommendations that were certainly in tension if not completely contradictory. In many ways, this was born of Saint Elizabeths' federal status and its location in the nation's capital. The advisory group highlighted a number of the institution's assets—its proximity to the NIMH, which was located in Bethesda, Maryland, and local universities; the robust psychiatric professional presence in the Washington area, including the national headquarters of the APA; and its history as a preeminent research and teaching hospital. All of these suggested that Saint Elizabeths should continue to serve as a federal center for research and training in mental health care delivery. On the other hand, the advisory group also recommended that the hospital be fully incorporated into the city's community mental health care system. From the advisory group's perspective, these recommendations were hardly incompatible; indeed they were interdependent. Given that the national policy was now based on comprehensive community mental health care, the group's chairman, Boisfeuillet Jones, made the argument that Saint Elizabeths and HEW would have to work closely with the District's Department of Public Health in order for the hospital to maintain its prominence in research and training.[17]

Critical to both of these conceptions of Saint Elizabeths' future was the reduction of the size of its inpatient population. The advisory group suggested that through the movement of elderly and chronically ill patients into nursing homes and long-term care facilities, the creation of a separate institution for male prisoner patients, and the transfer of young patients into residential psychiatric treatment units, the overall number of patients in the hospital could be cut from over 6,500 to 2,500. A decrease in the number of patients would bring the hospital in line with the community mental health model's emphasis on smaller treatment units while also continuing to provide HEW and NIMH with a "population laboratory" with which to conduct research. In order to optimize these research opportunities, the advisory group recommended that the hospital be transferred to the Public Health Service, a subagency of HEW, and administered by NIMH. Transfer of control of Saint Elizabeths to the District's government was out of the question, "for there is strong reason to believe [that it] would result in a prompt deterioration in the quality of the Hospital's professional staff," the advisory group counseled. Nonetheless the institution should continue to serve the District's population, both by providing medium- and long-term care for the entire city's mentally ill population and by offering intensive inpatient treatment for residents of Southeast DC.[18]

The advisory group's suggestion that Saint Elizabeths provide inpatient services to residents of the southeastern quadrant of the city was in keeping with its overarching recommendation that the hospital be integrated into the District's community mental health care program. The CMHC model was based on the principle of geographic distribution, in which CMHCs would be dispersed throughout a city or state so as to make the centers easily accessible to all of its residents. Cities or states were segmented into catchment areas, ideally—and arbitrarily, according to some critics—containing a population of between 75,000 and 200,000. Defining catchment areas in this limited way would put those in need of mental health care closer to treatment facilities and ensure that centers would not be stretched beyond their capacity.[19] Essentially the advisory group's recommendation was to turn part of Saint Elizabeths into a CMHC for one of the District's catchment areas.

Assisted by a $2 million federal grant, the District had begun planning its community mental health care system at the same time that the advisory group was assessing the future of Saint Elizabeths. District officials agreed with many of the advisory group's recommendations, including the importance of reducing the size of the hospital, although they were less sanguine about the ability to do so. They also concurred with the group's suggestion that Saint Elizabeths function as the CMHC for the catchment area for Southeast DC and continue to provide medium- and long-term care for all of the District's mentally ill residents. Where city officials dissented from the advisory group was in the latter's insistence that administration of Saint Elizabeths remain with the federal government. The officials designing the District's program countered the federal government's self-important claims by making an argument for the imperative of local control. Dr. Murray Grant, the District's director of public health, wrote to an HEW official in March 1964, "The possibility of developing Saint Elizabeths Hospital as a model for other jurisdictions in planning and implementing the transition from large custodial-type hospitals to community-based mental health centers rests on the premise that this transition be planned, directed and accomplished by local effort." District officials considered the dual objectives of turning Saint Elizabeths into a federal center for "research and development" and an integral part of a more locally based community mental health care system—objectives seen by the advisory group as mutually beneficial—as having the potential to undermine their own efforts.[20]

For the next two and a half years, federal and local officials continued to study the questions of how best to merge these two visions of Saint Elizabeths' future and how HEW and the District's Mental Health Authority could most effectively collaborate in the management of the hospital. These two and a half years represented a limbo for many on Saint Elizabeths' staff. The uncertainty of whether the institution would be a centerpiece for federal efforts to enhance research into mental disease and training of mental health care workers or primarily a CMHC serving the local community led to the departure of many on the hospital's clinical staff. The uncertainty also made it difficult for the hospital's administration to recruit employees, particularly qualified psychiatry residents.

In August 1967 HEW secretary John Gardner announced the decision to transfer control of Saint Elizabeths to NIMH. Even though on its face this reorganization suggested that federal officials viewed research and training to be the primary missions of the hospital, Gardner clearly indicated that the institution's integration into the District's mental health care system was high on his agenda. "This move will permit Saint Elizabeths to serve as a national demonstration for the conversion of a large, old-style mental institution into a modern, community-based mental health facility," he stated in a press release. To that end, he was supportive of the eventual transfer of Saint Elizabeths to the District's health department, and he announced that he would work with the District's Board of Commissioners to create an Advisory Committee on Hospital-Community Relationships in Mental Health. The *Washington Post* celebrated the move, opining that NIMH control of the hospital would elevate it to its once august stature. "St. Elizabeths was once the leader in the Nation's mental health program," the editorial board declared. "It now has the opportunity to take over that leadership again."[21]

By the following fall, NIMH had reorganized the structure of Saint Elizabeths. In November 1968 NIMH director Stanley Yolles announced the establishment of the National Center for Mental Health Services, Training, and Research (NCMHSTR). As the title suggested, the center had three core responsibilities, and it was structured as such. One division of the center was concerned primarily with clinical research, including "clinical neurology, personality assessment, and clinical behavior." The Division of Intramural Training focused on preparing professionals to utilize the most up-to-date treatment techniques as well as to engage the "new concepts of community-wide treatment and prevention services." Related to this was the third division, which remained the heart of the hospital's day-to-day operations: the Saint Elizabeths Hospital-Division of Clinical and Community Services. This division comprised the medium- and long-term treatment and care facilities that existed at the hospital prior to its reorganization. The division also included the CMHC that would serve the residents who lived south of the Anacostia River in Southeast and Southwest DC—otherwise known as Area D.[22]

"Special Needs of Ghetto Citizens": Area D Community Mental Health Center

Washington was one of the first cities to take advantage of the federal funding authorized by the Mental Retardation and Community Mental Health Centers Act, when it secured a $2 million grant in 1964. The Directorate for Mental Health, which was under the Department of Public Health, began planning for the development of CMHCs in the District. It established four catchment areas, but these did not correspond neatly to the District's quadrants. The first catchment area that the department targeted to receive a CMHC was Area C. Opened in 1966 and housed in the psychiatric services of DC General Hospital—Gallinger Hospital's name since 1953—the center served residents in Southwest and Southeast north of the Anacostia River and a significant portion of Northeast. After establishing Area C's center, the department turned its attention to Area B, which included the east-central section of Northwest and part of Northeast. Because of its location in Area B, Howard University partnered with the department to obtain an NIMH grant, but the relationship between the two fell apart over disputes as to which entity would control the center. Area B did not acquire a center until August 1969, when the city purchased and renovated a former Jewish nursing home just north of Howard's campus. Both Area B and Area C consisted of predominantly low-income communities of color, the former containing a large number of Latino residents. Area A was the last catchment area to acquire a center, which it did in 1972. However, Area A, which included Georgetown and upper Northwest, was also the most affluent catchment area, whose residents had greater access to private psychiatrists. As a *Washington Post* reporter quipped in 1967, "No one worries about Area A."[23]

Following the transfer of Saint Elizabeths to NIMH in the summer of 1967, a task force consisting of both District and federal officials was formed to begin planning Area D's CMHC. Consistent with the general principles of comprehensive community mental health care, the task force recognized that the CMHC had to be fully integrated into the existing services—both public and private—in the local area; had to be easily accessible to community residents, largely through satellite offices located in neighborhood clinics; had to offer individualized treatment plans; and had to contain a public education and advocacy component. In order to develop a center that was responsive to the community, it was imperative that its planners be especially familiar with the needs of that community and to work with local leaders and organizations. Although the area still had pockets of middle-class whites, significant outmigration by whites combined with in-migration of African Americans displaced by urban renewal projects in other parts of the city led to a predominantly black population by the late 1960s. A number of public housing projects dotted the landscape, and what had once been the area's chief appeal, its remoteness from the "mainstream of metropolitan D.C. life," was now a cause and symptom of urban blight. The Anacostia River functioned as a natural barrier, according to the task force, leading to the "particularly isolated, barren character of the Area D ghetto." The CMHC's core mission needed to be to meet the "special needs of ghetto citizens," including helping them deal with "emerging problems in the areas of drug abuse, delinquency, educational and vocational handicaps, relative mental retardation, illegitimacy, child neglect, alcoholism, adult crime and the exacerbation of all psychiatric conditions due to social isolation and poor community identity."[24]

In order to serve this population—as well as the "high-risk" groups that were already institutionalized at D. C. Village and the District's home for dependent children, Junior Village—Area D's center would need to have an extensive presence in the community and would need to be thoroughly staffed. The task force proposed a three-layered approach to community mental health care in Anacostia and Southwest, anchored at Saint Elizabeths and spreading out into the surrounding neighborhoods in concentric circles. At the core would be a community mental health center located at the Dix Building, with the capacity to house one hundred inpatients, including separate rooms for up to two dozen children and adolescents. The center would also provide twenty-four-hour emergency services. Extending out beyond Saint Elizabeths' campus, the Area D CMHC would have "subarea mental health satellites." The task force estimated that there should be one satellite center for every fifty thousand residents,

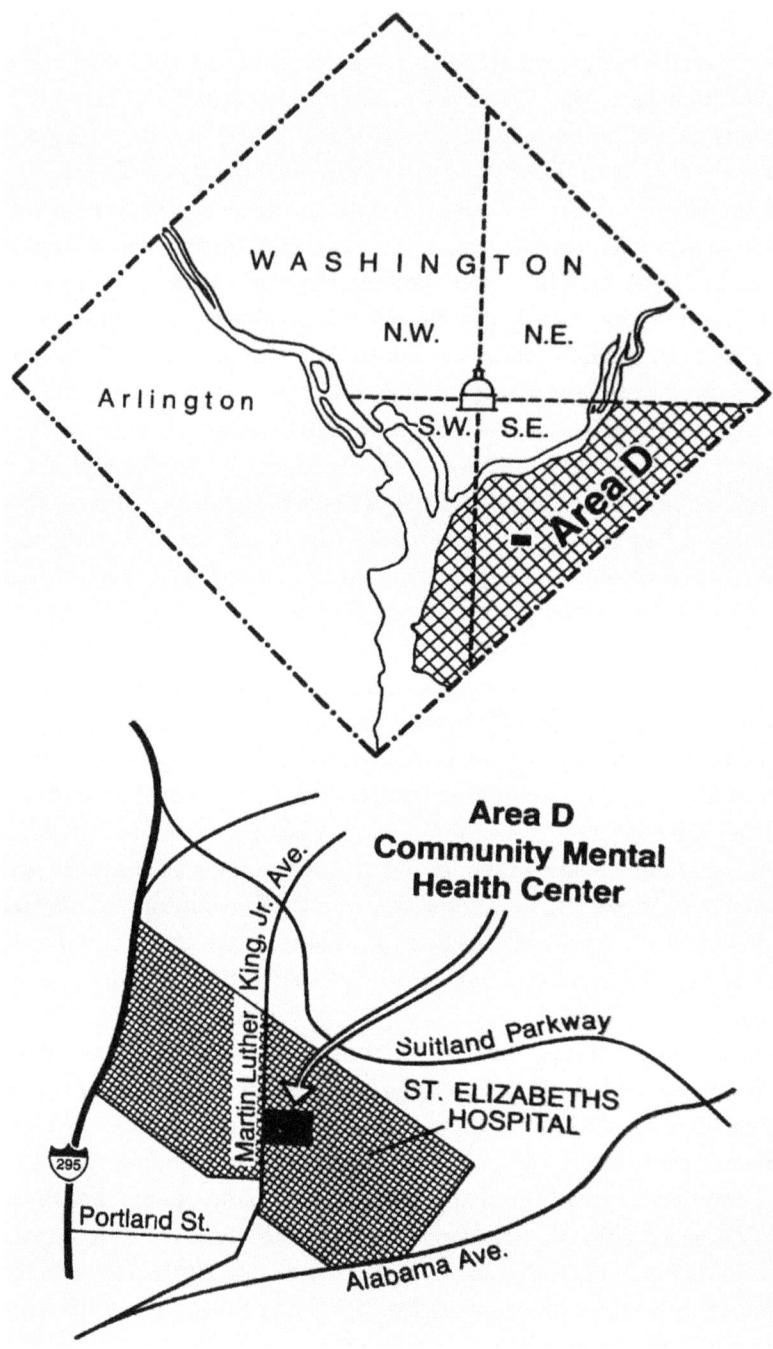

A map of Area D, a catchment area of the District of Columbia's community mental health care system, which comprised the portions of Southeast and Southwest DC that lay south of the Anacostia River. Area D's community mental health center, located on the Saint Elizabeths campus, served a predominantly black inpatient and outpatient population. *Department of Health, Education, and Welfare, Programs and Services of the Area D Community Mental Health Center (Washington, DC: US Department of Health, Education, and Welfare, 1971).*

and the centers should be located near welfare offices, social service organizations, and recreation and community centers. Each satellite center should be staffed with professionals who were capable of providing screening and treatment for outpatients as well as walk-ins. Finally, the outer appendages of the CMHC should be even more firmly embedded in community institutions. Satellite centers would be responsible for outreach, making contact with tenant associations, settlement houses, public clinics, and day care facilities.[25]

These secondary satellite centers required collaboration with community organizations. The task force felt confident that it could find neighborhood partners to work with, as it reported in May 1968 that there was a "'grass roots' movement pushing the development of a local community mental health center." The task force was most likely referring to residents of the Valley Green neighborhood, who approached Saint Elizabeths in February and requested that the hospital provide mental health services in the area. Some Saint Elizabeths staff members began meeting regularly with residents and established the Valley Green Counseling Center that spring. But task force members were also careful not to take community participation for granted. They acknowledged that there was still a fair amount of skepticism on the part of local residents due to Saint Elizabeths' "reputation as an 'end of the road,' remote state hospital." Indeed in its final report in early 1969, committee members continued to express concern that it was going to be difficult to obtain maximum community participation in the CMHC. To address this, they suggested that any CMHC should provide space for other resources that served the community but that were not necessarily explicitly related to mental health.[26]

The wariness with which Area D residents viewed Saint Elizabeths was paralleled by skepticism on the part of municipal officials and some hospital staff. District officials were concerned that the CMHC would prioritize the objectives of the NIMH—particularly research and training—over the delivery of mental health care to its citizenry. This skepticism was rooted in the seemingly incongruous recommendations of the 1964 advisory group and nurtured by the federal neglect of District sovereignty. But just as some members of the city's Department of Public Health felt that their partnership with the federal government might sacrifice the mental health care needs of local residents to the NIMH's research agenda, some on Saint Elizabeths' clinical staff were nervous that their professional interests might take a backseat to this new emphasis on community care. Speaking of the hospital staff's response to the formation of the Area D task force, Dr. Sherman Kieffer, the NCMHSTR's first director, noted that "for those whose work did not touch upon these immediate areas there was a perception of a setting of priorities which placed their needs at the bottom of a long and indefinite list, consequently with no prospects of any immediate relief for their concerns."[27] These staff members' fear that the presence of a CMHC on the grounds of Saint Elizabeths would be the initial step in turning the institution into just another municipal hospital was merely a different manifestation of the same anxiety that surrounded President Harry Truman's decision to cease the admission of military personnel in the mid-1940s. That the community the CMHC was intended to serve was increasingly black and poor most likely exacerbated those concerns.

In its final report, the task force sought to assuage the concerns of all of these interested parties by emphasizing the importance of collaboration and stressing the potential for the research agenda and community health care model to complement one another. The report's third recommendation was for the CMHC staff to collect data on the effects of its community programs and to partner where appropriate with the NCMHSTR staff in order to maintain a robust research agenda. But the task force also identified the training of Saint Elizabeths' staff in community-oriented mental health care practices as imperative to the success of the CMHC. As a way of alleviating local residents' skepticism, the task force recommended the development of a community services unit that would collaborate with the neighborhood health centers in the area. The committee made a number of other proposals for the structuring and operation of the CMHC. In addition to recommending the administrative and physical centralization of all mental health programs and services being provided in Area D, they urged a prioritizing of the enhancement of services specifically for children and adolescents. This was necessary because of the large proportion of local residents under the age of eighteen and an expressed interest among community residents in services for children.[28]

In April 1969 the Area D CMHC was established on the grounds of Saint Elizabeths. The CMHC staff was divided into eight units: an outpatient and an inpatient unit for four subareas within Area D. Each outpatient unit consisted of a psychiatrist, psychologist, social worker, mental health counselor, chaplain, and part-time vocational rehabilitation specialist. Inpatient units comprised physicians, mental health counselors, nurses, and nursing assistants. Both outpatient and inpatient units worked with more specialized programs that addressed childhood and adolescence, alcohol and narcotics addiction, and suicide.[29]

The CMHC incorporated existing inpatient services that had been operating since the summer of 1967. Mentally disturbed residents in Area D who needed to be hospitalized were admitted to units in either the Dix Division or the William A. White Division. Treatment in these units ranged from individual and family psychotherapy to group therapy, psychodrama to vocational rehabilitation. Each division also operated partial care (or day) units and community service clinics to assist outpatients and discharged patients. The William A. White Division sponsored a community nursing service through which psychiatric nurses and their assistants conducted home visits. The division also ran the Valley Green

Counseling Center, providing therapeutic services in public housing facilities and running a "training program for indigenous community workers." Within two years Area D CMHC had five satellite centers in Southeast and Southwest.[30]

The distribution of Area D patients across two divisions at the hospital was based on the individual's residence, essentially a more localized manifestation of the geographic distribution principle of comprehensive community health care. While this reflected a motivation to rationalize care and maintain parity in the delivery of services, there was criticism of the whole concept of catchment areas in general, if not the division of Area D into subareas in particular. In addition to feeling that the population criterion for determining catchment areas was arbitrary, critics pointed to the rigid borders that defined these areas and the detrimental effects that those barriers could have on people in need. Franklin D. Chu and Sharland Trotter recounted a disturbing example: "Even though one hospital might be closer than another for many people, catchment boundaries are rigidly enforced. This had tragic consequences not long ago, when a young black woman, having wandered around in the middle of the night for several hours, actively hallucinating and with her two small children in tow, finally made her way to St. Elizabeths. Because she did not belong in the catchment area assigned to that hospital, she was refused admission and told to go across town to D.C. General. She was killed by a car on the highway outside St. Elizabeths, with her children the only witnesses."[31]

In this particular case, Area D CMHC staff may have turned this young women and her children away because they perceived her request for admission as part of a larger pattern of other CMHCs attempting to pawn off their own inpatients. As Chu and Trotter noted, Saint Elizabeths' staff suspected that even though the other CMHCs had their own dedicated inpatient facilities, they tended to use the hospital as a "'dumping ground' for undesirables or 'hopeless' patients.'"[32] Although the medium- and long-term inpatient facilities at Saint Elizabeths were supposed to serve all of the District and the Area D CMHC was technically not connected to that part of the institution, the feeling that they were being taken advantage of may have contributed to the fatal decision that night. It would not have been the first time the Area D staff turned away a distressed woman. With limited access to the District's Detox Center and longer-term rehabilitation facility because the majority of beds were reserved for men, women alcoholics seeking help had to resort to CMHCs. Yet they were routinely denied admission, a result of "lack of space or the arbitrary opinion of an admitting doctor," according to a community service organization, Help Alcoholic Women. Dr. James M. Brown, an admitting physician at Area D, acknowledged that his staff often provided women who were seeking assistance but did not live in the catchment area cab or bus fare to DC General.[33] Regardless of the rationale for refusing service, the case of the woman who came to Saint Elizabeths with her children illustrates the bureaucratic wrangling that took place within an increasingly resource-starved environment and the very real human casualties that could result from it.

The opening of Area D CMHC facilitated the reduction of Saint Elizabeths' inpatient population, a process that had begun in earnest when the hospital was transferred to NIMH. Between November 1968 and June 1970, the number of residential patients declined by 25 percent, from 5,400 to 4,000. In addition to the homes of family members, they were being moved into foster homes and halfway houses. Although many of these patients had been readmitted during this year and a half, most were now being handled as outpatients at Area D CMHC. Officials who commented on the significant shift in the focus of Saint Elizabeths' care trumpeted the increasing number of patients being treated at the CMHC and the resulting reduction in the length of stay for those patients who had to be admitted to the hospital's inpatient services. An NIMH document, probably produced in 1970, commended the CMHC for its handling an average of one thousand cases a year, allowing the hospital to achieve its objective of "changing the whole thrust of its emphasis from long-term, in-patient care to out-patient care." Of course, this movement of patients outside the walls of the institution was not without its problems—for the community or for the patients themselves. There were not nearly enough residential facilities in the catchment area to provide space for all the patients being released. This particularly affected patients with acute medical conditions and chronic illnesses. It also disproportionately hurt poor patients, laying the groundwork for the epidemic of homelessness among mentally ill Americans that would occur as a result of full-blown deinstitutionalization.[34]

Still, Saint Elizabeths attempted to provide services to the local community and worked closely with grassroots organizations to do so. Perhaps what was most emblematic of the community orientation of Area D CMHC was the involvement of nonprofessional (at least in the area of mental health care) local residents in the operation of the center. When he referenced Area D CMHC in his announcement of the reorganization of Saint Elizabeths in November 1968, Yolles made a point of mentioning that community members would provide input through a formal advisory board. Although local residents were not involved in the planning of the center, a local councilman convened a provisional board in the fall of 1970. The board expressed a desire that the CMHC prioritize youth services, including special education, and alcohol and drug treatment, including a clinic specifically for female alcoholics. The Citizens Association of the Area D CMHC was incorporated the following spring. Consisting of community lay people, the association's board of directors assisted the CMHC director and staff members in making decisions regarding "major policy and direction, planning and operation of new programs, selection of sites for satellite center and ... the evaluation process of ongoing programs."[35]

The community was involved in the Area D CMHC in other ways. Saint Elizabeths partnered with the District's Department of Vocational Rehabilitation to provide workshops for patients in, among other things, furniture making, welding, upholstering, and cabinetmaking. Patients received small weekly payments in order to foster a sense of personal responsibility. The CMHC also collaborated with area mental health associations to find employment for individuals discharged from the hospital. Saint Elizabeths' staff offered "formal orientation in mental health concepts" to local residents and groups providing services to the community, including civic associations, law enforcement agencies, physicians, educators, and clergy. The hospital assisted Federal City College (which would merge with two other schools in 1976 to become the University of the District of Columbia) and a nonprofit organization, Washington Opportunities for Women, in training women from low-income backgrounds to become social work aides and health care workers. Saint Elizabeths' officials also sought to become integrated into the community by allowing Area D CMHC to become a civic space of sorts. It routinely hosted community conferences, including ones on exceptional children and the public school system; black families, which included a keynote address by the National Urban League's director of research; and teenage pregnancy.[36] Saint Elizabeths administrators, center staff, and community members clearly worked together to optimize their efforts in preventive mental health care as well as aftercare for discharged patients.

An investment in a community-oriented approach to mental health did not necessarily yield a positive experience for residential patients or community members seeking treatment, nor did it translate into a seamless transition back into the community for released patients. There is little documentary evidence available to assess how patients experienced or thought about their interaction with Area D CMHC. In their report on community mental health centers, Chu and Trotter compared the Area D CMHC favorably to the District's other CMHCs. In an overall critique of Washington's mental health care system, they pointed out that Area D was the only catchment area in which comprehensive services were provided. This is hardly surprising, given that Area D was already equipped with a nationally renowned mental hospital. But Chu and Trotter attributed Area D CMHC's success more to it being outside of municipal control than to any affirmative role by the federal government. "If Area D is better organized, more fully equipped, and its staff more unified than its counterparts in the rest of Washington," they judged, "it probably has more to do with its insulation from the D.C. Department of Human Resources (and its more secure financial situation) than with its ties to NIMH or St. Elizabeths." The implication of Chu and Trotter's report was that Area D was successful despite the "institutionalized insensitivity" of the NIMH and, moreover, that it could be considered successful only if compared to the utter debacles that were the CMHCs of Area B and Area C.[37]

The investigators did not provide any discussion of the qualitative experiences of patients and individuals seeking treatment at Area D CMHC. Nonetheless it is probable that they shared some of the same feelings that people in Area C had about their experiences with its center. A joint study of Area C's CMHC by Catholic University School of Social Services and the District's Department of Human Resources (DHR) in 1968 found that staff members and patients complained of understaffing, poor organization, and substandard facilities. One line of criticism exposed the fraught racial politics of community mental health care. "The problems created by a predominantly white staff's working in a black ghetto community were also identified by both [staff members and patients]," Chu and Trotter noted. "Said a staff member, 'Hire more black staff . . . who are sure of their racial identity, who can instill a sense of black identity among patients. More staff familiar with white racism, poverty, and the culture of patients.' A patient put it more poignantly: 'There is no place in the city of Washington where a poor black person can go and feel like a person. Educate secretaries and nurses in human behavior.'"[38] A profound statement. Although we do not have a comparable statement from an Area D CHMC patient, it is difficult to imagine a similar sentiment not being shared by some who utilized the center's services.

What we do have documentary evidence for are some of the structural problems that characterized Area D CMHC, and Saint Elizabeths more broadly, which would have negatively shaped the experiences of patients. One of these was racism in hiring and promotion practices at Saint Elizabeths. A personnel audit conducted at Area D CMHC found extensive "racial bias," including the passing over of qualified African American employees for promotions. Chu and Trotter's report corroborated the audit's findings. "Although nearly two-thirds of the staff is black, professional control is clearly white," they concluded.[39] More general charges against management for poor working conditions and racist supervisors came from other Saint Elizabeths employees. In the early 1970s, nursing assistants who belonged to District Council 20, Local 2095 of the American Federation of State, County and Municipal Employees went public with several grievances against the hospital administration. They complained of being "forced to work under 'hazardous' conditions." The work was so dangerous—including being threatened by patients with guns, having lye thrown at them, finding themselves in disorderly situations—that they deserved "hazard pay," they argued. The executive director of the District Council charged that the administration ran the hospital like a "plantation." He pointed to "rampant discrimination in all phases of employment" and "white supervisors who are totally insensitive to the problems of black workers." As government employees, the nursing assistants were prohibited from going on strike, and it is unclear whether the hospital responded to their main complaint: the dangerous conditions on the wards and the lack of hazard pay.[40]

It is hard to say definitively how such management-employee tensions would have affected the therapeutic relationships that existed in Saint Elizabeths and the Area D CMHC. At the very least, a less than optimal work environment threatened to hamper the effectiveness of the employees. Although committed to their patients and the hospital's mission, many black clinical, paraprofessional, and support staff who felt disrespected by their peers, administrators, and supervisors, or who deemed their workspace to be stressful or hostile, were more than likely to cut corners, pay less attention to detail, and ignore advice or directives. Without a belief that a concerted effort would result in professional advancement, many black employees probably did what was minimally needed to keep their job. From the patient's perspective, seeing a predominantly African American staff being dominated by white supervisors and administrators probably did not inspire a lot of confidence in the institution. This would have been particularly the case in the larger atmosphere of Black Power and community control that prevailed in African American neighborhoods in the 1970s. Ironically, when the nursing assistants challenged the administration, the acting superintendent at the time was none other than Luther D. Robinson. The first African American psychiatrist hired permanently at Saint Elizabeths in 1955, Robinson had worked his way up the administrative hierarchy, establishing one of the nation's first mental health programs for the deaf in the process.[41] But probably few patients utilizing the CMHC would have known who the superintendent was, and if they did, like many of the African Americans on the staff, it likely did not change their opinion that the hospital was at best a paternalist institution and, at worst, a racist tool of social control.

Equally problematic as the racist hiring and promotion practices, if not more so, was the fiscal starvation of the center. By the early 1970s, as the nation became increasingly mired in the Vietnam War, funding for social services was severely cut back. The financial support for CMHCs was not commensurate with the expectations that community mental health advocates attached to them. Dr. Roger Peele, Area D CMHC's director, claimed that the NIMH had not provided the necessary support to conduct any meaningful evaluation of their programs. An official connected to Area D CMHC provided even more scathing criticism of the loss of federal funding. In a set of handwritten notes to prepare someone for testimony before Congress, the author enumerated several problems with which staff members at Area D CMHC had to contend. One was the decimation of the staff itself. The author pointed out that two hundred temporary positions had been cut in June 1974 and, thanks to austerity cuts that reduced NIMH's budget by 2 percent, another eighty full-time positions were going to be eliminated by the summer of 1975. The cuts particularly affected the center's ability to conduct outreach and facilitate the integration of discharged patients into the community. Some of the eliminated part-time positions, for instance, were in the Community Placement Office. Other services negatively affected were the satellite centers. "Need for SATELLITE clinics (storefronts, outreach teams) for CMHC Area D," the author fumed. "All other CMHCs (Areas A, B, C) have these, but we have no $ for it, or staff, yet we're supposed to be community-oriented." It is not clear from these notes whether the official was complaining of a failure to open additional satellite centers over the five that had already been established by 1971, or if those original five had been closed due to staffing and funding shortages. Neither is it clear if the official was making a distinction between first-ring satellite centers that were housed in health clinics and staffed by professionals and the second-ring satellite centers that were supposed to be "closer" to the community in spaces like community centers and tenant associations. In their 1972 task force report, Chu and Trotter indicated that Area D CMHC had no satellite clinics, resulting in limited outreach to the community.[42] Whatever situation he or she was describing, the official's frustration is clear.

Lack of funding—at both the federal and local levels—certainly compromised the center's efforts to assist patients. Saint Elizabeths cooperated with the District's DHR to find suitable foster homes for inpatients deemed to be sufficiently improved to be provisionally released from the hospital. Hospital staff provided guidelines and established certain standards that had to be met by a sponsor before they could host an outpatient. They also offered training in basic care. Sponsors were generally private homeowners and were responsible for providing released patients with sleeping quarters, three meals a day, and clean linens and towels, as well as supervising their medication regimen. Foster home operators received a combined payment from the federal and local government. But by the mid-1970s, the amount—$146 from the federal Supplemental Security Income Program plus $24 from the DHR—was considered so meager that Saint Elizabeths had difficulty recruiting sponsors. Additionally the DHR did not have enough staff to provide follow-up services for provisionally released patients. This led Luther Robinson, who had become superintendent in 1972, to complain in 1975 that, since the opening of Area D CMHC six years earlier, the hospital had been able to discharge only a few patients who were living in foster care homes.[43]

One program aimed at helping released patients find homes of their own was run primarily by the Citizens Association, which raised money for security deposits and furnishings, cosigned leases, and took over rental payments in emergency situations. With an average of only $500 in its treasury by the end of the decade, however, the association rarely had sufficient funds to help with former patients' reentry into society. "Next to the problem of uncooperative landlords, the primary factor limiting the program's effectiveness is lack of money and furniture," a Washington journalist reported. "Between 15 and 25 patients are usually on the waiting list for an apartment."[44] Even though, over the course of the 1970s, the federal government had provided supplemental income and housing support for people with disabilities—including mental illness—by the beginning of the 1980s it was cutting back substantially on its funding for Section 8 rental housing and its Community Support Program.[45] These reductions in federal subsidies clearly shifted the burden of helping released patients reintegrate into the community to private and nonprofit social service organizations. With as limited a budget as the Citizens Association had, it could not provide the kind of support needed to make community mental health care—and its corollary, deinstitutionalization—as successful as its advocates envisioned.

While the reduction of the inpatient population had always been a central goal of the community mental health care approach, deinstitutionalization was very much accelerated by the courts. In February 1974 the Mental Health Law Project sued Saint Elizabeths on behalf of a patient, William Dixon. The case, which evolved into a class action suit, was one of many across the nation in the 1960s and 1970s that successfully challenged the constitutionality of involuntary commitment, set legal standards for a "minimally acceptable quality of care," and established rights of patients to receive individualized treatment plans and care in the "least restrictive setting." The plaintiffs in *Dixon v. Weinberger* were Saint Elizabeths patients who claimed that their mental conditions did not warrant their continued institutionalization; rather, they had improved enough to deserve outplacement into "alternative facilities" such as foster care homes, halfway houses, and nursing homes.[46]

The *Dixon* case unnerved many associated with Saint Elizabeths who had always thought about the institution as the gold standard of psychiatric care. Before the district judge rendered his decision, NIMH director Bertram Brown informed Congress that the hospital had been working hard to enhance its treatment of patients for years, including running its admissions services around the clock and increasing the numbers of psychologists with PhDs, psychiatric social workers, and board-certified psychiatrists on its staff. And in fact there was much for Saint Elizabeths to be proud of. In addition to the substance abuse programs and psychiatric services for juveniles that it provided for residents of Southeast and Southwest, the hospital also housed one of the only mental health programs for the deaf in the country. Still, there were deficiencies within the capacity of the hospital to treat its patients that could not be denied. As Dr. Thomas D. Reynolds, chief of service of the William A. White Division, confessed in 1972:

> If we examine the actual quality of the lives of these people we now return so easily to the community, in their homes and foster homes and halfway houses, taking their Thorazine tablets or their Prolixin

injections, we will discover that the great majority, while outwardly sane and tractable, are living utterly barren and blasted lives. . . . We have created a kind of slow spiritual euthanasia with chemical agents, whose primary function is to get the patients away from us so that by not seeing the poverty of their lives, we may cease feeling any responsibility for the matter.[47]

In part, Reynolds was attributing the direness of schizophrenics' lives to the profession's inability to comprehensively understand mental disease, yet he placed some responsibility on the hospital's hastiness in releasing patients and the substandard aftercare that it offered them.

In December 1975 US District Judge Aubrey E. Robinson Jr. ruled in favor of the plaintiffs and held that it was the joint responsibility of the federal and District of Columbia governments to provide "suitable care and treatment" to approximately 1,200 patients "under the least restrictive conditions." Robinson gave both governments forty-five days to submit a plan outlining how they would comply with his ruling. It would take close to five years for Robinson's ruling to be fully implemented, a process that was delayed by wrangling and turf battles between federal and local officials and the plaintiffs' rejection in 1977 of a plan they considered "too general." In April 1980 the court finally accepted a joint plan that laid out areas in which there would be a clear division of labor between the federal and local governments. The Department of Health and Human Services (HHS)—which, along with the Department of Education, replaced HEW in 1979—remained solely responsible for inpatient care and assumed a role in evaluating needs for outpatients and providing some aftercare. Overseeing community services and community residential facilities for outpatients became the main responsibility of the District. HHS and the District agreed to collaborate in the construction of a nursing facility and the development of additional housing for outpatients.[48]

Despite the plaintiffs' successful suit, only a fraction of the beneficiaries of the decision had been released into alternative facilities two years later. And even those who had been released—or who had been outpatients prior to the court case—could not necessarily count on suitable residential settings and efficiently delivered services. There were certainly some successful reentries, with released patients finding spaces in halfway houses run by social service organizations, entering vocational training and life skills programs, and forming their own support groups. But there were also many patients whose lives were scarcely improved, or even made worse, by deinstitutionalization. Like many other mental institutions, Saint Elizabeths was able to release significant portions of its geriatric patient population once Medicare and Medicaid's policy of mental health parity allowed poor, elderly, and disabled patients to get coverage for their treatment outside of mental hospitals. But for this class of patient, release from Saint Elizabeths often meant becoming residents of nursing homes.[49] With fewer foster homes available than were necessary to meet the housing demand, many patients also ended up in welfare hotels or privately run single-room occupancy hotels (SROs). As Congressman Ronald Dellums of California pointed out at a 1981 congressional hearing on deinstitutionalization, "At first, SRO's were run by caring and concerned people who were attempting to aid the former patients, but very shortly, it was discovered that a sizeable profit could be made at the expense of care."[50]

Importantly, the hearing was conducted by the fiscal affairs and health subcommittee of the Committee on the District of Columbia in part to spotlight the "enormous problems with deinstitutionalization in Washington and large urban centers." While the subcommittee heard testimony about the yeoman-like work many private mental health programs were doing in the District, it nonetheless came to the conclusion that a lack of planning and an inability to consistently assess outpatient programs led to many patients either being reinstitutionalized or dropping out of the system altogether. "Instead of finding hope and homes in the communities," DC's delegate Walter E. Fauntroy noted, "many former patients have become a part of a growing street community which exists in most major cities around the country." Fauntroy's claim was reinforced by John Dillingham, director of the Metropolitan Mental Health Skills Center, who estimated that 20 to 40 percent of the approximately five thousand homeless people in the District suffered from mental illness. Indeed some patients ended up being released directly into homeless shelters. As a 1982 *Washington Post* article noted, "When about two dozen patients were leaving the hospital . . . St. Elizabeths officials simply called workers at the Blair shelter, located at 6th and I streets NE, and asked if they had room for the people they were releasing."[51] The paucity of foster care homes no doubt contributed to these officials' decision. Given the declining public financing of social welfare programs and the lack of systematic coordination between the federal programs that served the mentally ill, decisions like these resulted in the release of patients with little more than treatment plans provided by Saint Elizabeths' staff but without access to the resources or services necessary to follow through on them.

A Hospital for Chocolate City: Transferring Saint Elizabeths to the District of Columbia

A year after Judge Aubrey Robinson rendered his decision, Saint Elizabeths lost its accreditation. There were telling signs that this would happen in the preceding years. Concerned about deficiencies in the hospital's infrastructure and management, the Joint Commission on Accreditation of Hospitals (JCAH) renewed Saint Elizabeths' accreditation for just one year in 1973 and did so again in 1974. When it conducted its survey in 1975, the JCAH cited more than a hundred problems that needed remediation, ranging from overcrowding to the poor conditions of some buildings, from the management of patient records to the quality of the food. The NIMH's appeal of the JCAH's decision lasted for more than a year before the commission handed down its final decision on December 18, 1976.[52]

There were diverse explanations for how such a reputable institution could be nearing what appeared to be such an ignominious end. Dr. E. Fuller Torrey, an expert on schizophrenia and a psychiatrist on the hospital's staff, blamed the neglectful attitude of NIMH officials. It was the inattention of the hospital's oversight agency that explained how Saint Elizabeths could lose its accreditation despite the fact that its funding from Congress was increasing at the same time that its patient population was decreasing.[53] What Torrey interpreted as neglect, Peele—by this point the hospital's acting superintendent—suggested was mixed messages from the executive branch. When he became president in 1969, Richard M. Nixon proposed transferring control of Saint Elizabeths to the District of Columbia since 85 percent of its patients were Washingtonians. No longer geared toward the rehabilitation or custodial care of members of the armed services, there was no reason for the federal government to continue to oversee the hospital. "With that kind of mandate from above," Peele remarked to a reporter, "it was difficult for NIMH to be planning the hospital's future in a constructive sort of way since they were told to get rid of us." NIMH director Brown expressed a similar opinion, partly attributing nonaccreditation to "the five-year impasse concerning the transfer of the Hospital to the District of Columbia."[54]

There had already been a diminishing of morale within some quarters of the hospital, going back to the decision in the late 1960s to transform part of Saint Elizabeths into a community mental health care center. The concern that mental health research was being compromised by a shifting of priorities to community care was no doubt exacerbated by nonaccreditation. Moreover, despite the fact that Saint Elizabeths' residency program was not affected by the decision of the JCAH, hospital and federal officials were anxious that nonaccreditation would make it that much more difficult to recruit and retain top-notch psychiatrists and other mental health care professionals. Confronted with the prospect of further deterioration of the hospital's reputation, President Gerald Ford stepped in and responded to Saint Elizabeths' "loss of face" by proposing a doubling of its budget for fiscal year 1977 and reallocating some federal funds so that 102 staff positions that had been cut the previous year could be reinstated. Within five years Saint Elizabeths had regained its accreditation.[55]

The path to reaccreditation was long and arduous. But Saint Elizabeths was hardly alone. A number of state mental hospitals lost their accreditation in the 1970s. What made Saint Elizabeths different, as Brown and Peele indicated, was the awkward relationship between the federal government and the District of Columbia. When HEW secretary John W. Gardner announced the movement of Saint Elizabeths under the umbrella of NIMH in August 1967, he pointed out that this was an "initial step toward future transfer" of the hospital to the District. Within two years the Nixon administration's official policy was for the immediate transfer of Saint Elizabeths, a policy influenced by the fact that the overwhelming majority of the hospital's patients were civilian residents of the District and by Nixon's support for home rule for the nation's capital.[56] In the summer of 1969 Nixon's HEW secretary, Robert H. Finch, and Mayor Walter Washington formed a committee to study the future of the hospital, including the "most effective means" of transferring control of Saint Elizabeths to the District. The committee, headed by Howard P. Rome, a psychiatrist from the Mayo Clinic, issued its report a year later.[57]

The Rome Committee made a number of recommendations, including establishing a general hospital on Saint Elizabeths' grounds that would serve the Anacostia community, converting a section of the institution into a hospital for chronically ill and geriatric patients, and removing the criminally insane to an as yet unbuilt separate facility. But perhaps the recommendation that received the most scrutiny and generated the greatest response was the committee's suggestion that the NIMH run Saint Elizabeths for five years, after which it would be turned over to an independent, municipally run agency. The five years were needed, according to the report, in order to turn Saint Elizabeths "from a snake pit into a first-rate psychiatric facility."[58] In general, there was cautious support among federal and local officials for the transfer of Saint Elizabeths to the District. Brown endorsed the Rome Committee's recommendation, albeit with the caveat that HEW continue to provide "financial and technical assistance" to local administrators. Dr. Francis Waldrop, the acting deputy director of the NIMH's research and training program at Saint Elizabeths, also supported the transfer, but criticized the five-year probationary period as a patronizing approach to mental health care professionals and government officials in the District. While he shared Brown's position that HEW and NIMH continue to offer help where they could, Waldrop was skeptical that a five-year delay in the transfer would make the transition any easier for local officials. In fact, he suggested, it would prolong the "ambiguity, turmoil, and misery which have become characteristic of Saint Elizabeths Hospital for nearly a decade." By December 1970 the District had established the Mental Health Administration, a constituent agency of the DHR, and was prepared for the "expeditious transfer" of the hospital from federal to municipal control.[59]

There was some resistance to the proposed move. Even before the Rome Committee was officially impaneled, the District of Columbia Mental Health Association (DCMHA), an advocacy organization, came out in opposition to HEW's stated policy of transfer. They argued it was an attempt to reduce federal costs by shifting the fiscal responsibility for the four-thousand-plus employees at Saint Elizabeths to the District. They also expressed concern that the transfer would solidify Saint Elizabeths' decline from "its status as an internationally famous and leading institution [to] just another municipal hospital."[60] Saint Elizabeths' employees themselves were deeply concerned about such a shift in administration. Even though some were no doubt fearful of the adverse impact that a transfer would have on the reputation of Saint Elizabeths, many were leery of the potential loss of civil service protections they possessed as federal employees. The Rome Committee's recommendation that the federal benefits for Saint Elizabeths' employees be preserved was not enough to assuage those concerns. In the months after the report was released, the Committee of 1,000, a group of hospital employees, began a lobbying campaign to keep Saint Elizabeths under the jurisdiction of the NIMH, which included one of its prominent members, Father Joseph O'Brien, testifying before Congress.[61]

Hospital employees and mental health advocates were not the only ones opposed to the transfer of the hospital to the District. Community activists were as well. Despite their support for home rule, members of the Southeast, Far-Southwest Health Steering Committee, which represented over fifty grass-roots organizations, cautioned against any move that would "be a prostitution of the manpower and resources" of the District's health department. In a letter to Mayor Washington written before the Rome Committee even issued its report, the steering committee's cochairs pointed out that the District was not in a position to take over the hospital when it could not even open health clinics in their neighborhoods. "The Anacostia–Congress Heights area needs health input NOW," William Sheffey and Reverend Shane MacCarthy wrote. "Mr. Mayor, it is inconceivable to us how you can expect the D.C. Health Department which presently is incapable of supplying even the necessary minimum services to our city and particularly to our community, of assuming the burdensome responsibility of running St. Elizabeths. Please, do not let the people of our community continue to suffer from a lack of adequate health facilities for the sake of the bureaucratic ideal of self-government."[62] These activists were not inflexible in their opposition to the transfer. They merely wanted the process to be a slow and orderly one that would allow for the NIMH to put the Area D CMHC on a firm footing and for the District's health department to build up a health care infrastructure in the city's most underserved communities.

Although it is not clear how much influence the Committee of 1,000, the DCMHA, or activists opposed to the transfer had with federal officials, their

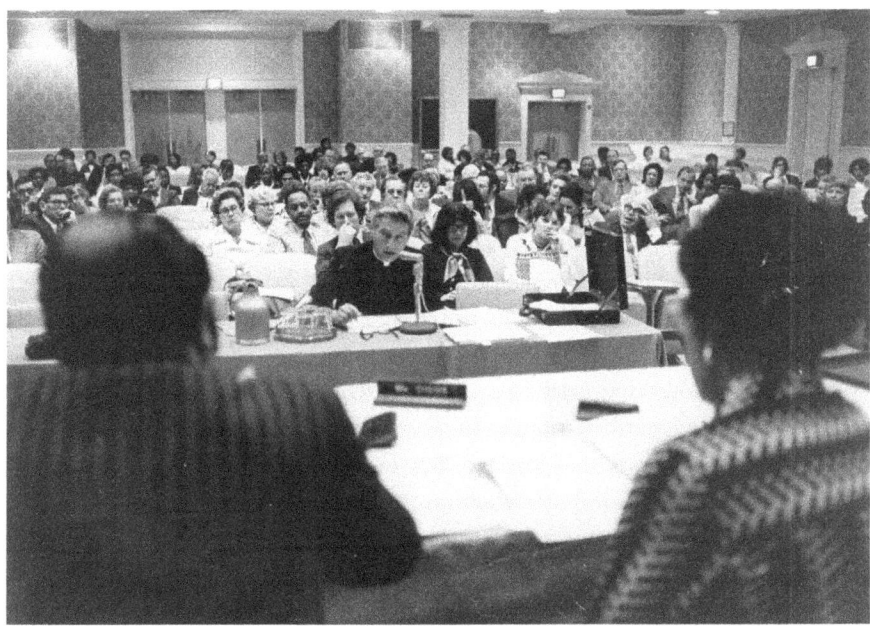

Father Joseph O'Brien, a Catholic priest and staff member at Saint Elizabeths, testifies before Congress in 1975 on the issue of transferring control of the hospital from the federal government to the District of Columbia. O'Brien represented the Committee of 1,000, a group of hospital employees; by the mid-1970s the group had pulled back from its opposition to the transfer and instead advocated for a minimum delay of ten years. *Washington Star Collection, Washingtoniana Division, DC Public Library. Reprinted with permission of the DC Public Library, Star Collection © Washington Post.*

preferred outcome, the status quo, persisted for several years. Authorized by a presidential reorganization directive in 1973, HEW was unable to coordinate a transfer before that authority lapsed at the end of the fiscal year. Congress was no more successful. Two companion bills introduced in the Senate and the House of Representatives in the summer of 1973 died the following December with the adjournment of the second session. Between January 1975 and the spring of 1977 discussions continued between HEW, the Office of Management and Budget, and the District government, but they did not result in the implementation of a transfer plan. The loss of accreditation in 1976 dealt a significant blow to the prospect of shifting control of the hospital to the District. As a federal hospital, Saint Elizabeths received its funding directly from the NIMH. As a municipally run hospital, however, it would have been reliant on reimbursements from Medicare and Medicaid, but with the loss of accreditation, the hospital would not have been eligible for those reimbursements. As such, it would have been impossible to maintain care of what was largely a poor and older inpatient population.[63]

During the latter part of these discussions, Representative Charles Diggs (D-MI), chair of the House Committee on the District of Columbia, introduced a bill to facilitate transfer of Saint Elizabeths to the District. H.R. 3335 would create a federal corporation that would oversee improvements at the hospital to bring it in line with accreditation standards, after which point it would transition into DC's Mental Health Administration. For three days in March and April 1977, the subcommittee on fiscal and government affairs, chaired by Ron Dellums (D-CA), held hearings during which they heard testimony from federal officials, District government officials, mental health care professionals, and community stakeholders.[64] There was no uniform position on H.R. 3335 even within groups that might be assumed to harbor similar opinions about local versus federal control, such as the laypeople involved with the community mental health care centers. Moreover few individuals who testified before the subcommittee were absolutist in their positions; most expressed some qualification in accordance with certain preconditions or in response to language in the bill that they may have found vague. In the end H.R. 3335 did not become law, and it would be another ten years before Saint Elizabeths would officially become a municipal hospital. But witness testimony and various statements from committee members on both sides of the issue illustrate the extent to which rights consciousness, the language of citizenship, and the politics of race shaped the debate over control of Saint Elizabeths.

Citizenship—whether cast as the rights of individual Washingtonians or the collective rights of residents who lived in a city in political and electoral limbo—became a lens through which government officials and community stakeholders assessed and opined about the hospital's transfer. Congress had finally extended home rule to the District four years earlier. However, while Washingtonians could now elect their city officials, Congress maintained control of the District's budget and court system and retained the authority to override municipal legislation. Home rule legislation also hampered the District's ability to raise revenue by prohibiting the local government from taxing suburban residents who commuted to their (largely) federal jobs in the city.[65]

In this context the subordinate relationship that the District and its residents had always had to the federal government became an important touchstone for evaluating the fate of Saint Elizabeths. Although she equivocated on the question of transferring the hospital to the District, Reverend Annie Woodridge, the chair of the Area B Community Mental Health Center Advisory Board, began her testimony by calling her city the nation's "last colony." James F. Dickson, an assistant secretary of HEW, was also circumspect about the most appropriate and effective way to proceed with the transfer. But he left little doubt that the transfer itself symbolized something much larger:

I think that no matter which road we go down, the road is not going to be an easy one. The basic reason, I think, is that while we are attending ourselves to considerations of health and mental health here, what we are really dealing with here is the process of what takes place on the road to self-determination in the District. This will not be an easy one, but I think that it has to be gotten on with in the spirit of a challenge both to leadership and to toil. I think it actually is out of messes like this, if you will, that the District will realize its destiny in time. I do not think either road will be easy.[66]

Dickson and Woodridge were not the only individuals involved in discussions about transfer who framed it within the context of home rule, replete with all its promises and challenges. While many merely raised home rule as one bureaucratic variable among others, Woodridge and Dickson spoke to the deeper historical and symbolic meaning that a District takeover of Saint Elizabeths would represent.

Others who testified before the congressional subcommittee evoked citizenship not so much in terms of District residents' formal relationship to the nation as in terms of the people's inherent right to shape the institutions that were the closest, most responsive, and most accountable to them. In this sense, they affirmed the principles of the community mental health care movement and the community control ethos of the radical social movements of the late 1960s and 1970s.[67] In some ways, this particular rhetoric transcended racial and class lines. Lawrence Schwartz and Debra Shore, respectively chairman and secretary of the advisory board of Area A CMHC, which included more affluent white neighborhoods in Northwest in its catchment area, advocated for "citizen input" into the operation of Saint Elizabeths and expressed hope that "this [would be] the first step toward full control of the mental health system by the citizens of the District of Columbia." Woodridge, whose support for the transfer was more cautious than others', nonetheless echoed her fellow witnesses' emphasis on the indispensability of community control. "Although many medical, religious and social welfare groups have previously taken interest in mental illness, it was the lay movement initiated by interested citizens that brought the scattered efforts into cohesive thrust," she pointed out to the subcommittee. Woodridge concluded her statement by reinforcing that it was the "courage, common sense and confidence" of ordinary community members that would "serve the District of Columbia's cause in their efforts to see that every man, woman, boy and girl in its jurisdiction be entitled to quality mental health services."[68]

Woodridge represented Area B, whose catchment area included neighborhoods with more low- and middle-income people of color, including a sizable Latino population. The demographics of Area D resembled those of Area B much more than Area A. So while the language of citizenship and community control might be used by community mental health care advocates throughout the city, it took on greater import when uttered by people working with predominantly African American and Latino communities. When Patricia Wells, the chair of the Area D CMHC Citizens Board of Directors, remarked that whatever happened with Saint Elizabeths, the end result should be the improvement of the "quality of life of residents of the area D and immediate community which surrounds" the hospital, she was implicitly invoking a history of racial neglect in the District's health care system. In other words, community control took on a completely different sense of urgency for a community that had far fewer private mental health resources than predominantly white neighborhoods in the city— and even less disposable income or robust insurance plans to afford them.[69]

While race only occasionally surfaced as an explicit line of questioning— when, for instance, the dearth of African Americans among the hospital's management staff was broached by a subcommittee staff assistant—an exchange toward the end of the hearings left little doubt that racism within the psychiatric profession and larger culture was a concern for some committee members and mental health experts. When asked about his confidence that the District could develop a "unified and competent delivery system," the president of the DCMHA, John L. Johnson, replied that the city's majority-black population and the tendency to overinstitutionalize African Americans posed particular challenges. "It seems to me," he stated, "there is something environmentally— there is an environmental problem of some kind that may be beyond the notion of just simply providing psychiatric treatment for people. People that happen to have characteristics that other people don't like and find themselves in hospitals, so it is a much broader question. We think it is a broader question, but the essence of it is going to be getting people together to talk about some of this in public and to have an adequate plan."[70] Johnson's point prompted a poignant back and forth between two representatives on the committee. Ron Dellums, the nephew of the African American labor organizer C. L. Dellums, took the prerogative to share his own professional trajectory and the role that racism and psychiatry played within it. "I would just on a personal note indicate that that is how I got to Congress," he told Johnson and his fellow committee members. "I started off as a psychiatric social worker and then, thinking that there were some other factors that dealt with people. I came to the Congress, and now I am probably more frustrated than I ever was, thinking that some day I would get to the basic place where you could come to grips with the ultimate problem." Connecticut Republican Stewart McKinney concurred with the problem identified by Johnson and his colleague. "I would suggest that one of the reasons you discuss your frustration with the difference between white and black admissions and outpatient treatment is one of the basic problems we have at St. Elizabeths," he stated. "The inability of a city in the United States to deal with these problems, because cities in this country, through Federal neglect, have been forced to deal with all the social problems that the country has refused to face up to."[71] McKinney's commiseration with Dellums and Johnson was likely influenced by his overall irritation at the inability of the federal government to manage its own mental institution at the same time that it was setting standards for care at state hospitals.[72] Still, the crisis unleashed by federal austerity, bureaucratic inertia, and deinstitutionalization—and its disproportionate impact on Washington's African American community—was patently obvious to everyone, regardless of their ideology or political persuasion.

By the time both the federal and District governments had agreed on the terms and timing of the transfer, Saint Elizabeths was a leaner institution, but a dysfunctional one as well. A $25 million cut in 1983 led to a reduction in staff by nearly one thousand people and the elimination of a dozen programs for patients. Three years later a deficit reduction package in Congress imposed a hiring freeze, leading to more than 350 vacancies on the staff. Even though patients were being released in accordance with the *Dixon* ruling, the relative staff shortage meant that much of inpatients' days was spent watching television and, as one told a *Washington Post* reporter, "buying cigarettes, smoking cigarettes, and hustling cigarettes." As hospital officials planned for the transition, they reorganized the wards, disrupting the relationships that patients had with staff and also using the space inefficiently. "The result [of the reorganization] is widespread confusion, demoralization and little more than custodial care," the *Post* reported in 1986. "Some wards have too few staff and nurses who do not know the patients, according to professional staff, while others have been so overcrowded that patients have had to sleep on cots in a conference room." Of course, overcrowding had been a perennial problem, one with which every single superintendent over the course of the hospital's history had to contend. What made this moment different was the parallel problem of increasing homelessness that deinstitutionalization produced. Another distinction was demographic in nature. On the eve of Saint Elizabeths' transfer in 1987, the majority of inpatients were "poor, black, uninsured, schizophrenic males over 45" who had been institutionalized multiple times.[73]

What began as a noble effort aimed at preventing mental illness, treating the mentally ill in their own communities, and investing therapeutic authority in communities themselves ended up foundering on the shoals of shifting priorities within the federal government. Funding for social welfare programs became the casualty of America's military adventurism, and by 1980 the national consensus had moved from a commitment to New Deal liberalism to a gospel of devolution of government power and responsibility to the states. This had profound effects for Saint Elizabeths and, even more important, for the communities it served. When John F. Kennedy decided to embrace the NIMH's model of community mental health care, Saint Elizabeths' administrators and HEW officials thought the hospital would be in a good position to continue to serve as a model for other institutions about how best to transition from custodial care to prevention and community treatment. Some within the organization thought they exhibited an unwarranted optimism and feared that the change in focus would lead to a diminution of the hospital's stature. While the skeptics did not necessarily predict the role of declining federal investment, they were correct in predicting that Saint Elizabeths would become just another municipal hospital. The institution went from being a model for enlightened care—idealized, to be sure—to an emblem of federal neglect. This new status only crystallized as control of Saint Elizabeths was transferred from the federal government to the District of Columbia in the late 1980s.

Conclusion

In an archival box in the Still Picture Division of National Archives II lies a page from an August 1941 edition of the *Washington Daily News*. Sepia-toned and ragged around the edges, the page is dominated by two images under the headline "Washington: Two Social Levels." The photograph that takes up almost the entire upper half of the page is a bird's-eye view of a sprawling complex of perfectly placed four- and five-story brick buildings, neatly manicured quadrangles, and winding drives and pathways. Labeled "High," the caption reads, "Taken from the air with a special $6000 camera, this exclusive photo illustrates the manner in which Washington is spreading out as the Government brings increasing numbers of workers here. Just across the river in Arlington are these modern, well-planned apartments. With their parks and playgrounds, they offer the perfect setting for rearing healthy, happy children."

Countering this pristine portrait of suburban Washington is an image with the label "Low." Everything about the photo is meant to put the optimism of its counterpart into stark relief. It occupies the entire lower half of the page and, contrary to the elevated position of the photographer in the superior image, the camera angle is at street level. The subject of the photograph is Logan Court, one of the many alleys that were home to black working-class Washingtonians. As opposed to the panoramic scene of Arlington, the photo is crammed with wooden structures, a littered street, sheets and garments suspended from clotheslines, laboring men, and unkempt children. The accompanying caption gives additional weight to this dystopic vision: "By contrast, this is Logan Court ('Clothesline Alley') which lies sufficiently near the Capitol (at North Capitol and L streets) to provide a constant reminder that democracy will never function freely until the least of her people have a fair opportunity to grow into useful citizens. These ragged children will have to fight for everything they need, and, failing that, may turn to crime. Clothesline Alley is a perfect incubator for reformatory inmates."[1]

For most readers in 1941, the parallels these images evoked could not have been clearer. Liberal readers would have certainly been sympathetic to the argument that it was a travesty that a generation of African Americans was in danger of being left behind despite the economic growth that was occurring within the region and the nation's self-promotion as a beacon of freedom and equality and a bulwark against totalitarianism. They would have lamented the gap between the aspirational and the real, the same gap that Charles Dickens had recognized some one hundred years earlier. And even those readers who were not in complete accord with the underlying argument about the necessity of racial equality to a fully functioning democracy would have found it difficult not to be struck by the juxtaposed images of hope and despair, progress and stagnation.

There were probably more than a few readers who stifled a laugh when seeing the photos, however, not because they were indifferent to the poverty represented in the Logan Court photograph but because they recognized that the image meant to depict suburban Washington was instead that of the east campus of Saint Elizabeths Hospital. It perhaps would have been easy for the photo editor of the *Washington Daily News* to confuse the newer part of the hospital's campus—separated from the original west campus, with its red brick Gothic Revival buildings—with a modern apartment complex in Arlington, Virginia. We can only imagine what Superintendent Overholser or the head of the Federal Security Agency thought when they saw the mistake. Someone surely thought it was noteworthy (or silly) enough to hold onto for posterity.

What was most likely an honest mistake actually serves as a fitting coda to this history of race and mental illness in Washington, DC. The paired photographs were aimed at alerting Washingtonians to the problem of growing inequality and the potential erosion of the nation's exceptionalism if "the least of her people" were not given a "fair opportunity to grow into useful citizens." Ironically Saint Elizabeths Hospital, the photograph of which was meant to represent the prosperous future of the nation's capital and its surroundings, would eventually become associated with urban decline. Initially envisioned as a "model of enlightened care" for the nation's soldiers and sailors, the institution had, by the mid-1980s, become what many employees, mental health experts, and federal officials in the 1960s and 1970s feared: "just another municipal hospital."[2] Even though it would be an exaggeration to say that Saint Elizabeths had ever become a model, it certainly occupied an important place in the fields of asylum medicine, neurology, and dynamic psychiatry from the mid-nineteenth century through the mid-twentieth.

Its transformation into an emblem of much of what was wrong with American culture and politics in the late twentieth century—the dissolution of the New Deal liberal consensus, the disinvestment in American cities, the prioritizing of military spending over social welfare, the persistent economic and social marginalization of people of color—was decades in the making. It began, arguably, five years after the photographic error in the *Washington Daily News*, when

President Harry Truman ordered the US Army and US Navy to stop sending their mentally ill service members there. With that decision, older, black civilian residents of the District gradually became the predominant share of the patient population. The fear that Saint Elizabeths would become "just another municipal hospital," then, had as its unspoken subtext the equally frightening prospect that it would become just another urban ghetto hospital. Race, in other words, was intimately connected to "the politics of decline" of what once was a preeminent research and teaching mental hospital.[3]

But race and racism had always been part of Saint Elizabeths' history. Because the District did not have a public asylum for its civilian residents—and because blacks served in the regular army and navy from the 1860s onward—African Americans were among the first patients at Saint Elizabeths, and they continued to constitute a significant portion of the patient population over the entire span of the hospital's 132-year operation as a federal institution. The presence of African Americans at the federal asylum presented important challenges and potential opportunities for the medical professionals tasked with healing the psychic wounds of soldier and civilian alike.

The institutional challenge of treating African American patients within a segregated facility was, in many ways, a product of the conceptual challenge that black madness posed to Saint Elizabeths' staff and the larger psychiatric profession. From nineteenth-century asylum medicine's association of insanity with civilization and civilized races to twentieth-century dynamic psychiatry's understanding of mental illness as individual maladjustment to society, mentally ill African Americans occupied an enigmatic space in the psychiatric imagination. If insanity was a disease of civilization that afflicted more cerebrally and culturally developed races, then what were Saint Elizabeths' physicians to make of blacks who, as a primitive people that enjoyed a presumed immunity to mental breakdown, nonetheless needed to be institutionalized? How were they to explain the apparent increase of black insanity in the postemancipation and post-Reconstruction era? Was it a product of an underdeveloped nervous system—the same biological trait that accounted for their supposed immunity during the antebellum era—or an underdeveloped culture? With the turn to dynamic psychiatry in the early twentieth century and its contemplation of the role of the more primitive unconscious in the development of psychopathology, how were Saint Elizabeths' psychiatrists to interpret psychopathological behavior in African Americans, whom they still largely believed to be closer to their primitive ancestors to begin with? All of these questions and more were predicated on the presumption of racial difference. The belief that whites and blacks had fundamentally different psyches contributed to a great deal of clinical ambiguity surrounding institutionalized African Americans. And this ambiguity contributed to their racially ambivalent and racist treatment—from confinement in inferior wards or with the most disturbed and pathological of white patients to coerced labor masquerading as therapy or little to no psychotherapeutic engagement.

But it was this purported racial difference, from the psychiatrists' perspective, that also provided them a rare opportunity. Working at a preeminent research and teaching mental hospital, Saint Elizabeths' staff could take advantage of the large African American patient population to conduct research into comparative psychology. Outside of a few psychiatrists at other institutions, clinicians at Saint Elizabeths were by far the most prolific producers of knowledge about the differences between the causes and symptoms of mental illness in whites and African Americans. Despite the fact that their empirical observations rarely confirmed their hypotheses, Saint Elizabeths' psychiatrists in the first third of the twentieth century continued to pursue research premised on the racial peculiarity of mentally ill African Americans. And it was this fundamental premise that connected the challenges and opportunities that African American patients posed for Saint Elizabeths' psychiatrists throughout much of the hospital's history. For endeavoring to comprehend the black psyche was motivated only in part by a desire to heal the mentally distressed African Americans who ended up in the institution. It was also driven by a quest to develop a better understanding of the abnormal white psyche. As such, the comparative psychology research conducted at the hospital continued to do what physicians at Saint Elizabeths had been doing since its founding in the mid-nineteenth century: placing the damaged white psyche at the center of their therapeutic vision and making the preservation of white mental health their primary mission.

As problematic as this stance was, Saint Elizabeths' staff, on the whole, certainly did not abandon their African American charges. Belief in racial difference, racist assumptions about black inferiority, and empathy for sufferers of mental illness coexisted on the segregated wards. Moreover, they continued to shape the clinical encounter between white staff and African American patients after the universalist turn in psychiatry—which rejected the premise of fundamental differences in black and white psyches—and the ascendancy of a more progressive social psychiatry after World War II. Racial friction persisted between patients, too, even after the wards were integrated in the 1950s. The bitter roots that were anchored by decades-long privileging of white sufferers at the hospital, and in the profession as a whole, could not be dug up so quickly.

Although racial ambivalence and racism characterized the black experience at Saint Elizabeths, the relationships that patients and their families and friends had with the hospital were not solely adversarial. Rather, like the attitudes of Saint Elizabeths' psychiatrists toward their African American patients, black sufferers of mental illness and the communities from which they came often felt their own ambivalence toward the institution. This ambivalence was perfectly captured by a patient interviewed by the *Washington Post* in the early 1980s: "St. Elizabeths, she said, 'was like a second home. Anything I needed, they kept giving it to me.' Still, would she rather be in St. Elizabeths?" the reporter asked. "'You got to be joking,' she responded instantly. 'You know I don't want to be on a ward.'"4

The history of the relationship between Saint Elizabeths and Washington's African American community serves as a window into African Americans' relationship with psychiatry more generally. For decades, medical and public health professionals have been confronted with the question of why African Americans—along with other people of color—have historically underutilized outpatient mental health services, often leading to their overrepresentation in inpatient services, and especially public mental health hospitals. Several explanations have been advanced for this reluctance to engage with mental health services, including African Americans' tendency to understand mental stress within a spiritual or religious framework and to rely on pastoral or extended family care in times of psychical and emotional crisis. Another explanation that has been offered is that black people believe psychiatry is "the product of white, European culture, shaped by research primarily on white, European populations."5 The Eurocentric nature of psychiatry—or the construction and constant reaffirmation of the white psyche as the norm—fundamentally shaped Saint Elizabeths' staff's approach to African American patients and these patients' experiences within the institution.

While these racial dynamics in treatment and treatment-seeking have certainly existed, we need to develop a more textured understanding of African Americans' relationship to the discipline and profession of psychiatry, one that moves beyond thinking about this relationship—at least up to the civil rights era—as either indifferent or antagonistic. African American sufferers of mental illness did not allow themselves to be transformed into mere objects of medical scrutiny and targets of institutional control. Nor did those who cared for and about them relinquish their own moral and familial authority to Saint Elizabeths. African American patients and their social networks engaged the hospital in ways that sought to manage their own therapeutic experience. For the sufferers themselves, these engagements were aimed at shaping the conditions of their institutionalized existence. For members of their social networks, these engagements were often efforts to affirm their own civic belonging during a period in which African Americans, and Washingtonians more broadly, did not fully share the fruits of citizenship. These endeavors ranged from individual acts of monitoring the treatment of their loved ones to collective struggles to desegregate the hospital and shape the evolution of community mental health care in their neighborhoods. Black Washingtonians were anything but agnostic about or hostile toward the role of psychiatry in addressing issues of mental illness, mental health, emotional well-being, and overall quality of life. The history of African American agency in the realm of mental health care—both collective activism and individual treatment-seeking—is still largely a history waiting to be told.

The history of Saint Elizabeths has been a history of intentions, magnificent and otherwise. The intention of reformers, superintendents, presidents, lawmakers, and federal bureaucrats over the years to elevate the institution to a "model of enlightened care" and a symbol of American genius was often thwarted by congressional parsimony when it came to funding. Even after the cessation of military admissions, advocates of Saint Elizabeths expressed an intention to transform it into an exemplar of community mental health care. Yet this, too, was undermined by federal neglect and the larger political struggle surrounding the District's unique relationship to the federal government. For their part, Saint Elizabeths' staff approached their work with the intention of caring for, if not treating, everyone who found themselves in the hospital's wards. Those intentions, however, were constrained by the racial blinders they wore, blinders that placed the white sufferer at the center and the black sufferer at the periphery. But African American patients and members of their social networks brought their own intentions with them into their interactions with Saint Elizabeths. At times these intentions were in accord with those who ran the institution; at others, they were in conflict. In the end, the history of race and mental illness in the nation's capital is this story of the distance between expectations and limitations, between medical altruism and racism, between medical objectification and sufferers' agency, and between the aspirational and the real.

NOTES

Abbreviations

BBP	Bertram Brown Papers, National Library of Medicine, Bethesda, Maryland
DCPL	Washingtoniana Division, D.C. Public Library, Washington, DC
DDC	Dorothea Dix Collection, Houghton Library, Harvard University, Cambridge, Massachusetts
DOI-LR	RG 48 Records of the Department of Interior, Entry 298 Letters and Other Records Relating to the Government Hospital for the Insane, 1851–1902, NARA
NA	National Archives, Washington, DC
NARA	National Archives II, College Park, Maryland
PWO	Papers of Winfred Overholser, Manuscript Division, Library of Congress, Washington, DC
SEH/AF	RG 418 Records of Saint Elizabeths Hospital, Records of the Superintendent, Entry 7, Administrative Files, ca. 1921–64, NA
SEH/ARSU	RG 418 Records of Saint Elizabeths Hospital, Records of the Superintendent, Entry 20, Annual Reports of Subordinate Units, 1919–66, NA
SEH/BOVC	RG 418 Records of Saint Elizabeths Hospital, Records of the Board of Visitors, 1855–1947, Correspondence and Other Records, 1857–1903, NA
SEH/BOVGC	RG 418 Records of Saint Elizabeths Hospital, Records of the Board of Visitors, 1855–1947, General Correspondence of the Secretary, NA
SEH/BOVM	RG 418 Records of Saint Elizabeths Hospital, Records of the Board of Visitors, 1855–1947, Minutes, 1855–1901, NA
SEH/BOVR	RG 418 Records of Saint Elizabeths Hospital, Records of the Board of Visitors, 1855–1947, NA
SEH/CFP	RG 418 Records of Saint Elizabeths Hospital, Records of the Medical Records Branch, Entry 66, Case Files of Patients, 1855–ca.1950, NA
SEH/Nichols	RG 418 Records of Saint Elizabeths Hospital, Records of Superintendent Charles H. Nichols, Entry 24, Records Concerning Hospital Administration, 1857–77, NA
SEH/RC	RG 418 Records of Saint Elizabeths Hospital, Records of the Medical Records Branch, Register of Cases, 1855–1941, NA
SEH/Super	RG 418 Records of Saint Elizabeths Hospital, Records of the Superintendent, NA

SEH/White   RG 418 Records of Saint Elizabeths Hospital, Records of the
             Superintendent, Records of Superintendent William A. White, Records
             Pertaining to the Investigations of 1926, NA
WFP   Walter Fauntroy Papers, Part II, Special Collections Research Center,
             George Washington University Libraries, Washington, DC

Introduction

1. "An Act to Organize an Institution for the Insane of the Army and Navy, and of the District of Columbia, in the Said District," March 3, 1855, reprinted in *By-Laws of the Government Hospital for the Insane, Etc. September 1855* (Washington, DC: G. S. Gideon, 1855), in DOI-LR, box 1, NARA; Charles H. Nichols to Dorothea Dix, September 20, 1852, DDC, entry 474, folder 2; William A. White, "The New Government Hospital for the Insane," *American Journal of Insanity* 66 (April 1910): 526; William A. White, "The New Saint Elizabeth's Hospital," *American Journal of Psychiatry* 81 (January 1924): 513; Advisory Group on the Future of Saint Elizabeths Hospital, "Final Report of the Advisory Group on the Future of Saint Elizabeths Hospital," May 1964, 24, 27, BBP, container 30, folder 4.
2. The other hospital was the Canton Asylum for Insane Indians in South Dakota, which operated from 1902 to 1934. For a general history, see Diane T. Putney, "The Canton Asylum for Insane Indians, 1902–1934," *South Dakota History* 14 (Spring 1984): 1–30; Carla Joinson, *Vanished in Hiawatha: The Story of the Canton Asylum for Insane Indians* (Lincoln: University of Nebraska Press, 2016).
3. Godding quoted in Thomas Otto, *St. Elizabeths Hospital: A History* (Washington, DC: US General Services Administration, 2013), 89.
4. "Report of the Board of Visitors of the Government Hospital for the Insane, for the year ending June 30th 1856," entry 1, box 1, folios 30–31, SEH/BOVR, NA.
5. Charles Dickens, *American Notes* (New York: John W. Lovell, 1883), 695, 698.
6. It would take too much space to provide a comprehensive inventory of scholarship that constitutes, or has influenced, the cultural turn in medical history. The works that have been most formative for me are Byron J. Good, *Medicine, Rationality, and Experience: An Anthropological Perspective* (New York: Cambridge University Press, 1994); Frank Huisman and John Harley Warner, eds., *Locating Medical History: The Stories and Their Meanings* (Baltimore, MD: Johns Hopkins University Press, 2004); Charles E. Rosenberg and Janet Golden, *Framing Disease: Studies in Cultural History* (New Brunswick, NJ: Rutgers University Press, 1992); and Megan Vaughan, *Curing Their Ills: Colonial Power and African Illness* (Stanford, CA: Stanford University Press, 1991). My debt to other scholars will become apparent in the notes throughout this book.
7. Perhaps the most well-known and prolific historian of the humanitarian interpretation is Gerald Grob. See *The State and the Mentally Ill: A History of Worcester State Hospital in Massachusetts, 1830–1920* (Chapel Hill: University of North Carolina Press, 1966); *Mental Institutions in America: Social Policy to 1875* (New York: Free Press, 1972); *Mental Illness and American Society, 1875–1940* (Princeton, NJ: Princeton University Press, 1983); *The Mad among Us: A History of the Care of America's Mentally Ill* (New York: Free Press, 1994). See also Norman Dain, *Concepts of Insanity in the United States, 1789–1865* (New Brunswick, NJ: Rutgers University Press, 1964). Emerging almost concurrently with this interpretation was a revisionist literature that attributed more self-interested motives to the formation of the asylum. Influenced by Michel Foucault's theoretical formulations of the relationships among reason, madness, and power, these scholars looked at asylums and saw instruments of social control. See David Rothman, *The Discovery of the Asylum: Social Order and Disorder in the New Republic* (Boston: Little, Brown, 1971); Andrew T. Scull, "Madness and Segregative Control: The Rise of the Insane Asylum," *Social Problems* 24 (February 1977): 337–49; Andrew T. Scull, "Psychiatry and Social Control in the Nineteenth and Twentieth Centuries," *History of Psychiatry* 2 (1991): 149–69; Robert Castel, "Moral Treatment: Mental Therapy and Social Control in the Nineteenth Century," trans. Peter Miller, in *Social Control and the State: Historical and Comparative Essays*, ed. Stanley Cohen and Andrew Scull (Oxford: Martin Robinson, 1983), 248–66. See also Michel Foucault, *Madness and Civilization: A History*

of Insanity in the Age of Reason, trans. Richard Howard (New York: Random House, 1965); Michel Foucault, *Discipline and Punish: The Birth of the Prison*, trans. Alan Sheridan (New York: Random House, 1977). Writing mainly in the mid- to late 1980s, a group of post- or counterrevisionist historians offered a corrective to earlier studies that many regarded as ideologically motivated and theory-bound. Rather than addressing macro-level themes such as the social function of the asylum or the relationship between asylums and the state, postrevisionists turned to individual asylums as case studies. Influenced by the "new social history," these historians looked inside the asylum experience by examining administrative records, case files, census data, and patient-doctor-family correspondence. Their micro-level analyses led to not only greater understanding of the internal dynamics of particular hospitals; they also led to a rejection of sweeping generalizations of the function of the asylum. See Constance M. McGovern, "The Myths of Social Control and Custodial Oppression: Patterns of Psychiatric Medicine in Late Nineteenth-Century Institutions," *Journal of Social History* 20 (Fall 1986): 3–23; Ellen Dwyer, *Homes for the Mad: Life inside Two Nineteenth-Century Asylums* (New Brunswick, NJ: Rutgers University Press, 1987); Nancy Tomes, *A Generous Confidence: Thomas Story Kirkbride and the Art of Asylum-Keeping, 1840–1883* (Cambridge, UK: Cambridge University Press, 1984); Peter McCandless, *Moonlight, Magnolias, and Madness: Insanity in South Carolina from the Colonial Period to the Progressive Era* (Chapel Hill: University of North Carolina Press, 1996). For a thorough overview of the literature, see Thomas E. Brown, "Dance of the Dialectic? Some Reflections (Polemic and Otherwise) of the Present State of Nineteenth-Century Asylum Studies," *Canadian Bulletin of Medical History* 11 (1994): 267–95.

8. Norman Dain, *Disordered Minds: The First Century of Eastern State Hospital in Williamsburg, Virginia, 1766–1866* (Williamsburg, VA: Colonial Williamsburg Foundation, 1971), esp. 108–13; Gerald N. Grob, "Class, Ethnicity, and Race in American Mental Hospitals, 1830–75," *Journal of the History of Medicine and Allied Sciences* 28 (July 1973): 222–29; Todd L. Savitt, *Medicine and Slavery: The Diseases and Health Care of Blacks in Antebellum Virginia* (Urbana: University of Illinois Press, 1978), 247–79; Leland Bell, *Treating the Mentally Ill: From Colonial Times to the Present* (New York: Praeger, 1980), 58–73; Steven Noll, "Southern Strategies for Handling the Black Feeble-Minded: From Social Control to Profound Indifference," *Journal of Policy History* 3 (1991): 130–51; Dain, *Concepts of Insanity*, 104–8; Grob, *Mental Illness and American Society*, 38, 220–21; Grob, *Mad among Us*, 88–90; McCandless, *Moonlight, Magnolias, and Madness*.

9. John S. Hughes, "Labeling and Treating Black Mental Illness in Alabama, 1861–1910," *Journal of Southern History* 58 (August 1992): 435–60; Elizabeth Lunbeck, *The Psychiatric Persuasion: Knowledge, Gender, and Power in Modern America* (Princeton, NJ: Princeton University Press, 1994), 124–25, 205; Kirby Ann Randolph, "Central Lunatic Asylum for the Colored Insane: A History of African Americans with Mental Disabilities, 1844–1885" (PhD diss., University of Pennsylvania, 2003); Ellen Dwyer, "Psychiatry and Race during World War II," *Journal of the History of Medicine and Allied Sciences* 61 (April 2006): 117–43; Matthew Gambino, "'These Strangers within Our Gates': Race, Psychiatry and Mental Illness among Black Americans at St. Elizabeths Hospital in Washington, D.C. 1900–1940," *History of Psychiatry* 19 (2008): 387–408; Matthew Gambino, "Mental Health and Ideals of Citizenship: Patient Care at St. Elizabeths Hospital in Washington, D.C., 1903–1962" (PhD diss., University of Illinois at Urbana-Champaign, 2010); Dennis Doyle, "'Where the Need Is Greatest': Social Psychiatry and Race-Blind Universalism in Harlem's Lafargue Clinic, 1946–1958," *Bulletin of the History of Medicine* 83 (Winter 2009): 746–74; Dennis Doyle, "'Racial Differences Have to Be Considered': Lauretta Bender, Bellevue Hospital, and the African American Psyche, 1936–52," *History of Psychiatry* 21 (2010): 206–23; Jonathan Metzl, *The Protest Psychosis: How Schizophrenia Became a Black Disease* (Boston: Beacon Press, 2010); Mical Raz, *What's Wrong with the Poor? Psychiatry, Race, and the War on Poverty* (Chapel Hill: University of North Carolina Press, 2013). See also the recent book by Dennis A. Doyle, *Psychiatry and Racial Liberalism in Harlem, 1936–1968* (Rochester, NY: University of Rochester Press, 2016), in which he points out that nineteenth- and early twentieth-century psychiatrists often used race-neutral language but nonetheless "equated human normality with whiteness" (27).

10. For an excellent study that examines how biomedicine constructs racial categories, see Keith Wailoo, *Drawing Blood: Technology and Disease Identity in Twentieth-Century America* (Baltimore, MD: Johns Hopkins University Press, 1997), esp. 134–61.
11. Edward Jarvis, "Causes of Insanity," *Boston Medical and Surgical Journal* 45 (November 12, 1851): 291–92, 302–4; Amariah Brigham, *An Inquiry concerning the Diseases and Functions of the Brain, the Spinal Cord, and the Nerves* (1840; repr., New York: Arno Press, 1973), 203, 213, 286; A. P. Merrill, "An Essay on Some of the Distinctive Peculiarities of the Negro Race," *Southern Medical and Surgical Journal* 12 (January–March 1856): 23, 84; Daniel H. Tuke, "Does Civilization Favour the Generation of Mental Disease?," *Journal of Mental Science* 4 (October 1857): 96–97, 105–6; John Charles Bucknill and Daniel H. Tuke, *A Manual of Psychological Medicine: Containing the History, Nosology, Description, Statistics, Diagnosis, Pathology, and Treatment of Insanity, with an Appendix of Cases* (Philadelphia: Blanchard and Lea, 1858), 56; C. B. Hayden, "On the Distribution of Insanity in the U. States," *Southern Literary Messenger* 10 (March 1844): 180. On nineteenth-century physicians' ideas regarding the relationship between mind and body, see Charles E. Rosenberg, "Body and Mind in Nineteenth-Century Medicine: Some Clinical Origins of the Neurosis Construct," *Bulletin of the History of Medicine* 63 (Summer 1989): 185–97.
12. John S. Haller Jr., "The Physician versus the Negro: Medical and Anthropological Concepts of Race in the Late Nineteenth Century," *Bulletin of the History of Medicine* 44 (1970): 154–67; John S. Haller Jr., "Race and the Concept of Progress in Nineteenth Century American Ethnology," *American Anthropologist* 73 (1971): 710–23.
13. White American psychiatrists' constant grappling with the presumed "normal abnormality" of their African American patients bears striking similarities to the difficulties that colonial psychiatrists had in diagnosing and evaluating Africans. See Vaughan, *Curing Their Ills*, 100–128; Lynette Jackson, *Surfacing Up: Psychiatry and Social Order in Colonial Zimbabwe, 1908–1968* (Ithaca, NY: Cornell University Press, 2005). For an articulation of this ambiguous and contradictory construction of the Negro in the New South, see Andrew Zimmerman, *Alabama in Africa: Booker T. Washington, the German Empire, and the Globalization of the New South* (Princeton, NJ: Princeton University Press, 2010), 39–40.
14. William A. White, *Outlines of Psychiatry* (New York: Journal of Nervous and Mental Disease, 1907), 18.
15. My thinking on the complex imbrication of medical and racial objectification, on the one hand, and the desire to heal, on the other, in the intimacy of the clinical encounter is influenced by the following works: Good, *Medicine, Rationality, and Experience*, esp. 65–87; Ann Laura Stoler, "Tense and Tender Ties: The Politics of Comparison in North American History and (Post)Colonial Studies," *Journal of American History* 88 (December 2001): 829–65; Ann Laura Stoler, *Carnal Knowledge and Imperial Power: Race and the Intimate in Colonial Rule*, rev. ed. (Berkeley: University of California Press, 2010); Steven M. Stowe, *Doctoring the South: Southern Physicians and Everyday Medicine in the Mid-Nineteenth Century* (Chapel Hill: University of North Carolina Press, 2004).

    My use of the term "racialist" here follows Susan Reverby, author of *Examining Tuskegee: The Infamous Syphilis Study and Its Legacy* (Chapel Hill: University of North Carolina Press, 2009), who distinguishes between racialism as "the use of racial categories without emphasis on hierarchy" and racism as "a set of beliefs and behaviors and individual and institutional structures used to disempower and keep African Americans from equality" (6–7). Although not explicitly, Dennis Doyle, in *Psychiatry and Racial Liberalism in Harlem*, refuses that distinction when he defines racialism as "the premise that biological race determines an individual's personal capabilities" (4). Throughout this book I will use racialism sparingly. Through at least the mid-twentieth century, psychiatric thought was grounded in the belief in racial difference, so to speak of a racialist psychiatric thought is redundant. I also want to reserve the term *racist* for ideas that reflected or reinforced the belief in white superiority and black inferiority and practices and policies that produced unequal conditions and distribution of resources within Saint Elizabeths.
16. Nate Haseltine, "Woman's Campaign Started St. Elizabeths a Century Ago," *Washington Post and Times-Herald*, March 3, 1955, 17.

17. My own use of citizenship as a category of historical analysis differs from that of Matthew Gambino, who, in his astute dissertation on Saint Elizabeths, argues that a gendered and racialized conception of citizenship shaped the hospital staff's understanding of mental health and their therapeutic approaches to the institutionalized population. See Gambino, "Mental Health and Ideals of Citizenship," esp. 1–20.
18. For a study that explores the connection between access to medical care and citizenship within the context of emancipation, see Jim Downs, *Sick from Freedom: African-American Illness and Suffering during the Civil War and Reconstruction* (New York: Oxford University Press, 2012).
19. Beatrix Hoffman, *Health Care for Some: Rights and Rationing in the United States since 1930* (Chicago: University of Chicago Press, 2012), xii. See also Susan L. Smith, *Sick and Tired of Being Sick and Tired: Black Women's Health Activism in America, 1890–1950* (Philadelphia: University of Pennsylvania Press, 1995).
20. Susan Schweik, *The Ugly Laws: Disability in Public* (New York: New York University Press, 2009), 11.

Chapter 1

1. "Report of the Board of Visitors of the Government Hospital for the Insane, for the year ending June 30th 1856," entry 1, box 1, folios 30–31, SEH/BOVR.
2. "Fifth Annual Report of the Board of Visitors of the Government Hospital for the Insane, 1859–60," 10, in *Reports of the Government Hospital for the Insane*, vol. 1, 1855–1874, DOI-LR.
3. "Fifth Annual Report," 13.
4. Savitt, *Medicine and Slavery*, 258–79; Grob, "Class, Ethnicity, and Race," 223; McCandless, *Moonlight, Magnolias, and Madness*, 75–77.
5. For a detailed list of mental hospitals in the United States in the nineteenth century, see Grob, *Mental Institutions in America*, 374–95.
6. Grob, *Mental Institutions in America*, 7–10; Rothman, *Discovery of the Asylum*, 30–43; Dain, *Disordered Minds*, 5; Robert William Schoeberlein, "Mental Illness in Maryland: Public Perception, Discourse, and Treatment, from the Colonial Period to 1964" (PhD diss., University of Maryland, 2006), 2–10.
7. William Waller Hening, *The Statutes at Large: Being a Collection of All the Laws of Virginia, from the First Session of the Legislature, in the Year 1619* (Richmond, VA: J. & G. Cochran, 1821), 8:378–81; Dain, *Disordered Minds*, 37, 40.
8. William Kitty, comp., *The Laws of Maryland, to Which Are Prefixed the Original Charter . . . the Bill of Rights, and the Constitution. Revised and Collected, under the Authority of the Legislature*, vol. 2 (Annapolis, MD: n.p., 1799–[1800]), chaps. 102 and 114; Schoeberlein, "Mental Illness in Maryland," 10–13, 32–33.
9. Betty L. Plummer, "A History of Public Health in Washington, D.C., 1800–1890" (PhD diss., University of Maryland, 1984), 21–22, 25; Constance McLaughlin Green, *Washington: Village and Capital, 1800–1878* (Princeton, NJ: Princeton University Press, 1962), 41–42.
10. Green, *Washington: Village and Capital*, 42, 75–76; Charles W. Richardson and Edwin Melvin Williams, "Hospitals," in *Washington Past and Present: A History*, ed. John Clagett Proctor (New York: Lewis Historical Publishing, 1930), 2:669–70.
11. Green, *Washington: Village and Capital*, 164–65; *Laws of the Corporation of the City of Washington: Passed by the Thirtieth Council* (Washington, DC: Way and Gideon, 1833), 11.
12. *Intelligencer*, April 21, 1835, quoted in Richardson and Williams, "Hospitals," 683; Frank Rives Millikan, "Wards of the Nation: The Making of St. Elizabeths Hospital, 1852–1920" (PhD diss., George Washington University, 1990), 21; Plummer, "History of Public Health," 83–84.
13. "Message from the President of the United States," H.R. Doc. No. 25-96, at 1–2 (1838); "Richard Lawrence and Others," H.R. Rep. No. 25-923 (1838); "Memorial of the Corporate Authorities of the City of Washington, Praying the Improvement and Repair of Certain Streets, and the Establishment of an Hospital and Lunatic Asylum, in Said City," S. Doc. No. 26-98, at 2 (1840).

14. Schoeberlein, "Mental Illness in Maryland," 33–39; Millikan, "Wards of the Nation," 21; Albert Deutsch, *The Mentally Ill in America: A History of Their Care and Treatment from Colonial Times*, 2nd ed., rev. and exp. (New York: Columbia University Press, 1949), 106.
15. T. Hartley Crawford to Robert McClelland, August 14, 1855, DOI-LR, box 1.
16. "Pauper Lunatics, District of Columbia," H.R. Doc. No. 27-81 (1843); Deutsch, *Mentally Ill in America*, 106; Cong. Globe, 28th Cong., 1st Sess. 212 (1844).
17. Cong. Globe, 28th Cong., 1st Sess. 212, 231, 251–52, 592, 660 (1844); Richardson and Williams, "Hospitals," 669; Millikan, "Wards of the Nation," 22; Plummer, "History of Public Health," 85; Green, *Washington: Village and Capital*, 165; Schoeberlein, "Mental Illness in Maryland," 46.
18. Grob, *Mental Institutions in America*, 82, 246; Schoeberlein, "Mental Illness in Maryland," 39, 46. On the number of African Americans at Maryland Hospital in 1852 and the racial differential in the hospital's charge, see Charles H. Nichols to Dorothea Dix, December 5, 1852, DDC, entry 474, folder 2.
19. For general discussions of noninstitutionalized care of the insane in this period, see James E. Moran, "Asylum in the Community: Managing the Insane in Antebellum America," *History of Psychiatry* 4 (1998): 217–40; Samuel B. Thielman, "Community Management of Mental Disorders in Antebellum America," *Journal of the History of Medicine and Allied Sciences* 44 (July 1989): 351–74; Tomes, *A Generous Confidence*, esp. 103–8.
20. Green, *Washington: Village and Capital*, 21 (table 1); Letitia Woods Brown, *Free Negroes in the District of Columbia, 1790–1846* (New York: Oxford University Press, 1972), 41–49.
21. Mary Elizabeth Corrigan, "A Social Union of Heart and Effort: The African-American Family in the District of Columbia on the Eve of Emancipation" (PhD diss., University of Maryland, 1996), 219–79; Constance McLaughlin Green, *The Secret City: A History of Race Relations in the Nation's Capital* (Princeton, NJ: Princeton University Press, 1967), 16. See also Chris Myers Asch and George Derek Musgrove, *Chocolate City: A History of Race and Democracy in the Nation's Capital* (Chapel Hill: University of North Carolina Press, 2017), 32, 39–44.
22. For a discussion of lay treatments for insanity and other nervous diseases, see Thielman, "Community Management of Mental Disorders"; Kay K. Moss, *Southern Folk Medicine, 1750–1820* (Columbia: University of South Carolina Press, 1999), 145–47.
23. Sharla M. Fett, *Working Cures: Healing, Health, and Power on Southern Slave Plantations* (Chapel Hill: University of North Carolina Press, 2002), 169–92; John W. Blassingame, *The Slave Community: Plantation Life in the Antebellum South*, rev. and enlarged ed. (New York: Oxford University Press, 1979), 298–99; Dea H. Boster, "An 'Epeleptick' Bondswoman: Fits, Slavery, and Power in the Antebellum South," *Bulletin of the History of Medicine* 83 (Summer 2009): 276, 290–301. See also Dea H. Boster, *African American Slavery and Disability: Bodies, Property, and Power in the Antebellum South, 1800–1860* (New York: Routledge, 2013), 95–118; Marli F. Weiner with Mazie Hough, *Sex, Sickness, and Slavery: Illness in the Antebellum South* (Urbana: University of Illinois Press, 2012), 168–74.
24. Brown, *Free Negroes*, 24; Barbara Jeanne Fields, *Slavery and Freedom on the Middle Ground: Maryland during the Nineteenth Century* (New Haven, CT: Yale University Press, 1985), 32; Fett, *Working Cures*, 26; Leslie Howard Owen, *This Species of Property: Slave Life and Culture in the Old South* (New York: Oxford University Press, 1976), 44–46; Mary Tremain, *Slavery in the District of Columbia: The Policy of Congress and the Struggle for Abolition* (1892; repr., New York: Negro Universities Press, 1969), 31.
25. Corrigan, "Social Union of Heart and Effort," 309–10.
26. Leonard P. Curry, *The Free Black in Urban America, 1800–1850: The Shadow of the Dream* (Chicago: University of Chicago Press, 1981), 17–18, 21, 258–60; Green, *Secret City*, 15–16, 28, 37; Corrigan, "Social Union of Heart and Effort," 123–24, 175–218. The restrictions on free blacks were passed after a race riot that followed an enslaved man's attempt to murder his white mistress, an attempt that white Washingtonians attributed to the circulation of abolitionist literature in the District.
27. Corrigan, "Social Union of Heart and Effort," 159–60.
28. Green, *Washington: Village and Capital*, 91; Corrigan, "Social Union of Heart and Effort," 87–88n71.
29. The data and the explanation are provided by Leonard Curry in *Free Black in Urban America*, 123–26.

30. Thomas Miller to William Easby, January 24, 1852, DOI-LR, box 1 (emphasis in the original); Millikan, "Wards of the Nation," 23.
31. "Memorial of D. L. Dix, Praying a Land Grant for the Relief and Support of the Indigent Curable and Incurable Insane in the United States," June 27, 1848, 30th Congress, 1st Session, Miscellaneous Senate Document No. 150, 21, 24 (italics in the original), reprinted in Dorothea L. Dix, *On Behalf of the Insane Poor: Selected Reports* (New York: Arno Press and New York Times, 1971).
32. Cong. Globe, 32nd Cong., 1st Sess. 2133 (1852); Schoeberlein, "Mental Illness in Maryland," 45; Millikan, "Wards of the Nation," 24–25.
33. Cong. Globe, 32nd Cong. 1st Sess. 2133 (1852).
34. Cong. Globe, 32nd Cong., 1st Sess. 2133 (1852).
35. Richard Wallach to Alexander H. H. Stuart, December 21, 1850, in "Report of the Secretary of the Interior," S. Doc. No. 31-8 (1850).
36. Cong. Globe, 32nd Cong., 1st Sess. 2133, 2341, 2419 (1852); Cong. Globe, 32nd Cong., 1st Sess. xvii (1852) index; Cong. Globe, 32nd Cong., 2nd Sess. 9 (1853).
37. Miller to Easby, January 24, 1852, DOI-LR, box 1.
38. Fillmore to Dix, October 21, 1852 (emphasis in the original), in *The Lady and the President: The Letters of Dorothea Dix and Millard Fillmore*, ed. Charles M. Snyder (Lexington: University Press of Kentucky, 1975), 140. Superintendent was often a plum government position, and their appointment as well as their removal could be an intensely politically partisan affair. For more on the patronage politics surrounding the nineteenth-century asylum, see Grob, *Mental Institutions in America*, 142–43.
39. On Nichols's Quakerism, see Stephen A. Chase et al. to Baltimore Monthly Meeting of Friends, May 10, 1860, box 1, SEH/Nichols. On the influence of Quakerism in the development of the colonial and antebellum asylum, see Grob, *Mental Institutions in America*, 17–19, 47–48.
40. Charles H. Nichols to Thomas S. Kirkbride, March 3 and March 30, 1852, box 137, file 76, Thomas Story Kirkbride Material, Series 2, Subseries A, Institute of Pennsylvania Hospital Archives, Pennsylvania Hospital Historic Collections, Philadelphia; Nichols to Dix, February 23, 1852, DDC, entry 474, folder 1 (emphasis in the original).
41. Nichols to Dix, September 11, 18, and 20, 1852, DDC, entry 474, folder 2 (emphasis in the originals).
42. "Report of the Secretary of the Interior," S. Doc. No. 32-11, at 13 (1852).
43. "Report of the Secretary of the Interior," 2; Nichols to Dix, September 20, 1852, DDC, entry 474, folder 2.
44. "Report of the Secretary of the Interior," 3; John P. H. Murphy, "Progress, Science and the Mind: A History of Saint Elizabeths Hospital," *Medical Annals of the District of Columbia* 7 (October 1938): 316–17; Louise Daniel Hutchinson, *The Anacostia Story: 1608–1930* (Washington, DC: Smithsonian Institution Press, 1977), 49–53.
45. "Report of the Secretary of the Interior," 3–5, 8–11.
46. "Report of the Secretary of the Interior," 5 (emphasis in the original).
47. Savitt, *Medicine and Slavery*, 17–26, 240–46; Conevery Bolton Valenčius, *The Health of the Country: How American Settlers Understood Themselves and Their Land* (New York: Basic Books, 2002), 79–80, 114; James Borchert, *Alley Life in Washington: Family, Community, Religion, and Folklife in the City, 1850–1970* (Urbana: University of Illinois Press, 1980), 5, 13; Curry, *Free Black in Urban America*, 139.
48. Historian Conevery Bolton Valenčius refers to this as a "geography of health" producing a "racial topography." See Valenčius, *Health of the Country*, 88.
49. "Report of the Secretary of the Interior," 7.
50. Isaac Ray, "American Hospitals for the Insane," *North American Review* 79 (July 1854): 72. See also Carla Yanni, *The Architecture of Madness: Insane Asylums in the United States* (Minneapolis: University of Minnesota Press, 2007), esp. chap. 1.
51. "Report of the Secretary of the Interior," 11.
52. Savitt, *Medicine and Slavery*, 266–71.
53. John M. Galt to Samuel B. Woodward (n.d.), box 1, folder 1, Samuel B. Woodward Papers, American Antiquarian Society, Worcester, Massachusetts.

54. John M. Galt, "Asylums for Colored Persons," *American Psychological Journal* 1 (January 1853): 84–86.
55. Galt, "Asylums for Colored Persons," 85.
56. See, for example, Samuel A. Cartwright, "Report on the Diseases and Physical Peculiarities of the Negro Race," *New Orleans Medical and Surgical Journal* 7 (1851), reprinted in *The Nature of Difference: Sciences of Race in the United States from Jefferson to Genomics*, ed. Evelynn M. Hammonds and Rebecca M. Herzig (Cambridge, MA: MIT Press, 2008). Cartwright wrote, "There is partial insensibility of the skin, and so great a hebetude of the intellectual faculties as to be like a person half asleep, that is with difficulty aroused and kept awake" (81). See also Mark M. Smith, *How Race Is Made: Slavery, Segregation, and the Senses* (Chapel Hill: University of North Carolina Press, 2006), esp. 11–28.
57. Galt, "Asylums for Colored Persons," 87.
58. For similar arguments made with respect to other southern asylums, see Randolph, "Central Lunatic Asylum," 51; Savitt, *Medicine and Slavery*, 270–71; Dain, *Disordered Minds*, 109–13; McCandless, *Moonlight, Magnolias, and Madness*, 274.
59. Nichols to Kirkbride, April 24, 1855, quoted in Grob, "Class, Ethnicity, and Race," 225; Nichols to Dix, January 1, 1853, DDC, entry 474, folder 2.
60. On Kirkbride's opposition to the racial integration of Eastern Lunatic Asylum, see Dain, *Disordered Minds*, 109.
61. "Proceedings of the Tenth Annual Meeting of the Association of Medical Superintendents of American Institutions for the Insane," *American Journal of Insanity* 12 (July 1855): 88–89.
62. Yanni, *Architecture of Madness*, 24.
63. Ray, "American Hospitals for the Insane," 80.
64. "Asylum for the Insane of the Army and Navy and the District of Columbia," *American Journal of Insanity* 9 (April 1853): 385; "Report of the Secretary of the Interior," 4; Nichols to Dix, July 24, 1853, DDC, entry 474, folder 3.
65. "Report of the Secretary of the Interior," S. Doc. No. 33-35, at 3 (1854); Dix to Fillmore, February 9, [1854], and July 13, [1854], in Snyder, *Lady and the President*, 171–72, 198–99.
66. Nichols to Dix, April 7, 1855, DDC, entry 474, folder 3.
67. Cong. Globe, 33rd Cong., 2nd Sess. Appendix 391 (1855).
68. "Notice for the Annual Report of 1877 of the retirement of Dr. C. H. Nichols," entry 2, box 1, SEH/BOVR, 1855–1947, Correspondence and Other Records, 1857–1903; "Report of the Superintendent of the Government Hospital for the Insane," October 1, 1855, 3, 10, pamphlet in vertical file, "Hospitals, St. Elizabeth's Legislation," DCPL.
69. Nichols to Dix, October 29, 1855, DDC, entry 474, folder 4; L. F. Tasistro, *Morrisons' Stranger's Guide for Washington City; with Etiquette to be Observed in Calling Upon the President, Officers of the Government, Foreign Ministers, &c.* (Washington, DC: W. H. & O. H. Morrison, 1866), 40; "Report of the Superintendent," 5.
70. "Report of the Superintendent," 5.
71. Nichols to Dix, April 7, 1855, DDC, entry 474, folder 3. For more on the process of constructing Saint Elizabeths, see Millikan, "Wards of the Nation," 40–56.

Chapter 2

1. "Letter from the Secretary of the Interior," H.R. Doc. No. 33-24, at 1 (1854); *By-Laws of the Government Hospital for the Insane*, 6–7.
2. Cong. Globe, 33rd Cong., 2nd Sess. Appendix 400 (1855); "Letter from the Secretary of the Interior," 3–4.
3. C. H. Nichols to Dr. Gunnell, May 20, 1886, copy, entry 1, box 1, folios 414–16, SEH/BOVM.
4. "Report of the Superintendent of the Government Hospital for the Insane," October 1, 1855, 3, pamphlet in vertical file, "Hospitals, St. Elizabeth's Legislation," DCPL.
5. All five were born in the District of Columbia and were listed as "civil indigent," which was synonymous with the category "pauper insane." See Hospital Register, box 1, vol. 1, entries 52–56, SEH/RC.
6. SEH/RC, box 1, vol. 1, entry 97.

7. "No. 749, W.H.D.," Journal of the Reception of Convicts Received into the Penitentiary for the District of Columbia, n.p., Entry 474, Records Relating to the US Penitentiary for the District of Columbia, Registers of Convicts, 1831–1862, vol. 1; March 13, 1858–March 22, 1859, Register of Punishments, Entry 475, Records Relating to the US Penitentiary for the District of Columbia, Register of Punishments, 1831–1862, box 1, Record of Punishment—US Penitentiary, 1854 to 1860. Both in RG 48 Records of the Department of the Interior, NARA. SEH/RC, box 1, vol. 1, entry 250.
8. Quoted in David K. Sullivan, "Behind Prison Walls: The Operation of the District Penitentiary, 1831–1862," *Records of the Columbia Historical Society, Washington, D.C.* 71-72 (1971): 262.
9. *By-Laws of the Government Hospital for the Insane*, 19, 22.
10. SEH/RC, box 1, vol. 1, entries 66, 67, and 180.
11. SEH/RC, box 1, vol. 1, entries 281, 283, and 369.
12. Clement Dorsey, *The General Public Statutory Law and Public Local Law of the State of Maryland, from the Year 1692 to 1839 Inclusive: With Annotations Thereto, and a Copious Index* (Baltimore, MD: John D. Toy, 1840), 1:338–39.
13. Thomas D. Morris, *Southern Slavery and the Law, 1619–1860* (Chapel Hill: University of North Carolina Press, 1996), 354–68.
14. SEH/RC, box 1, vol. 1, entry 283; George Waters to Charles H. Nichols, December 24, 1859, SEH/Nichols.
15. Tomes, *A Generous Confidence*, 122–23. For a different argument that emphasizes the conflict between lay communities and asylum physicians over insanity, see Moran, "Asylum in the Community," 217–40.
16. Cong. Globe, 33rd Cong., 2nd Sess., Appendix 400 (1855).
17. Charles H. Nichols to Robert McClelland, July 30, 1855, DOI-LR, box 1.
18. Tomes, *A Generous Confidence*, 118–19; Rothman, *Discovery of the Asylum*, 143–44. Nichols did not attempt to resolve the contradiction of advocating for a procedure in criminal court as a way of stripping commitment of "the odor of criminal detention."
19. "Report of the Board of Visitors of the Government Hospital for the Insane, For the Year Ending 1857," 739–40, in *Reports of the Government Hospital for the Insane*, vol. 1, *1855–1874*, DOI-LR, box 6; Cong. Globe, 34th Cong. 3rd Sess. 560 (1857).
20. William Miller, Daniel Ratcliffe, and C. H. Nichols to Gentlemen, July 1, 1857, entry 2, box 1, SEH/BOVR.
21. Cong. Globe, 34th Cong., 3rd Sess. 560 (1857); Minutes, n.d. [1861], entry 1, box 1, folio 128, SEH/BOVM (quote).
22. July 1, 1856 minutes, entry 1, box 1, folio 15, SEH/BOVM; "Fifth Annual Report of the Board of Visitors of the Government Hospital for the Insane, 1859–60," 7, in *Reports of the Government Hospital for the Insane*, vol. 1, *1855–1874*, DOI-LR, box 6.
23. Suryabala Kanhouwa and Jogues R. Prandoni, "The Civil War and St. Elizabeths Hospital: An Untold Story of Services from the First Federal Mental Institution in the United States," *Journal of Civil War Medicine* 9 (January–March 2005): 12–13; Green, *Washington: Village and Capital*, 247, 254, 261.
24. Charles H. Nichols to Dorothea Dix, May 9, 1861, DDC, entry 474, folder 6; "Reports of the Board of Visitors and the Superintendent of Construction of the Government Hospital for the Insane, For the year 1861–62," 25–26, in *Reports of the Government Hospital for the Insane*, vol. 1, *1855–1874*, DOI-LR, box 6; Otto, *St. Elizabeths Hospital*, 77.
25. Kanhouwa and Prandoni, "Civil War and St. Elizabeths Hospital," 2–3.
26. S. Preston Jones to Charles H. Nichols, July 1, 1863, SEH/Nichols; Tomes, *A Generous Confidence*, 166.
27. Minutes, n.d. [1861], entry 1, box 1, folios 134–35, SEH/BOVM.
28. By the end of the 1864–65 fiscal year, military patients made up 86 percent of total admissions to Saint Elizabeths (443 of 515). For every civilian admission, there were approximately six military admissions. These figures include African Americans. See Kanhouwa and Prandoni, "Civil War and St. Elizabeths Hospital," 7–8. For a discussion of the postcombat stress experienced by African American soldiers, see Joseph T. Glatthaar, *Forged in Battle: The Civil War Alliance of Black Soldiers and White Officers* (New York: Free Press, 1990), 238–42.
29. Minutes, n.d. [1861], entry 1, box 1, folios 134–35, SEH/BOVM.

30. Fields, *Slavery and Freedom*, 92–108, 115; Kate Masur, *An Example for All the Land: Emancipation and the Struggle over Equality in Washington, D.C.* (Chapel Hill: University of North Carolina Press, 2010), 24–25; Green, *Washington: Village and Capital*, 274 (quote); Asch and Musgrove, *Chocolate City*, 109–15. No serious colonization of freed slaves was ever undertaken.
31. Fields, *Slavery and Freedom*, 111; Masur, *Example for All the Land*, 30. Fugitive slave laws were not abrogated until June 1864, although they were routinely challenged by legal and extralegal tactics by African Americans and sympathetic whites.
32. Allan Johnston, *Surviving Freedom: The Black Community of Washington, D.C., 1860–1880* (New York: Garland, 1993), 108–11.
33. "Contraband of war" was a designation given to fugitive slaves by the Union military early in the conflict in order to allow them to avoid returning slaves to their Confederate masters—and later to actually confiscate enslaved people—without appearing to threaten general emancipation. The use of the term "contraband" to refer to escaping slaves eventually became widespread in the press, political circles, and popular culture. See Kate Masur, "'A Rare Phenomenon of Philological Vegetation': The Word 'Contraband' and the Meanings of Emancipation in the United States," *Journal of American History* 93 (March 2007): 1050–84.
34. Green, *Washington: Village and Capital*, 275–76; Johnston, *Surviving Freedom*, 121; Plummer, "History of Public Health," 101–2; Masur, *Example for All the Land*, 55.
35. Masur, *Example for All the Land*, 44; Plummer, "History of Public Health," 103; Joseph P. Reidy, "'Coming from the Shadows of the Past': The Transition from Slavery to Freedom at Freedmen's Village, 1863–1900," *Virginia Magazine of History and Biography* 95 (October 1987): 407–13; Johnston, *Surviving Freedom*, 122.
36. R. A. Abbott to Secretary of the Interior, June 29, 1863, DOI-LR, box 1.
37. Chief Clerk of the Department of the Interior to J. P. Sherburn, September 26, [1863?], copy in Letter Book, p. 51, RG 48 Records of the Department of the Interior, Entry 301, Letters Sent concerning the Government Hospital for the Insane, 1857–1866, NARA; Cong. Globe, 36th Cong., 2nd Sess. 1246 (1861). Nichols proposed this change in the admissions policy. See Charles H. Nichols to Moses Kelly, February 11, 1861, DOI-LR, box 1.
38. "Reports of the Board of Visitors and the Superintendent of Construction of the Government Hospital for the Insane, For the year 1862–63," 4, in *Reports of the Government Hospital for the Insane*, vol. 1, 1855–1874, DOI-LR, box 6.
39. Charles H. Nichols to James Harlan, August 7, 1865, DOI-LR, box 1.
40. Elias Greene to J. P. Usher, June 3, 1864; Charles H. Nichols to Usher, June 6, 1864. Both in DOI-LR, box 1.
41. Amos Pettijohn to Upsher [sic], July 21, 1864; [F. W.?] Mead to Upsher [sic], July 25, 1864; Nichols to Usher, July 27, 1864. All in DOI-LR, box 1.
42. Nichols to Usher, June 6, 1864, DOI-LR, box 1.
43. Lois E. Horton, "The Development of Federal Social Policy for Blacks in Washington, D.C. after Emancipation" (PhD diss., Brandeis University, 1977), 93–97.
44. Downs, *Sick from Freedom*, 146–52.
45. On camps in northern Virginia, see Johnston, *Surviving Freedom*, 122.
46. Of the 146 admissions between 1855 and 1866, 92 inmates were diagnosed with either mania, chronic mania, or acute mania. One individual was diagnosed with epileptic mania. The next category of disease that was most commonly diagnosed in African Americans was dementia, including chronic, acute, and epileptic dementia. Only 3 of the 146 inmates were diagnosed with some form of melancholia. There was no diagnostic information for five of the individuals admitted. See SEH/RC, box 1, vol. 1.
47. SEH/RC, box 1, vol. 1, entry 2212. While there was no bright line between the two, physicians tended to group physiological phenomena contributing to insanity under the broad category of physical or remote causes and psychological phenomena under the category of moral or inciting causes. Physical or remote causes were rarely enough to induce mental derangement by themselves. Rather, they had an enervating effect on the mental faculties, thereby making the mind more susceptible to psychological disturbances.
48. Henry Maudsley, *The Physiology and Pathology of the Mind* (London: Macmillan, 1867), 303–4.

49. Frank Rives Millikan suggests that Nichols placed a premium on gathering knowledge about incoming inmates. This was reflective of a larger dynamic that existed between the nineteenth-century psychiatric profession and lay communities. Ellen Dwyer argues, "While certainly through their diagnostic schema asylum doctors did their best to medicalize popular notions of insanity, asylum doctors most often simply acquiesced in a diagnosis made outside the institution. Families, neighbors, and employers usually were first to label as 'insane' markedly eccentric or threatening behavior, and committing doctors' papers most often parroted their observations." Dwyer, *Homes for the Mad*, 117–18; Millikan, "Wards of the Nation," 71.
50. William B. Carpenter, *Principles of Mental Physiology, with Their Application to the Training and Discipline of the Mind, and the Study of Its Morbid Conditions*, 4th ed. (London: Henry S. King, 1876), 658–63; Maudsley, *Physiology and Pathology of the Mind*, 311–19. Nichols did believe in the phenomenon of moral insanity, however. See "Annual Meeting of the Association of Medical Superintendents of American Institutions for the Insane," *American Journal of Insanity* 20 (July 1863): 60–106.
51. Maximilian Leidesdorf, "Lehrbuch der psychischen Krankheiten" (1865), cited in William A. Hammond, *A Treatise on Insanity and Its Medical Relations* (New York: D. Appleton, 1883), 288.
52. Maudsley, *Physiology and Pathology of the Mind*, 320–24; "Annual Meeting of the Association of Medical Superintendents of American Institutions for the Insane," 63–64.
53. Maudsley, *Physiology and Pathology of the Mind*, 323, 320.
54. Bucknill and Tuke, *Manual of Psychological Medicine*, 222, 293.
55. Dwyer, *Homes for the Mad*, 119; Grob, *Mental Institutions in America*, 224.
56. "Eleventh Annual Report of the Board of Visitors and the Fourteenth Annual Report of the Superintendent of Construction, of the Government Hospital for the Insane, for the Year 1865–'66," 578–79, in *Reports of the Government Hospital for the Insane*, vol. 1, *1855–1874*, DOI-LR, box 6. Not all physicians and asylum superintendents were sanguine about the curability of insanity through this therapeutic model. Pliny Earle, who worked at Saint Elizabeths during the Civil War before becoming superintendent of Northampton Lunatic Hospital in Massachusetts, thought the asymptomatic nature of mental illness prevented early intervention in many cases. For his position and for a discussion of the various medical remedies of the mid-nineteenth century, see Pliny Earle, *The Curability of Insanity* (Boston: Albert J. Wright, 1876), 17–19, 28. Another physician, Charles A. Lee, took issue with moral treatment, both in what he felt was its inattention to distinguishing forms of insanity and its rationale of sequestration. See Charles A. Lee, *On Provision for the Insane Poor of the State of New York* (Albany, NY: Van Benthuysen's Steam Printing House, 1866), 10.
57. John M. Galt, *Essays on Asylums for Persons of Unsound Mind* (Richmond, VA: H. K. Ellyson's Power Press, 1850), 9.
58. Nichols to Dix, January 28, 1856, DDC, entry 474, folder 4.
59. "Remarks of Hon. John G. Davis," Cong. Globe, 33rd Cong., 2nd Sess. 202 (1855) (quote); C. H. Nichols to William Gunton, August 2, 1862, entry 2, box 1, SEH/BOVR.
60. See the Inspection Reports for August 1, 1876, November 6, 1877, and December 2, 1873, folios 303–4, 342, and 265, SEH/BOVM. Erving Goffman referred to this as "looping," in which the "inmate's reaction to his own situation is collapsed back into this situation itself." Erving Goffman, *Asylums: Essays on the Social Situation of Mental Patients and Other Inmates* (New York: Anchor Books, 1961), 35–37.
61. My thinking on this has been influenced by Steven M. Stowe, who, in his study of nineteenth-century southern doctors, argues that, "even though utilitarian daybooks might seem to stand outside ideology, their unselfconscious practicality and their baseline medical judgments gave them an essentially ideological power to reinscribe and naturalize fundamental social relations" between physicians and patients. Stowe, *Doctoring the South*, 104.
62. Alexander Robertson, "Notes of a Visit to American Asylums," *Journal of Mental Science* 15 (1869): 68; "Government Hospital for the Insane," *New National Era*, March 20, 1873, 2.
63. "Eleventh Annual Report," 582.
64. "Proceedings of the Association of Medical Superintendents," *American Journal of Insanity* 30 (October 1873): 179.

65. "Report of the Board of Visitors of the Hospital for the Insane, Accompanying the Annual Report of the Secretary of the Interior For the Year 1859," 12, 15, in *Reports for the Government Hospital for the Insane*, vol. 1, *1855–1874*, DOI-LR, box 6; "Fifth Annual Report," 3; "Bibliographical Reports of American Asylums," *American Journal of Insanity* 18 (January 1862): 274; Minutes, July 2, 1861, entry 1, box 1, folio 117, SEH/BOVM; "Eleventh Annual Report," 584.
66. John Curwen, "Proceedings of the Association of Medical Superintendents," *American Journal of Insanity* 32 (January 1876): 319; Charles H. Nichols to the Board of Visitors, January 5, 1875, in "Letter from the Secretary of the Interior, relative to the erection of a new building to be devoted solely to the detention and treatment of female patients at the Insane Asylum," S. Doc. 43-136 (1875), in DOI-LR, box 1.
67. "Report of the Board of Visitors of the Hospital for the Insane . . . For the Year 1859," 15. On the colored lodges' lack of forced-air ventilation, see "Reports of American Asylums, 1875–1876," *American Journal of Insanity* 33 (January 1877): 431. On the importance of forced-air ventilation and the quote, see Charles H. Nichols, "On the Best Mode of Providing for the Subjects of Chronic Insanity," in *Transactions of the International Medical Congress* (Philadelphia: Printed for the Congress by John Ashurst Jr., 1877), 1129.
68. Racist opposition to the construction of a colored lodge was discussed in chapter 1. For the quote, see Nichols to Dix, April 7, 1855, DDC, entry 474, folder 3.
69. Isaac Ray, *Ideal Characters of the Officers of a Hospital for the Insane* (Philadelphia: J. B. Chandler, 1873), 12, 32.
70. *By-Laws of the Government Hospital for the Insane*, 13; George F. Shrady, "Proceedings of the Fifteenth Annual Meeting of the Association of Medical Superintendents of American Institutions for the Insane," *American Journal of Insanity* 17 (July 1860): 57, 60.
71. For a discussion of the use of slave labor in southern asylums, see Grob, *Mental Institutions in America*, 214–15.
72. Charles H. Nichols to C. B. Poulson, May 15, 1858, quoted in Millikan, "Wards of the Nation," 63. Nichols did hire African Americans to work in positions that would not require contact with patients, such as mowers, cowboys, plowmen, and ox drivers. See "Complete Alphabetical List of All the Employes of the Government Hospital for the Insane, whose Salaries are paid by the Superintendent with the amount of salary paid each," ca. 1865, DOI-LR, box 1.
73. Lee, *On Provision for the Insane Poor*, 10. For a good discussion of the restraint-nonrestraint debate, see Grob, *Mental Institutions in America*, 206–10.
74. For examples, see C. H. Nichols to T. S. Kirkbride, August 14, 1861, folder "Letters Received from Dorothea Dix, 1858–1868," SEH/Nichols; Nichols to Kirkbride, May 13,1855, box 137, file 76, Thomas Story Kirkbride Material, Series 2, Subseries A, Institute of Pennsylvania Hospital Archives, Pennsylvania Hospital Historic Collections, Philadelphia.
75. John Charles Bucknill, "Notes on Asylums for the Insane in America," *American Journal of Insanity* 33 (July 1876): 39; Robertson, "Notes of a Visit," 66.
76. In fact Nichols argued that "all rules of classification in American institutions are, and should be, regarded as generalizations" except "the rule, which should be inflexibly adhered to, that the violent and turbulent should be entirely separated from the quiet and orderly." See Nichols, "On the Best Mode," 1135.
77. How this manifested at Saint Elizabeths will be discussed at greater length in chapter 4. An example of this dynamic outside of the United States is Cape Colony. In Robben Island Lunatic Asylum in southern Africa in the late nineteenth century, for instance, the most violent white inmates were housed with the majority of coloured inmates in the *kraal* (Dutch for animal pen), and the few "respectable" coloured inmates were placed in the predominantly white section, which was known as "Lunatic Square." See Harriet Jane Deacon, "Madness, Race and Moral Treatment: Robben Island Lunatic Asylum, Cape Colony, 1846–1890," *History of Psychiatry* 7 (1996): 292.
78. Nichols, "On the Best Mode," 1134 (emphasis in the original).
79. Millikan, "Wards of the Nation," 61; "Report of the Superintendent of the Government Hospital for the Insane [1855]," 6; Robertson, "Notes of a Visit," 66.

80. Charles Nichols to Thomas Kirkbride, October 27, 1858, box 137, file 76, Thomas Story Kirkbride Material, Series 2, Subseries A, Institute of Pennsylvania Hospital Archives, Pennsylvania Hospital Historic Collections, Philadelphia.
81. John M. Galt, *Essays on Asylums for Persons of Unsound Mind*, 2nd series (Richmond, VA: Ritchies and Dunnavant, 1853), 15–16.
82. Robertson, "Notes of a Visit," 66; 1863 Diary of Pliny Earle, box 9, Pliny Earle Papers, American Antiquarian Society, Worcester, Massachusetts; *Memoirs of Pliny Earle, M.D.*, ed. F. B. Sanborn (1898; repr., New York: Arno Press, 1973), 246; Minutes, June 19, 1867, November 2, 1875, entry 1, box 1, folios 174 and 294, SEH/BOVM.
83. Robertson, "Notes of a Visit," 66; Galt, *Essays on Asylums*, 2nd series, 19.
84. Segregation, and the eventual integration, of recreational and leisure spaces at Saint Elizabeths in the twentieth century will be addressed in chapters 8 and 9.
85. 1864 Diary of Pliny Earle, box 9, Earle Papers.
86. For a fascinating study that examines how minstrelsy was used in the New York State Lunatic Asylum by staff to maintain order and by white patients to position themselves as rational actors in relation to blacks, see Benjamin Reiss, *Theaters of Madness: Insane Asylums and Nineteenth-Century American Culture* (Chicago: University of Chicago Press, 2008), 51–77. See also Philip Cushman, *Constructing the Self, Constructing America: A Cultural History of Psychotherapy* (Reading, MA: Addison-Wesley, 1995), 41–52.
87. Samuel F. to C. H. Nichols, August 11, 1873, Case File No. 3322, box 12, SEH/CFP; SEH/RC, box 1, vol. 1, entry 3322.
88. Julius H. Nelson (pseudonym) to C. H. Nichols, December 10, 1875, November 1876, Case File No. 3345, box 12, SEH/CFP.
89. Archibald Lester (pseudonym) to C. H. Nichols, July 31, 1874, August 5, 1874, Case File No. 3057, box 9, SEH/CFP.
90. Jacob Foster (pseudonym) to "Sir," November 5, 1875, Case File No. 4320, box 20, SEH/CFP.
91. Lucinda Callaway (pseudonym) to C. H. Nichols, August 30, 1875, January 1878, Case File No. 3780, box 15, SEH/CFP.
92. SEH/RC, box 1, vol. 1, entry 4117; Randolph, "Central Lunatic Asylum," 117; McCandless, *Moonlight, Magnolias, and Madness*, 231; G. S. Palmer to Columbus Delano, June 30, 1875, box 1, RG 48 Records of the Department of the Interior, Letters Received and Other Records relating to the Freedmen's Hospital, 1872–1910, NARA. Given Harris's prominence as a black physician and fledgling Reconstruction politician, I have chosen not to shield his identity.
93. Mrs. Dr. Harris to Dr. Witmer, July 19, 1877; Harris to W. W. Godding, November 28, 1878. Both in Case File No. 4117, box 19, SEH/CFP (emphasis in the original).
94. Joseph D. Harris to Charles H. Nichols, November 27, 1876, February 24, 1876, Case File No. 4117, box 19, SEH/CFP (emphasis in the original).
95. Joseph D. Harris to Charles H. Nichols, March 26, 1877, Case File No. 4117, box 19, SEH/CFP (emphasis in the original).
96. "Charges and Specifications against Dr. C. B. Purvis, Surgeon-in-Charge of Freedmen's Hospital [1890]"; Thomas H. Musick to W. W. Godding, copy, June 25, 1890; Affidavit of W. W. Godding, copy, June 26, 1890. All in box 3, RG 48 Records of the Department of the Interior, Letters Received and Other Records relating to the Freedmen's Hospital, 1872–1910, NARA.
97. I take the term "prerogative power" from political scientist Wendy Brown, who defines it as the "legitimate arbitrary power in policy making and legitimate monopolies of internal and external violence in the police and military." Wendy Brown, *States of Injury: Power and Freedom in Late Modernity* (Princeton, NJ: Princeton University Press, 1995), 176.
98. "The Insane Asylum. Grave Allegations. Mismanagement—Corruption," *Saturday Evening Visitor*, November 6, 1869, 1; "The Insane Asylum. An Investigation Progressing," *Saturday Evening Visitor*, November 27, 1869, 1; "The Insane Asylum Investigation," *Saturday Evening Visitor*, December 4, 1869, 1; Nichols to Dix, November 26, 1869, DDC, entry 474, folder 9.

99. "Cruelty to Insane Persons," *New York Times*, August 17, 1875, 1. Another episode was further evidence of corruption, according to the *Times*, in which the escorting and abandonment of two patients had been a ruse for a Metropolitan police officer to travel to a prizefight outside of the District. The boondoggle was allegedly aided by Nichols, who happened to be vice president of the Police Board at the time.
100. "House Investigations," *New York Times*, April 21, 1876, 1; "The Government Insane Asylum," *New York Times*, April 23, 1876, 2. For a good discussion of the 1876 investigation, see Millikan, "Wards of the Nation," 84–96.
101. For examples, see "Proceedings of the Association of Medical Superintendents," *American Journal of Insanity* 33 (October 1876): 215; Morris to the editor, *New York Times*, May 20, 1876, 3.
102. "Notes from the Capital," *New York Times*, July 31, 1876, 1; Millikan, "Wards of the Nation," 92–94.
103. J. K. Barnes et al. to William Windom, February 26, 1877, Joseph Meredith Toner Collection, container 87, Manuscript Division, Library of Congress, Washington, DC.
104. "Summary," *American Journal of Insanity* 34 (July 1877): 113; "Notes and Comments," *American Journal of Insanity* 46 (January 1890): 408.

Chapter 3

1. G. A. Tucker, *Lunacy in Many Lands; Being an Introduction to the Reports on the Lunatic Asylums of Various Countries Visited in 1882–5* (Sydney: Charles Potter, 1887), 60–61.
2. Tucker, *Lunacy in Many Lands*, 61.
3. George M. Fredrickson, *The Black Image in the White Mind: The Debate on Afro-American Character and Destiny, 1817–1914* (1971; repr., Hanover, NH: Wesleyan University Press, 1987), 198–227; Joel Williamson, *A Rage for Order: Black-White Relations in the American South Since Emancipation* (New York: Oxford University Press, 1986).
4. There is a large body of scholarship on post-Reconstruction rhetoric about African American criminality and susceptibility to disease. Some representative titles are Tera W. Hunter, *To 'Joy My Freedom: Southern Black Women's Lives and Labors after the Civil War* (Cambridge, MA: Harvard University Press, 1997); Khalil G. Muhammad, *The Condemnation of Blackness: Race, Crime, and the Making of Modern Urban America* (Cambridge, MA: Harvard University Press, 2011); and Smith, *Sick and Tired of Being Sick and Tired*.
5. Grob, *Mental Illness and American Society*, 50–62; Rosenberg, "Body and Mind in Nineteenth-Century Medicine," 194–95. There was, however, a rather high-profile dispute over what, in effect, constituted insanity when asylum physician and editor of the *American Journal of Insanity* John P. Gray and New York neurologist Edward C. Spitzka testified on opposing sides in the trial of Charles Guiteau, the assassin of President James A. Garfield. See Gerald Grob, "Psychiatry's Holy Grail: The Search for the Mechanisms of Mental Diseases," *Bulletin of the History of Medicine* 72 (Summer 1998): 199–200.
6. For general discussions about the influence of Darwinian biology and hereditarianism on psychiatric thought, see Grob, *Mental Illness and American Society*, 167–69; Charles E. Rosenberg, "The Bitter Fruit: Heredity, Disease, and Social Thought," in *No Other Gods: On Science and American Social Thought*, rev. and expanded ed. (Baltimore, MD: Johns Hopkins University Press, 1997), 25–53.
7. Hughes, "Labeling and Treating Black Mental Illness," 441; Randolph, "Central Lunatic Asylum," 62–63.
8. A classic study that makes the same argument, although not in the context of African Americans and mental illness, is Richard W. Fox, *So Far Disordered in Mind: Insanity in California, 1870–1930* (Berkeley: University of California Press, 1978).
9. Hoffman, *Health Care for Some*, xii. For a similar argument that access to federal medical care reflected an expanding "notion of political rights" for freedpeople during Reconstruction, see Downs, *Sick from Freedom*, 9. My use of the term "engagement" is deliberate, as it suggests a greater degree of initiative than "response."
10. A. O. Kellogg, "Shakespeare's Delineations of Mental Imbecility as Exhibited in His Fools and Clowns," *American Journal of Insanity* 19 (October 1862): 176–85. That same year the superintendent of the Eighth Census, Joseph Camp Kennedy, made the prediction that

emancipation would lead to the extinction of the Negro race. See Haller, "Physician versus the Negro," 154.
11. US Census Office, *Report on the Defective, Dependent, and Delinquent Classes of the Population of the United States, as Returned at the Tenth Census (June 1, 1880)* (Washington, DC: Government Printing Office, 1888), vii, ix–x.
12. Judson B. Andrews, "The Distribution and Care of the Insane in the United States," *American Journal of Insanity* 44 (October 1887): 193; *Report of the Government Hospital for the Insane to the Secretary of the Interior* (1894), 16, DOI-LR, box 4.
13. US Census Office, *Report on the Defective, Dependent, and Delinquent Classes*, xix.
14. J. F. Miller, "The Effects of Emancipation upon the Mental and Physical Health of the Negro of the South," *North Carolina Medical Journal* 38 (November 20, 1896): 285–94; Theophilus O. Powell, "The Increase of Insanity and Tuberculosis in the Southern Negro Since 1860, and Its Alliance, and Some of the Supposed Causes," *Journal of the American Medical Association* 27 (December 5, 1896): 1185–88; J. Allison Hodges, "The Effect of Freedom upon the Physical and Psychological Developments of the Negro," *Richmond Journal of Practice* 14 (June 1900): 161–71.
15. Hammond, *A Treatise on Insanity*, 121; Grob, *Mental Illness and American Society*, 51.
16. James G. Kiernan, "Race and Insanity," *Journal of Nervous and Mental Disease* 12 (1885): 174–75 (emphasis in the original). See also J. D. Roberts, "Insanity in the Colored Race," *North Carolina Medical Journal* 12 (November 1883): 256–57; J. M. Buchanan, "Insanity in the Colored Race," *New York Medical Journal* 44 (July 17, 1886): 67–70.
17. Andrews, "Distribution and Care," 193. This close connection between the institutions of advanced culture and insanity had been a mainstay in Western medical thought for some time and extended beyond discussions of mental illness in the United States. See, for instance, Daniel H. Tuke, "Does Civilization Favour the Generation of Mental Disease?," *Journal of Mental Science* 4 (October 1857): 106.
18. "Notes and Comments," *American Journal of Insanity* 43 (October 1886): 279.
19. Henry M. Hurd, "The Relation of General Paresis and Syphilitic Insanity," *American Journal of Insanity* 43 (July 1886): 2. General paresis was discovered in the 1910s to be the result of tertiary syphilis. See Grob, *Mental Illness and American Society*, 112, 132.
20. Miller, "Effects of Emancipation," 292.
21. A. H. Witmer, "Insanity in the Colored Race in the United States," *Alienist and Neurologist* 12 (January 1891): 25, 30.
22. For two examples, see T. Duncan Greenlees, "A Contribution to the Statistics of Insanity in Cape Colony," *American Journal of Insanity* 50 (April 1894): 519–29; T. Duncan Greenlees, "Insanity among the Natives of South Africa," *Journal of Mental Science* 41 (January 1895): 71–78.
23. Hammond, *Treatise on Insanity*, 120, 119.
24. Edward C. Spitzka, *Insanity: Its Classification, Diagnosis and Treatment*, 2nd ed. (New York: E. B. Treat, 1889), 17. For Spitzka's assessment of the problems with current classification schemes, see 113–18. See also Grob, *Mental Illness and American Society*, 49–55; S. D. Lamb, *Pathologist of the Mind: Adolf Meyer and the Origins of American Psychiatry* (Baltimore, MD: Johns Hopkins University Press, 2014), 17–19.
25. Charles E. Rosenberg, *The Trial of the Assassin Guiteau: Psychiatry and the Law in the Gilded Age* (Chicago: University of Chicago Press, 1968), 69, 100; Stephen T. Casper, "The Patient's Pitch: The Neurologist, the Tuning Fork, and Textbook Knowledge," in *The Neurological Patient in History*, ed. L. Stephen Jacyna and Stephen T. Casper (Rochester, NY: University of Rochester Press, 2012), 27–28; Rothman, *Discovery of the Asylum*, 126.
26. Janet Oppenheim, *"Shattered Nerves": Doctors, Patients, and Depression in Victorian England* (New York: Oxford University Press, 1991), 265–92, esp. 288. For discussions of degeneration in the United States and Latin America, see, respectively, Kristin L. Hoganson, *Fighting for American Manhood: How Gender Politics Provoked the Spanish-American and Philippine-American Wars* (New Haven, CT: Yale University Press, 1998); Julia Rodriguez, *Civilizing Argentina: Science, Medicine, and the Modern State* (Chapel Hill: University of North Carolina Press, 2006). By the early twentieth century, anxieties about "race suicide" contributed to eugenic measures such as the sterilization of the feebleminded and

insane. There is no evidence that forced sterilizations occurred at Saint Elizabeths, however. On debates over and utilization of sterilization in mental institutions and homes for the mentally disabled, see Fox, *So Far Disordered in Mind*, 29–32; Edward J. Larson, *Sex, Race, and Science: Eugenics in the Deep South* (Baltimore, MD: Johns Hopkins University Press, 1995), 27–29, 45–49; Alexandra Minna Stern, *Eugenic Nation: Faults and Frontiers of Better Breeding in Modern America* (Berkeley: University of California Press, 2005), 82–114.
27. For a general discussion, see Fredrickson, *Black Image in the White Mind*, 228–55.
28. Faculty psychology was a central component of eighteenth-century Scottish commonsense philosophy, which posited a tripartite division of the mind into various faculties: intellect, moral affect, and passions.
29. R. M. Bucke, "The Origin of Insanity," *American Journal of Insanity* 49 (July 1892): 56–66 (quote on 65); Oppenheim, "Shattered Nerves," 272–77. For a more detailed discussion of Bucke's thought, see S. E. D. Shortt, *Victorian Lunacy: Richard M. Bucke and the Practice of Late Nineteenth-Century Psychiatry* (Cambridge, UK: Cambridge University Press, 1986), esp. 97–99.
30. Spitzka, *Insanity*, 178–84, 243–47 (quote on 182). On the hypothesizing of the relationship between general paresis and syphilis, see Grob, *Mental Illness and American Society*, 188; G. E. Berrios, "Dementia," in *A History of Clinical Psychiatry: The Origin and History of Psychiatric Disorders*, ed. German Berrios and Roy Porter (New York: New York University Press, 1995), 39.
31. Kiernan, "Race and Insanity," 290–93; James G. Kiernan, "Race and Paretic Dementia," *Journal of Nervous and Mental Disease* 13 (1886): 108–9. Kiernan included in the Aryan race Teutonic peoples (German, Dutch, Anglo-Saxon, and Scandinavian), Celtic, Latin (including French and French Canadian), and "Sclavonic" (specifically Polish, although he presumably meant all Slavs).
32. Haller, "Race and the Concept of Progress," 710–23.
33. R. M. Bucke, "Sanity," *American Journal of Insanity* 47 (July 1890): 22.
34. J. W. Babcock, "The Colored Insane," *Alienist and Neurologist* 15/16 (1895): 427–28. On the early theorizations on the relationship between mania and melancholia, such as Jules Baillarger's *folie à double forme* and Jean-Pierre Falret's *folie circulaire*, see David Healy, *Mania: A Short History of Bipolar Disorder* (Baltimore, MD: Johns Hopkins University Press, 2008), 52–88.
35. Buchanan, "Insanity in the Colored Race," 69. See also Thomas J. McKie, "A Brief History of Insanity and Tuberculosis in the Southern Negro," *Journal of the American Medical Association* 28 (March 20, 1897): 537–38, in which he discusses "religious frenzy" as a causative agent in black insanity.
36. Roberts, "Insanity in the Colored Race," 254, 258.
37. On the rarity of the diagnosis of melancholia among people of African descent, see Hughes, "Labeling and Treating Black Mental Illness," 447–49; Sally Swartz, "Changing Diagnoses in Valkenberg Asylum, Cape Colony, 1891–1920: A Longitudinal View," *History of Psychiatry* 6 (1995): 441–42.
38. In 1890 dementia constituted 29 percent of diagnoses; mania made up 26 percent; and melancholia constituted 30 percent. In 1895 the percentage of dementia, mania, and melancholia diagnoses were 30, 34, and 24, respectively. Mania made up 31 percent of diagnoses in 1900, followed by melancholia at 27 percent and dementia at 23 percent. This is a blunt characterization, which does not account for the more refined diagnoses that physicians actually made, such as chronic dementia, epileptic dementia, senile dementia, chronic melancholia, acute melancholia, simple melancholia, chronic mania, acute mania, recurrent mania, and so on. Diagnosis data are gathered from Hospital Register, box 1, vols. 1–2, and box 2, vols. 3–4, SEH/RC.
39. US Bureau of the Census, *Historical Statistics of the United States, Colonial Times to 1970*, pt. 1 (Washington, DC: Government Printing Office, 1975), 26, http://www2.census.gov/prod2/statcomp/documents/CT1970p1-01.pdf (accessed March 27, 2010). For admission statistics, see "Report of the Board of Visitors and Superintendent of Construction,

1870," in *Reports of the Government Hospital for the Insane*, vol. 1, 1855–74, DOI-LR, box 6; *Annual Report of the Operations of the Government Hospital for the Insane for the Fiscal Year Ending June 30, 1880; Report of the Government Hospital for the Insane to the Secretary of the Interior* (1890). The 1880 and 1890 reports are in DOI-LR, box 4.
40. For examples, see Return of Precinct No. 6, August 19, 1871, vol. 31; January 23, 1877, vol. 37; Return of Precinct No. 7, February 26, 1878, vol. 38, RG 351 Records of the Government of the District of Columbia, Records Pertaining Primarily to Law Enforcement, Records of the Metropolitan Police, Entry 125 Daily Returns of Precincts, 1861–78 and 1887, NA; George L. Harrison, *Legislation on Insanity: A Collection of All the Lunacy Laws of the States and Territories of the United States to the Year 1883, Inclusive. Also the Laws of England on Insanity, Legislation in Canada on Private Houses, and Important Portions of the Lunacy Laws of Germany, France, Etc.* (Philadelphia: n.p., 1884), 117–25.
41. Return of Precinct No. 2, April 14, 1870, vol. 29; Return of Precinct No. 3, February 5, 1877, vol. 37; Return of Precinct No. 8, February 1, 1877, vol. 37, RG 351 Records of the Government of the District of Columbia, Records Pertaining Primarily to Law Enforcement, Records of the Metropolitan Police, Entry 125 Daily Returns of Precincts, 1861–78 and 1887, NA.
42. "A Mecca for Cranks," *Washington Evening Star*, March 31, 1888, 2. "Across the branch" was a reference to the Anacostia River, also called the Eastern Branch of the Potomac. Saint Elizabeths was on the other side of the Anacostia River from the most populated part of the District.
43. Return of Precinct No. 8, August 7, 1871, vol. 31; Return of Sanitary Company, January 13, 1872, vol. 32; Arrest Book, entries for August 8, 1871, vol. 31 and January 13, 1872, vol. 32. All in RG 351 Records of the Government of the District of Columbia, Records Pertaining Primarily to Law Enforcement, Records of the Metropolitan Police, Entry 125 Daily Returns of Precincts, 1861–78 and 1887, NA.
44. See Randolph, "Central Lunatic Asylum," 86–87, in which she writes, "These asylums had high mortality rates. They were total institutions where whites had ultimate authority and African-Americans were infantilized. Another reason is that African-Americans had distinctly different understandings of the causes and treatments for mental illness than those of the institution. Given the antipathy with which asylum personnel treated them, patients and their families had little reason to adopt their definitions of disease."
45. For a discussion of collective "claims-making" within the realm of public health, see Smith, *Sick and Tired of Being Sick and Tired*.
46. C. Arlene Bullock (pseudonym) to A. H. Witmer, April 20, 1894, Case File No. 5529, box 39, SEH/CFP (emphasis in the original). On respectability and concerns about racial degeneracy within the African American community in the post-Reconstruction period, see Michele Mitchell, *Righteous Propagation: African Americans and the Politics of Racial Destiny after Reconstruction* (Chapel Hill: University of North Carolina Press, 2004), esp. 76–107.
47. Daniel H. Williams, *Report of the Freedmen's Hospital to the Secretary of the Interior* (1895), box 3, RG 48 Records of the Department of the Interior, Letters Received and Other Records Relating to the Freedmen's Hospital, 1872–1910, NARA; Gladys-Marie Fry, *Night Riders in Black Folk History* (1975; repr., Chapel Hill: University of North Carolina Press, 2001), 182–211; Thomas Holt, Cassandra Smith Parker, and Rosalyn Terborg-Penn, *A Special Mission: The Story of Freedmen's Hospital, 1862–1962* (Washington, DC: Howard University Press, 1975), esp. 19–20, 25. The medical abuse of African Americans and the resulting black mistrust of professional medicine have been covered extensively. Representative works include Robert L. Blakely and Judith M. Harrington, *Bones in the Basement: Post-Mortem Racism in Nineteenth-Century Medical Training* (Washington, DC: Smithsonian Institution Press, 1997); Todd L. Savitt, "The Use of Blacks for Medical Experimentation and Demonstration in the Old South," *Journal of Southern History* 48 (1982): 331–48; Harriet A. Washington, *Medical Apartheid: The Dark History of Medical Experimentation on Black Americans from Colonial Times to the Present* (New York: Doubleday, 2006).

48. Fry, *Night Riders in Black Folk History*, 177–78, 183–84. According to Fry's ethnography, these hospitals were the old Naval Hospital, the Homeopathic Hospital, and, interestingly, Freedmen's Hospital (largely because of its connection to Howard University's medical school).
49. Case File No. 5449, box 37, SEH/CFP.
50. L. Count Cook to "Doctor," March 9, 1882, Case File No. 5340, box 35, SEH/CFP. On Cook, see Willard B. Gatewood, *Aristocrats of Color: The Black Elite, 1880–1920* (Bloomington: Indiana University Press, 1990), 40.
51. Mrs. E. C. W. Chubb to Dr. Godding, March 1, 1883, Case File No. 5340, box 35, SEH/CFP.
52. Letter from Miss M. Anderson, May 8, 1883, Case File No. 5140, box 32, SEH/CFP. This letter is in the case file of a patient who has an almost identical name to the patient assigned case file no. 5340. It is clear from the content, however, that the letter had been misfiled and concerns Margaret W.
53. Kenneth G. Alfers, *Law and Order in the Capital City: A History of the Washington Police, 1800–1886* (Washington, DC: George Washington University, 1976), 9, 28, 33–35, 47.
54. Letter to "Doctor," May 26, 1884, Case File No. 5991, box 48, SEH/CFP. The writer of the letter was the superintendent of the Metropolitan Police.
55. David Holloway (pseudonym) to Dr. Gorden [Godding], May 8, 1882; Martha Addison (pseudonym) to "Doctor," December 29, 1885. Both in Case File No. 5357, box 36, SEH/CFP.
56. Patients' family members could also play the other angle. One husband approached a sanitary officer about retrieving his wife, who he claimed was not insane, from Saint Elizabeths. The officer wrote a note to the staff informing them of the husband's intention. Although the officer did not attempt to persuade the staff to release the patient, she was discharged as "recovered" on the day the husband went to the hospital. See D. H. Teeple to "Dr.," August 12, 1884, in Case File No. 6070, box 49, SEH/CFP; SEH/RC, box 2, vol. 2, entry 6070.
57. Constance M. McGovern, "The Community, the Hospital, and the Working-Class Patient: The Multiple Uses of Asylum in Nineteenth-Century America," *Pennsylvania History* 54 (January 1987): 20–21; Dwyer, *Homes for the Mad*, 86–87.
58. Borchert, *Alley Life in Washington*, 167–70; Johnston, *Surviving Freedom*, 14, 54.
59. "In the Matter of the Lunacy of [S.J.H.]," Case No. 11169, Equity Case Files, RG 21 Records of District Courts of the United States, District of Columbia, NA; SEH/RC, box 2, vol. 2, entry 7293.
60. SEH/RC, box 2, vol. 2, entry 5741; John L. to "My Dear Friend," October 18, 1883; Special Order No. 37, Adjutant General's Office, February 13, 1884. Both in Case File No. 5741, box 42, SEH/CFP.
61. SEH/RC, box 2, vol. 2, entry 6771; Theresa J. to A. H. Whitmer, n.d., in Case File No. 6771, box 67, SEH/CFP.
62. SEH/RC, box 2, vol. 2, entry 6644; William M. to Dr. Stack, August 22, 1887, in Case File No. 6644, box 63, SEH/CFP.
63. For a discussion of this dynamic in nineteenth-century asylums more generally, see Mark Finnane, "Asylums, Families and the State," *History Workshop* 20 (Autumn 1985): 138–39; Dwyer, *Homes for the Mad*, 94.
64. Finnane, "Asylums, Families and the State," 136.
65. E. T. Easley, "The Sanitary Condition of the Negro," *American Medical Weekly* 3 (July 31, 1875): 49–51.

Chapter 4

1. Masur, *Example for All the Land*, 18, 194; Robert Harrison, "From Biracial Democracy to Direct Rule: The End of Self-Government in the Nation's Capital, 1865–1878," *Journal of Policy History* 18, no. 2 (2006): 242–45; William Tindall, "The Executives and Voters of Georgetown, District of Columbia," *Records of the Columbia Historical Society, Washington, D.C.* 24 (1922): 90; Howard Gillette, Jr., *Between Justice and Beauty: Race, Planning, and the Failure of Urban Policy in Washington, D.C.* (Philadelphia: University of Pennsylvania Press, 2006), 59–60.

2. Green, *Washington: Village and Capital*, 336–37; Masur, *Example for All the Land*, 216–17; Harrison, "From Biracial Democracy to Direct Rule," 250–54; Gillette, *Between Justice and Beauty*, 58–59, 66.
3. Gillette, *Between Justice and Beauty*, 82; Constance McLaughlin Green, *Washington: Capital City, 1879–1950* (Princeton, NJ: Princeton University Press, 1963), 28–31; Green, *Secret City*, 163; Masur, *Example for All the Land*, 221.
4. Green, *Secret City*, 119–54. On Washington's black elite, see Gatewood, *Aristocrats of Color*, 39–68.
5. C. B. Purvis, "A Reply to 'Appropriations,'" *Washington Evening Star*, March 12, 1889, 8. For information on Purvis, see Holt, Smith Parker, and Terborg-Penn, *A Special Mission*, esp. 20, 25–27.
6. *Annual Report of the Operations of the Government Hospital for the Insane for the Fiscal Year Ending June 30, 1880*, 3, DOI-LR, box 6; Murphy, "Progress, Science and the Mind," 318.
7. Rosenberg, *Trial of the Assassin Guiteau*, 226–30; Surya Kanhouwa and Kenneth Gorelick, "A Century of Pathology at Saint Elizabeths Hospital, Washington, DC," *Archives of Pathology and Laboratory Medicine* 121 (January 1997): 84–86 (quote from Blackburn on 84).
8. Grob, *Mental Illness and American Society*, 57–58.
9. W. W. Godding, "Our Insane Neighbor: His Rights and Ours—Rights in Hospitals," *American Psychological Journal* 1 (July 1883): 123–34 (quote on 127).
10. Godding, "Our Insane Neighbor," 131–32.
11. Nichols quoted in John Curwen, "Proceedings of the Association of Medical Superintendents," *American Journal of Insanity* 35 (July 1878): 106.
12. J. K. Barnes to J. D. C. Atkins, February 17, 1879, entry 2, box 1, SEH/BOVC; Minutes, April 1, 1879, entry 1, box 1, folio 357, SEH/BOVM; Millikan, "Wards of the Nation," 118–20.
13. Millikan, "Wards of the Nation," 118; Deutsch, *Mentally Ill in America*, 212.
14. W. W. Godding, "Progress in Provision for the Insane, 1844–1884," *American Journal of Insanity* 41 (October 1884): 138–47; Grob, *Mental Illness and American Society*, 11, 64, 101–2.
15. Godding, "Progress in Provision," 147.
16. [John P. Gray], "Dr. Godding on Progress in Provision for the Insane for the Past Forty Years in America," *American Journal of Insanity* 41 (October 1884): 248; W. W. Godding, "A Vindication of History," *Alienist and Neurologist* 6 (January 1885): 71.
17. For information on black patients at Utica State Lunatic Asylum, see Dwyer, *Homes for the Mad*, 106–7; Grob, "Class, Ethnicity, and Race," 224.
18. W. W. Godding to J. C. Atkins, [1879], folios 15835–36, Joseph Meredith Toner Collection, Medical Correspondence, Physicians Letters, container 77, Manuscript Division, Library of Congress, Washington, DC; *Thirtieth Annual Report of the Government Hospital for the Insane to the Secretary of the Interior* (1885), 19, DOI-LR, box 4.
19. Minutes, October 3, 1882, folios 386–87; Minutes, April 3, 1883, folio 391, both in entry 1, box 1, SEH/BOVM; D. Hack Tuke, *The Insane in the United States and Canada* (1885; repr., New York: Arno Press, 1973), 164.
20. Tuke, *Insane in the United States and Canada*, 97, 164.
21. Tuke, *Insane in the United States and Canada*, 164; *Thirty-First Annual Report of the Government Hospital for the Insane to the Secretary of the Interior* (1886), 19, DOI-LR, box 4.
22. J. D. Harris to Dr. Godding, January 14, 1880, Case File No. 4117, box 19, SEH/CFP.
23. *Thirty-Second Annual Report*, 17.
24. *Report of the Government Hospital for the Insane to the Secretary of the Interior* (1889), 15–16, DOI-LR, box 4.
25. Minutes, April 1, 1890, entry 1, box 1, folio 446, SEH/BOVM.
26. *Report of the Government Hospital for the Insane* (1892), 17; *Report of the Government Hospital for the Insane to the Secretary of the Interior* (1890), 15, DOI-LR, box 4.
27. "Report of the Government Hospital for the Insane to the Secretary of the Interior (1897)," 19–21, in *Reports of the Government Hospital for the Insane*, vol. 4, *1892–97*, DOI-LR, box 4; "Report of the Government Hospital for the Insane to the Secretary of the Interior (1899)," 18, in *Reports of the Government Hospital for the Insane*, vol. 5, *1898–1900*, DOI-LR, box 6.

28. Millikan, "Wards of the Nation," 134–35; W. W. Godding to Secretary Carl Schurz, December 19, 1877; Charles H. Nichols to Secretary Columbus Delano, January 30, 1875, both in DOI-LR, box 1.
29. *Annual Report of the Government Hospital for the Insane* (1884), 20; W. W. Godding, "The Recognition of Classes of the Insane in Asylum Construction," *Alienist and Neurologist* 6 (July 1885): 363. Congress passed a law in 1882 authorizing the US attorney general to commit insane convicts and criminally insane individuals to Saint Elizabeths.
30. *Thirty-Second Annual Report*, 19; W. W. Godding, "The State in the Care of the Insane," *American Journal of Insanity* 46 (January 1890): 324; *Report of the Government Hospital for the Insane* (1889), 15–16; *Report of the Government Hospital for the Insane to the Secretary of the Interior* (1891), 15–16, DOI-LR, box 4. See also Millikan, "Wards of the Nation," 135.
31. Hunter McGuire and G. Frank Lydston, "Sexual Crimes among the Southern Negroes: Scientifically Considered," *Virginia Medical Monthly* 20 (1893): 105–25, quoted in Haller, "Physician versus the Negro," 162. On the Amok, see W. Gilmore Ellis, "The Amok of the Malays," *Journal of Mental Science* 39 (July 1893): 325–38; "Running Amuck," *American Journal of Insanity* 51 (October 1894): 239.
32. Charles K. Mills, "Arrested and Aberrant Development of Fissures and Gyres in the Brains of Paranoiacs, Criminals, Idiots, and Negroes: Description of a Chinese Brain," *Journal of Nervous and Mental Disease* 13 (September and October 1886): 517–50 (quotes on 529 and 544).
33. The historian Ellen Dwyer writes of New York State's Willard Asylum for the Chronic Insane, "Wards intended for one type of patient quickly became mixed owing to overcrowding and shifts in behavior. Thus . . . neither the daily lives of the insane nor the details of their environment were fixed and stable, despite doctors' best efforts to make them so." Dwyer, *Homes for the Mad*, 139.
34. *Report of the Government Hospital for the Insane to the Secretary of the Interior* (1894), 16, DOI-LR, box 4.
35. *Thirty-First Annual Report*, 18; "Report of the Government Hospital for the Insane (1897)," 60–62; W. W. Godding, "Active Treatment in General Paralysis of the Insane," *British Medical Journal* 2 (November 13, 1897): 1407–9.
36. Henry M. Hurd, ed., *The Institutional Care of the Insane in the United States and Canada*, vol. 2 (1916; repr., New York: Arno Press, 1973), 147; Joel Braslow, *Mental Ills and Bodily Cures: Psychiatric Treatment in the First Half of the Twentieth Century* (Berkeley: University of California Press, 1997), 40. Because the hospital had not yet developed a patient case file system and annual reports did not provide race-based statistics on the use of hydrotherapy, it is impossible to determine whether the administering of this form of treatment during Godding's tenure favored (or targeted) one racial group over the other. Hydrotherapy will be discussed in more detail in chapter 6.
37. *Thirtieth Annual Report*, 18.
38. Murphy, "Progress, Science and the Mind," 318; *Report of the Government Hospital for the Insane* (1889), 20.
39. *Report of the Government Hospital for the Insane* (1889), 20; *Thirty-First Annual Report*, 17.
40. *Report of the Government Hospital for the Insane* (1894), 16–17; Millikan, "Wards of the Nation," 145–47.
41. Howard Watt to "Dear Sir," August 22, 1891, in Case File No. 8066, box 102, SEH/CFP; SEH/RC, box 2, vol. 3, entry 8066. On pensions and disabled veterans, see Schweik, *Ugly Laws*, 79.
42. *Thirty-First Annual Report*, 17.
43. McCandless, *Moonlight, Magnolias, and Madness*, 273–74. For other studies that examine the reproduction of racial hierarchies within the insane asylum, see Randolph, "Central Lunatic Asylum," esp. 51; Hughes, "Labeling and Treating Black Mental Illness," 441–43.
44. Francis Harding (pseudonym) to W. W. Godding, February 20, 1888, in Case File No. 6103, box 50, SEH/CFP; SEH/RC, box 1, vol. 2, entry 6103.
45. Horace Timmons (pseudonym) to "Doctor," March 9, 1883, in Case File No. 5486, box 38, SEH/CFP. The connections between conjure and mental illness in black vernacular thought will be explored in more detail in chapter 6.

46. Lorna Crump (pseudonym) to "Dr.," November 3, [1882], in Case File No. 5483, box 38, SEH/CFP; SEH/RC, box 1, vol. 2, entry 5483.
47. J. A. Bowman (pseudonym) to Dr. Patterson, n.d., in Case File No. 7218, box 80, SEH/CFP.
48. In this sense, archival evidence of family members' interactions with Saint Elizabeths does not conform to the conclusions drawn by Ellen Dwyer, who, in her work on asylums in New York, claimed, "Once families had made the painful decision to send disturbed members to a state asylum, they were reluctant to investigate the therapeutic and custodial deficiencies of their relatives' new homes." Dwyer, *Homes for the Mad*, 28.
49. Winston Allen (pseudonym) to Doctor Godding or Doctor Stack, August 18, 1885, in Case File No. 6247, box 53, SEH/CFP.
50. Godfrey Smart (pseudonym) to W. W. Godding, November 13, 1885, in Case File No. 6296, box 55, SEH/CFP.
51. A. E. Winslow (pseudonym) to Godding, n.d. and April 4, 1885, in Case File No. 4459, box 22, SEH/CFP.
52. Sam J. Randall to W. W. Godding, April 29, 1882, in Case File No. 5350, box 36, SEH/CFP.
53. Martha Addison (pseudonym) to "Doctor," December 29, 1885, in Case File No. 5357, box 36, SEH/CFP.
54. Lily Grant (pseudonym) to Dr. Lyons, April 19, 1885, in Case File No. 6005, box 48, SEH/CFP.
55. Lily Grant (pseudonym) to Dr. Lyons, April 19, 1885; Godding to Mrs. Lee, March 7, 1887. Both in Case File No. 6005, box 48, SEH/CFP.
56. John S. to "Dear Sir," August 28, 1888, in Case File No. 7217, box 80, SEH/CFP; SEH/RC, box 1, vol. 2, entry 7217.
57. Henrietta Stoughton (pseudonym) to Dr. Godding, March 1893; Isadora Simpson (pseudonym) to Alonzo B. Richardson, 1901. Both in Case File No. 6384, box 57, SEH/CFP. SEH/RC, box 1, vol. 2, entry 6384.
58. SEH/RC, box 1, vol. 2, entry 6325; C. M. S. to W. W. Godding, June 28, 1885, August 15, 1885, September 19, 1885, October 6, 1885. All in Case File No. 6325, box 55, SEH/CFP.
59. Frank O. to Doctor Witmer, June 26, 1890, in Case File No. 7557, box 88, SEH/CFP.
60. E. W. Denison to W. W. Godding, February 15, 1884, in Case File No. 5800, box 43, SEH/CFP; SEH/RC, box 1, vol. 1, entry 5800.
61. Henrietta Stoughton to Dr. Godding, n.d., Case File No. 6384, box 57, SEH/CFP.
62. Henry J. to W. W. Godding, May 12, 1884, May 26, 1884, September 28, 1884, March 28, 1887. All in Case File No. 5354, box 36, SEH/CFP.
63. Henry is listed as married to Catherine in both the 1870 and 1880 censuses, so Catherine must have died sometime between 1880 and 1884. In the 1870 census, they and their five children are listed as mulatto. In the 1880 census, they and their seven children are listed as white. See 1870 US Census (Schedule 1), Washington City, Washington County, District of Columbia; p. 113, family 880, dwelling 839, lines 36–40; 1880 US Census (Schedule 1), Washington City, Washington County, District of Columbia; p. 29, family 318, dwelling 236, lines 29–37. Both accessed June 7, 2010, www.ancestry.com.
64. Dennis M. to Isaac M., August 12, 1889, in Case File No. 6958, box 73, SEH/CFP; SEH/RC, box 1, vol. 2, entry 6958.
65. SEH/RC, box 1, vol. 2, entries 6270 and 6351; Maria C. to Dr. Stack, November 13, 1885 and December 13, 1885, in Case File No. 6270, box 54, SEH/CFP.
66. W. W. Godding, "Aspects and Outlook of Insanity in America," *American Journal of Insanity* 47 (July 1890): 1–16; Ian Robert Dowbiggin, *Keeping America Sane: Psychiatry and Eugenics in the United States and Canada, 1880–1940* (Ithaca, NY: Cornell University Press, 2003), 24–64; Richard Noll, *American Madness: The Rise and Fall of Dementia Praecox* (Cambridge, MA: Harvard University Press, 2011), 19.
67. "Report of the Government Hospital for the Insane (1896)," 18, in *Reports of the Government Hospital for the Insane*, vol. 4, *1892–97*; "Report of the Government Hospital for the Insane (1899)," 25–26; 32 Cong. Rec. 2543-46 (1899); 33 Cong. Rec. 6216-19 (1900).
68. "Report of the Government Hospital for the Insane to the Secretary of the Interior (1900)," 4, 8, in *Reports of the Government Hospital for the Insane*, vol. 5, *1898–1900*.

69. On the history of the use of gender differentiation—the extent to which gender roles had been properly delineated—as a measure of a race's evolution in civilizationist discourse, see Gail Bederman, *Manliness and Civilization: A Cultural History of Gender and Race in the United States, 1880–1917* (Chicago: University of Chicago Press, 1995); Melissa N. Stein, *Measuring Manhood: Race and the Science of Masculinity, 1830–1934* (Minneapolis: University of Minnesota Press, 2015).
70. A. H. Witmer, "Insanity in the Colored Race in the United States," *Alienist and Neurologist* 12 (January 1891): 25.
71. "Report of the Government Hospital for the Insane (1900)," 8. See also Otto, *St. Elizabeths Hospital*, 167–68.

Chapter 5

1. William A. White, *William Alanson White: The Autobiography of a Purpose* (1938; repr., New York: Arno Press, 1980), 31–79 (quote on 39); Dowbiggin, *Keeping America Sane*, 106.
2. William A. White, untitled manuscript, April 1926, entry 48, box 1, folder "A," SEH/White.
3. William A. White, "The New Government Hospital for the Insane," *American Journal of Insanity* 66 (1910): 524–25; "Semi-Annual Report," October 2, 1906, 8–9, 13–15, box 1, folder "R, 1906–08," SEH/BOVGC. The pathologist diagnosed disease through gross anatomical examination, the histopathologist through microscopic observation (mainly of cerebral tissue), and the clinical pathologist through the testing of bodily fluids. Among other diseases, researchers in the scientific department were generally concerned with epilepsy, general paresis, pellagra, and syphilis.
4. *By-Laws and Rules and Regulations of the Board of Visitors of the Government Hospital for the Insane, 1900* (Washington, DC: Government Printing Office, 1900), 8, in entry 3, box 5, folder "1943–47," SEH/BOVGC; White to Medical Staff, December 22, 1905, entry 42, Instructions to Staff and Other Records, 1883–1908, box 1, folder 2, SEH/Super; Millikan, "Wards of the Nation," 144n54.
5. "Half-Year Summary," *American Journal of Insanity* 65 (April 1909): 773–74; "Semi-Annual Report," October 2, 1906, 10; William A. White to Members of the Board of Visitors, October 1, 1912, 6, entry 3, box 2, folder "R, 1908–12," SEH/BOVGC.
6. Alonzo B. Richardson was the first superintendent of Massillon State Hospital in Ohio and had served as the White House physician during the McKinley administration before he was appointed to replace Godding in October 1899. He died of a stroke in June 1903. White, *Autobiography*, 82; Hurd, *Institutional Care of the Insane*, 2:148–49.
7. "Medicine and Law Join in Organization," *Washington Times*, June 1, 1903, 10; "Care for the Insane," *Washington Post*, January 20, 1906, 1; "Asylum Scored by a Committee," *Washington Post*, February 19, 1906, 1, 5.
8. Special Comm. on Investigation of the Government Hospital for the Insane, H.R. Rep. No. 59-7644, at 1:iv, 1:17–41, 1:77–96, 1:149, 1:188–92, 2:1064, 2:1067–68 (1907). See also "Tell of Cruelties," *Washington Post*, May 16, 1906, 1–2.
9. H.R. Rep. 59-7644, at 1:670, 673–74, 904–5.
10. "I can best illustrate this by saying that our language has changed in this respect by the substitution of a consideration of things, organs, tissues, descriptions, classifications, by the consideration of events, processes, relations, meanings, purposes." William A. White, *Twentieth Century Psychiatry: Its Contribution to Man's Knowledge of Himself* (New York: Norton, 1936), 79–80.
11. Lamb, *Pathologist of the Mind*, 162. Lamb's excellent study is a history of the Phipps Clinic in Baltimore.
12. Noll, *American Madness*, 13; Grob, *Mental Illness and American Society*, 30–71, 108; William A. White, *Outlines of Psychiatry*, 10th ed. (Washington, DC: Nervous and Mental Disease, 1924), 6. Noll argues that this triadic conception of insanity was the result of a near universal belief that there was only one mental disease, with variant manifestations. This theory, known as the "unitary psychosis concept," was not subscribed to by all psychiatrists, and there was even disagreement among those sympathetic to the theory over questions of etiology and

classification. See German E. Berrios and Dominic Beer, "Unitary Psychosis Concept," in Berrios and Porter, ed., *History of Clinical Psychiatry*, 313–35.
13. Noll, *American Madness*, 58–66; Lunbeck, *Psychiatric Persuasion*, 128–30.
14. Noll, *American Madness*, 106, 162, 232–75.
15. William A. White to Medical Staff, July 11, 1905, box 1, folder 1, SEH/Super. The remaining categories were infection-exhaustion psychoses; paranoia and paranoid states (not otherwise classified); psychoses associated with other diseases; involution melancholia; constitutional inferiority; imbecility; idiocy; unclassified; and not insane.
16. William A. White, *Outlines of Psychiatry*, 1st ed. (New York: Journal of Nervous and Mental Disease, 1907), 16. The diagnostic confusion between dementia praecox and manic-depressive psychosis was a common concern among American psychiatrists. See Lunbeck, *Psychiatric Persuasion*, 144–45.
17. William A. White to E. Stanley Abbot, November 4, 1920, in *The Inner World of American Psychiatry, 1890–1940: Selected Correspondence*, ed. Gerald N. Grob (New Brunswick, NJ: Rutgers University Press, 1985), 108. The 10th edition of White's textbook illustrates just how pessimistic he had become: "Any attempt at grouping mental disorders under separate heads must now, *as always*, be but tentative and incomplete." See White, *Outlines of Psychiatry*, 10th ed., 25 (emphasis mine). See also William A. White, "Some Considerations Bearing on the Diagnosis and Treatment of Dementia Praecox," *American Journal of Psychiatry* 78 (October 1921): 193–98.
18. C. Macfie Campbell, "The Treatment of Dementia Praecox and Allied Conditions," in *The Modern Treatment of Nervous and Mental Diseases*, ed. William A. White and Smith Ely Jelliffe (Philadelphia: Lea and Febiger, 1913), 1:592. On therapeutic pessimism, see Dowbiggin, *Keeping America Sane*, 64; and Nathan G. Hale Jr., *Freud and the Americans: The Beginnings of Psychoanalysis in the United States, 1876–1917* (New York: Oxford University Press, 1971), 75–76.
19. Noll, *American Madness*, 116–24; Grob, *Mental Illness and American Society*, 108–12.
20. I thank Dennis Doyle for making this observation.
21. Lamb, *Pathologist of the Mind*; Grob, *Mental Illness and American Society*, 112–16. For a critical evaluation of Meyer, see Edward Shorter, *A History of Psychiatry: From the Era of the Asylum to the Age of Prozac* (New York: John Wiley and Sons, 1997), esp. 111–112.
22. One of the main contributions Meyer made to American psychiatry, his most recent biographer writes, was the idea that "the pathological processes underlying mental disorder took place not exclusively at the level of brain tissues or metabolism but also at the level of adaptive behavior and individual experience." See Lamb, *Pathologist of the Mind*, 4.
23. White, *Autobiography*, 252–53; White, *Outlines of Psychiatry*, 10th ed., 28; William A. White, "Life and Death Instincts," *Medical Annals of the District of Columbia* 2 (April 1933): 71.
24. Noll, *American Madness*, 55; Hale, *Freud and the Americans*, 54–55.
25. Adolf Meyer, "The Role of Habit-Disorganizations" (1905), in *The Commonsense Psychiatry of Dr. Adolf Meyer: Fifty-Two Selected Papers*, ed. Alfred Lief (New York: McGraw-Hill, 1948), 181.
26. Noll, *American Madness*, 168–73; Lamb, *Pathologist of the Mind*, 153–58.
27. White, *Outlines of Psychiatry*, 10th ed., 18–19 (emphasis in the original).
28. White, *Twentieth Century Psychiatry*, 20–21; White, *Outlines of Psychiatry*, 10th ed., 21.
29. John C. Burnham, *Psychoanalysis and American Medicine, 1894–1918: Medicine, Science, and Culture* (New York: International Universities Press, 1967), 19, 159–61; Grob, *Mental Illness and American Society*, 116; Lamb, *Pathologist of the Mind*, 225–26; Ruth Leys, "Meyer, Jung, and the Limits of Association," *Bulletin of the History of Medicine* 59 (Fall 1985): 356.
30. William A. White, "Fundamentals of the Freudian Psychology," *New York Medical Journal* 95 (May 11, 1912): 969–70; William A. White to W. A. Robinson, March 6, 1917, in Grob, *Inner World of American Psychiatry*, 107; Arcangelo R. T. D'Amore, "William Alanson White—Pioneer Psychoanalyst," in *William Alanson White: The Washington Years, 1903–1937*, ed. Arcangelo R. T. D'Amore (Washington, DC: US Department of Health, Education, and Welfare, 1976), 69. By World War I psychoanalysts had split into different factions: orthodox Freudians, adherents to Carl Jung, and followers of Alfred Adler. For a thorough history, see

George Makari, *Revolution in Mind: The Creation of Psychoanalysis* (New York: HarperCollins, 2008).
31. White, *Outlines of Psychiatry*, 1st ed., 18. On dynamic psychiatry's emphasis on the individualistic nature of psychoses more generally, see Noll, *American Madness*, 175; and Burnham, *Psychoanalysis and American Medicine*, 161.
32. Andrew Abbott, *The System of Professions: An Essay on the Division of Expert Labor* (Chicago: University of Chicago Press, 1988), 288; Dowbiggin, *Keeping America Sane*, 54, 71–86.
33. Makari, *Revolution in Mind*, 34–37; Larry Stewart, "Freud before Oedipus: Race and Heredity in the Origins of Psychoanalysis," *Journal of the History of Biology* 9 (Fall 1976): 215–28.
34. The name change reflected both the changing constituency of the organization (assistant physicians, not just superintendents, were now eligible for membership) and the increasing scientific and clinical orientation of the profession.
35. E. M. Green, "Manic-Depressive Psychosis in the Negro," *American Journal of Insanity* 73 (April 1917): 620–23.
36. Green, "Manic-Depressive Psychosis in the Negro," 625; George H. Kirby, "A Study in Race Psychopathology," *State Hospitals Bulletin* 1 (1909): 663–70.
37. Arrah B. Evarts, "Dementia Precox in the Colored Race," *Psychoanalytic Review* 1 (October 1914): 388n1; D'Amore, "William Alanson White," 69–70. White also joined the American Psychoanalytic Association in 1912, a year after it was founded, and served as its third president from 1915 to 1917.
38. William A. White, "The New Saint Elizabeths Hospital," *American Journal of Psychiatry* 81 (January 1924): 508. For an important historical examination of ideas about racial difference and race relations at Saint Elizabeths during White's administration, see Gambino, "'These Strangers within Our Gates.'"
39. D'Amore, "William Alanson White," 71; Donald L. Burnham, "Orthodoxy and Eclecticism in Psychoanalysis: The Washington-Baltimore Experience," in *American Psychoanalysis: Origins and Development*, ed. Jacques M. Quen and Eric T. Carlson (New York: Brunner/Mazel, 1978), 89.
40. "Dr. Nolan D. C. Lewis Dies at 90; Psychiatrist Was Leader in Field," *New York Times*, December 19, 1979; Nolan D. C. Lewis, "Discussion of Paper by Dr. D'Amore," in D'Amore, *William Alanson White*, 93; Smith Ely Jelliffe to Sigmund Freud, November 26, 1929, quoted in D'Amore, "William Alanson White," 89.
41. Edward J. Kempf, "Autobiographical Fragment," in *Edward J. Kempf: Selected Papers*, ed. Dorothy Clarke Kempf and John C. Burnham (Bloomington: Indiana University Press, 1974), 7.
42. Edward J. Kempf, *The Autonomic Functions and the Personality* (New York: Nervous and Mental Disease, 1918), 1.
43. Edward J. Kempf, *Psychopathology* (St. Louis: C. V. Mosby, 1920), 55.
44. Kempf, *Psychopathology*, 3; Lamb, *Pathologist of the Mind*, 88–97.
45. Kempf, *Psychopathology*, 4, 500, 29, 746–49.
46. In this sense, Kempf's racialized nonracialism resembled that of the most prominent psychoanalyst, Sigmund Freud. As Celia Brickman persuasively argues, "Given the invidious racial situation of his day, Freud attempted to transcend the racial taxonomies of his time by creating a model of the psyche as held in common by all humans. But his universalist solution shared with the project of modernity, of which it was a part, the problems of deep-seated connections to racism and colonization." See Celia Brickman, *Aboriginal Populations in the Mind: Race and Primitivity in Psychoanalysis* (New York: Columbia University Press, 2003), 11.
47. Kurt Danziger, *Naming the Mind: How Psychology Found Its Language* (London: Sage, 1997), 87–94; Charles W. Tolman, "Theories of Mental Evolution in Comparative Psychology: Darwin to Watson," in *Historical Perspectives and the International Status of Comparative Psychology*, ed. Ethel Tobach (Hillsdale, NJ: Lawrence Erlbaum Associates, 1987), 15–23.
48. See the work of Luise White, who, in writing about colonial medicine, defines genre as "formulaic stories structured by set elements and conventions" that "[access] all the fantasies,

paraphernalia, and technologies with which medical power was presented and represented." In the case of the comparative psychology research literature, the medical power was the power to rhetorically establish the foundational and irreconcilable differences between the white and black psyche. Luise White, *Speaking with Vampires: Rumor and History in Colonial Africa* (Berkeley: University of California Press, 2000), 92–93.

49. On the response of African Americans to degeneracy theory, see Mitchell, *Righteous Propagation*, esp. 122–24, 210–11; Samuel Kelton Roberts Jr., *Infectious Fear: Politics, Disease, and the Health Effects of Segregation* (Chapel Hill: University of North Carolina Press, 2009), 100.
50. Evarts, "Dementia Precox in the Colored Race," 388n1, 389.
51. John E. Lind, "Phylogenetic Elements in the Psychoses of the Negro," *Psychoanalytic Review* 4 (July 1917): 306. On Ellis, see "Obituary Notes," *Popular Science Monthly* 45 (June 1894): 288.
52. Lind, "Phylogenetic Elements," 305.
53. Richard Noll, *The Jung Cult: Origins of a Charismatic Movement* (Princeton, NJ: Princeton University Press, 1994), 47–48; Bederman, *Manliness and Civilization*, 77–120.
54. Bederman, *Manliness and Civilization*, 109–10.
55. White, *Outlines of Psychiatry*, 10th ed., 8. See also Dorothy Ross, *G. Stanley Hall: The Psychologist as Prophet* (Chicago: University of Chicago Press, 1972), 368–94; Hamilton Cravens and John C. Burnham, "Psychology and Evolutionary Naturalism in American Thought, 1890–1940," *American Quarterly* 23 (December 1971): 643.
56. Evarts, "Dementia Precox in the Colored Race," 388; W. M. Bevis, "Psychological Traits of the Southern Negro with Observations as to Some of His Psychoses," *American Journal of Psychiatry* 78 (July 1921): 69; Mary O'Malley, "Psychoses in the Colored Race: A Study in Comparative Psychiatry," *American Journal of Insanity* 71 (October 1914): 310–11. See also Arrah B. Evarts, "The Ontogenetic against the Phylogenetic Elements in the Psychoses of the Colored Race," *Psychoanalytic Review* 3 (July 1916): 272–87.
57. John E. Lind, "The Dream as a Simple Wish-Fulfilment in the Negro," *Psychoanalytic Review* 1 (1913–14): 295–96; O'Malley, "Psychoses in the Colored Race," 310, 312.
58. Bevis, "Psychological Traits of the Southern Negro," 70; Lind, "Dream as a Simple Wish-Fulfilment," 295.
59. O'Malley, "Psychoses in the Colored Race," 315–16. See also Bevis, "Psychological Traits of the Southern Negro," 72 ("In no other trait or peculiarity do we find more plainly the imprint of primitive African life and customs"); Evarts, "Dementia Precox in the Colored Race, 391 ("As to the religion of the native African, it is but a belief in witchcraft. Of ethics he has no conception"); Nolan D. C. Lewis and L. D. Hubbard, "Epileptic Reactions in the Negro Race," *American Journal of Psychiatry* 88 (January 1932): 654 ("*Magical or superstitious interpretations in connection with convulsions*, were of very common occurrence").
60. Lind, "Phylogenetic Elements," 304.
61. Makari, *Revolution in Mind*, 270–74.
62. Noll, *American Madness*, 183. Initially influenced by Freud, Jung split with his theory of psychoanalysis over its emphasis on the libido and psychosexual conflict as the root of all psychic turmoil. Jung ceased to identify as a psychoanalyst and referred to his theory and psychotherapeutic method as analytical psychology. According to John C. Burnham, most American psychoanalysts remained in the Freud camp after the split. This does not appear to be true in the case of Saint Elizabeths' psychiatrists. See Henri F. Ellenberger, *The Discovery of the Unconscious: The History and Evolution of Dynamic Psychiatry* (New York: Basic Books, 1970), 694–703; Burnham, *Psychoanalysis and American Medicine*, 43; Makari, *Revolution in Mind*, 266–79.
63. Deirdre Bair, *Jung: A Biography* (Boston: Little, Brown, 2003), 231, 338.
64. William A. White to Adolf Meyer, November 5, 1919, in Grob, *Inner World of American Psychiatry*, 36.
65. White, "Some Considerations," 193–94, 196. On Freud and phylogeny, see Brickman, *Aboriginal Populations in the Mind*, 51–89.
66. William A. White, "Primitive Mentality and the Racial Unconscious," *American Journal of Psychiatry* 82 (April 1925): 663, 669.

67. Evarts, "Ontogenetic against the Phylogenetic Elements," 272–73. See also Lind, "Phylogenetic Elements," 323.
68. Bevis, "Psychological Traits of the Southern Negro," 74; "Report of the St. Elizabeths Hospital to the Secretary of the Interior, 1926," 20–21 and "Report of the St. Elizabeths Hospital to the Secretary of the Interior, 1928," 19–20, both in *Government Hospital for the Insane: Reports, 1917–1932*, William A. White Collection, Saint Elizabeths Hospital Archives, Saint Elizabeths Hospital Library, Washington, DC. The next most commonly diagnosed disease was general paralysis (or general paresis).
69. Nolan D. C. Lewis, *The Constitutional Factors in Dementia Precox* (New York: Nervous and Mental Disease, 1923). On this point, I take issue with Jonathan Metzl's excellent book on the racially inflected evolution of the disease concept of schizophrenia. Metzl argues that psychiatrists explained the prevalence of dementia praecox among African Americans by utilizing a Kraepelinian etiological framework. They claimed, in essence, that African Americans were constitutionally predisposed toward the disease. This emphasis on the biological causes of dementia praecox, Metzl argues, fit nicely with residual nineteenth-century discourses of the constitutional incapacity of African Americans to adapt to their lives as freedpeople. He points to Arrah Evarts's article on dementia praecox as evidence: "Following Kraepelin's emphasis on brain biology, Evarts wrote that dementia praecox was 'essentially a deteriorating psychosis,' caused by 'lipoid degeneration, reticular degeneration of the ganglion cells, proliferation of neurogliar tissue, and Kornchen cells.'" Metzl, *Protest Psychosis*, 31. But Evarts actually identified these cellular changes as the *pathology* associated with dementia praecox; in other words, the damaging biological *effects* of the disease. Evarts departed from Kraepelin in her discussion of the cause of the disease, employing a more dynamic model: "We are beginning to think of insanity as a failure on the part of the individual to adjust to the demands of his environment." Evarts, "Dementia Precox in the Colored Race," 394, 395.
70. O'Malley, "Psychoses in the Colored Race," 323–24. My thinking about the psychiatric profession's assumptions about the "normal abnormality" of African Americans has been influenced by Jackson, *Surfacing Up*, 99–109; Vaughan, *Curing Their Ills*, 100–128.
71. Evarts, "Dementia Precox in the Colored Race," 394, 396.
72. Lind, "Phylogenetic Elements," 330; Evarts, "Dementia Precox in the Colored Race," 397. See also O'Malley, "Psychoses in the Colored Race," 335.
73. Evarts, "Dementia Precox in the Colored Race," 400. The therapeutic regime during White's administration will be covered in the next chapter.
74. Lind, "Dream as a Simple Wish-Fulfilment," 300.
75. Philip S. Graven, "Case Study of a Negro," *Psychoanalytic Review* 17 (April 1930): 275.
76. Graven, "Case Study of a Negro," 274, 279.
77. O'Malley, "Psychoses in the Colored Race," 310, 326.
78. Lewis, *Constitutional Factors*, 101. On the emergence of endocrinology as a field that contributed to discussions about psychology, and particularly gender identity, see Mark S. Micale, *Hysterical Men: The Hidden History of Male Nervous Illness* (Cambridge, MA: Harvard University Press, 2008), 172–76.
79. Lewis, *Constitutional Factors*, 126, 122–23.
80. Lewis, *Constitutional Factors*, 18. Of the 601 autopsies that formed the basis of his study, Lewis broke them down into eight groups: colored males with and without tuberculosis, colored females with and without tuberculosis, white males with and without tuberculosis, and white females with and without tuberculosis. Within these broad racial groups, he identified individual patients as African, Filipino, Danish, Scandinavian, and American.
81. Lewis would go on, some ten years later, to reinforce this distinction even more firmly in a discussion of a research study on epileptic reactions among African Americans that he conducted with his colleague, Lois D. Hubbard. "The negro is different from the standpoint of nurture and culture and his reactions at these levels should be carefully studied," he wrote. "I think that Garth and others who have done a great deal of psychometric testing feel that there are no very great fundamental differences in any of the races so far as those measurements are concerned. What I fear is that they are not measuring the important things." Lewis and Hubbard, "Epileptic Reactions in the Negro Race," 676.

82. John Carson, "Minding Matter/Mattering Mind: Knowledge and the Subject in Nineteenth-Century Psychology," *Studies in History and Philosophy of Biological and Biomedical Sciences* 30 (September 1999): 345–76.
83. As the historian of psychiatry George Makari points out about psychoanalysis, "If empirical observation was to be the foundation of the field, this was a terrible problem. It meant there were no rules for amassing the evidence that led to inferences about the unconscious. It was difficult enough to achieve consensus on unconscious processes that were neither directly observable nor quantifiable. But if the object of analysis was itself hard to grasp, it was paramount that the observers themselves be stable, uniform, and of course they were not." Makari, *Revolution in Mind*, 329.
84. For an excellent history that explores "how varying kinds of assumptions about race can fill in the uncertainty that is central to medicine," see Reverby, *Examining Tuskegee* (quote on p. 5).
85. Green, "Manic-Depressive Psychoses in the Negro," 626.

Chapter 6

1. Quote is from White, *Twentieth Century Psychiatry*, 32.
2. William A. White, "Some Considerations Bearing on the Diagnosis and Treatment of Dementia Praecox," *American Journal of Psychiatry* 78 (October 1921): 197.
3. *Report of the Government Hospital for the Insane to the Secretary of the Interior* (1904), in DOI-LR, box 4; William White to Members of the Board of Visitors, April 3, 1917, General Correspondence of the Secretary, entry 3, box 3, folder "R (1), 3/21/16–10/31/19"; "Semi-Annual Report," April 2, 1907, 5–6, box 1, folder "R, 1906–08"; "Semi-Annual Report of the Superintendent to the Board of Visitors," April 11, 1911, entry 3, box 2, folder "R, 1908–12," all in SEH/BOVGC.
4. William A. White to Rev. U. G. B. Pierce, July 25, 1919, copy, entry 3, box 3, folder "M–Q, 3/21/16–10/31/19," SEH/BOVGC.
5. William A. White to E. Stanley Abbot, November 4, 1920, in Grob, *Inner World of American Psychiatry*, 108; White, *Outlines of Psychiatry*, 10th ed., 128–29, 294–313.
6. *Annual Report of the St. Elizabeths Hospital to the Secretary of the Interior for the Fiscal Year Ended June 30, 1932* (Washington, DC: Government Printing Office, 1932), 14; *Annual Report of the Department of the Interior 1934* (Washington, DC: Government Printing Office, 1934), 376. The annual reports do not specify whether the same patients received psychotherapy each month or the monthly averages consisted of different patients.
7. See Fett, *Working Cures*, esp. 37–38, for an excellent discussion of the "contrasting notions of power underlying conflicts over slave illness."
8. On the importance of the case history to psychotherapy, see Eric Caplan, *Mind Games: American Culture and the Birth of Psychotherapy* (Berkeley: University of California Press, 1998), 109; Lamb, *Pathologist of the Mind*, 130–60.
9. Steven Noll, "Patient Records as Historical Stories: The Case of Caswell Training School," *Bulletin of the History of Medicine* 68 (Fall 1994): 413; John Harley Warner, "The Uses of Patient Records by Historians—Patterns, Possibilities and Perplexities," *Health and History* 1 (1999): 101–11. See also Guenter B. Risse and John Harley Warner, "Reconstructing Clinical Activities: Patient Records in Medical History," *Social History of Medicine* 5 (August 1992): 183–205; Warwick Anderson, "The Case of the Archive," *Critical Inquiry* 39 (Spring 2013): 532–47.
10. Thomas Laqueur, "Bodies, Details, and the Humanitarian Narrative," in *The New Cultural History*, ed. Lynn Hunt (Berkeley: University of California Press, 1989), 176–204. In interpreting records of the clinical encounters in the hospital's wards, I have avoided just pulling out instances in which white staff members make derogatory comments about African American patients as being indicative of some overarching racism. As Steven Noll and John Harley Warner have both pointed out, case files are full of negative remarks about patients, regardless of their race, ethnicity, gender, or class background. Instead my approach has been to analyze the racial content of the comments made about African American patients. I also want to assess any derogatory remarks about patients within the context of the larger case file, recognizing that there were many authors who contributed to the overall narratives about

patients and their illness experiences. These case files, then, reflect what Risse and Warner refer to as the "discrepancy between ideology and action." That is, when read carefully, we can discern the coexistence of therapeutic nihilism and care, the troubling commixture of medical altruism and racism. See Risse and Warner, "Reconstructing Clinical Activities," 202, 197–99; Warner, "Uses of Patient Records," 110; Noll, "Patient Records as Historical Stories," 424–27.

11. The distinction between sufferer and patient reminds us of the importance of recognizing the differences (and similarities) between how the individual who is afflicted with disease understands and experiences his or her illness and how the inhabitant of the diseased body is understood and approached by the physician. See Roy Porter, "The Patient's View: Doing Medical History from Below," *Theory and Society* 14 (March 1985): 175–98.

12. St. Elizabeths Hospital, *Book of Rules, Approved by the President of the Board of Visitors February 5, 1912, Revised November 22, 1920* (Washington, DC: Government Printing Office, 1920), 7, entry 3, box 4, folder "R(1), 10/31/19–12/15/23," SEH/BOVGC; Investigation of St. Elizabeths Hospital, H.R. Doc. No. 69-605, at 41–42 (1927), in "SEH Reports, Misc.," William A. White Collection, Saint Elizabeths Hospital Archives, Saint Elizabeths Hospital Library, Washington, DC.

13. White, *Outlines of Psychiatry*, 10th ed., 323.

14. Questionnaire enclosed in Assistant Physician to Mrs. C. A. Truman (pseudonym), n.d., copy; Case history, 1–6. Both in Case File No. 28129, box 448, SEH/CFP.

15. Case history, 6–6d, in Case File No. 28129, box 448, SEH/CFP.

16. John E. Lind, "Diagnostic Pitfalls in the Mental Examination of Negroes," *New York Medical Journal* 99 (June 27, 1914): 1286–87.

17. Constitutive of the case record is the examination, which Michel Foucault identified as productive of power relations: "In all the mechanisms of discipline, the examination is highly ritualized. In it are combined the ceremony of power and the form of the experiment, the deployment of force and the establishment of truth. At the heart of the procedures of discipline, it manifests the subjection of those who are perceived as objects and the objectification of those who are subjected." Foucault, *Discipline and Punish*, 184–85.

18. For examples, see Clinical notes, July 23, 1910, entry, in Case File No. 2706, box 7; Clinical notes, December 1, 1910, entry, in Case File No. 3985, box 17, both in SEH/CFP.

19. Clinical notes, June 1, 1906, entry, in Case File No. 4431, box 22; Clinical notes, August 18, 1921, entry, in Case File No. 7228, box 80; Clinical notes, April 15, 1911, entry, in Case File No. 5461, box 37. All in SEH/CFP.

20. On the dialogical nature of medicine as a whole, see Byron J. Good, "How Medicine Constructs Its Objects," in *Medicine, Rationality, and Experience*, 65–87.

21. Case history, 1–2, in Case File No. 27229, box 372, SEH/CFP.

22. Clinical notes, August 15, 1919, entry, in Case File No. 15105, box 248, SEH/CFP.

23. Medical Certificate, 1–2; Case history, 1–4. Both in Case File No. 27592, box 401, SEH/CFP.

24. SEH/RC, box1, vol. 2, entry 7228; Clinical notes, July 29, 1913, March 25, 1915, and December 10, 1915 entries, in Case File No. 7228, box 80, SEH/CFP.

25. Lind, "Diagnostic Pitfalls." See also O'Malley, "Psychoses in the Colored Race," 313; E. M. Green, "Psychoses among Negroes—A Comparative Study," *Journal of Nervous and Mental Disease* 41 (November 1914): 706.

26. Mical Raz, "Between the Ego and the Icepick: Psychosurgery, Psychoanalysis, and Psychiatric Discourse," *Bulletin of the History of Medicine* 82 (Summer 2008): 395, 407–408; Gambino, "Mental Health and Ideals of Citizenship," 168–70. The quote is from an article by White's successor, Winfred Overholser, in the 1949 issue of the *Digest of Neurology and Psychiatry*.

27. Grob, *Mental Illness and American Society*, 293; Braslow, *Mental Ills and Bodily Cures*, 74–75.

28. Matthew Gambino, "Fevered Decisions: Race, Ethics, and Clinical Vulnerability in the Malarial Treatment of Neurosyphilis, 1922–1953," *Hastings Center Report* 45 (2015): 2–3. Gambino attributes the disproportionate diagnosis of cerebral syphilis to lower rates among military admissions and the "underlying epidemiological reality" confronting African American communities, including "poverty, lack of education, and inadequate access to health care."

29. Convulsive therapies, such as insulin, metrazol, and electroshock, were not used with any regularity until the late 1930s and 1940s and therefore will not be dealt with in this chapter.

30. "Half-Yearly Summary," *American Journal of Insanity* 53 (April 1897): 611–13; "Half-Yearly Summary," *American Journal of Insanity* 54 (April 1898): 666–67 (quote).
31. John E. Lind, "Treating Maniacs with Water," *Popular Science Monthly* 90 (March 1917): 401–4; "Semi-Annual Report," April 2, 1907, 9, and "Annual Report to the Board of Visitors," October 8, 1907, 3, both in box 1, folder "R, 1906–08," SEH/BOVGC.
32. Lind, "Treating Maniacs with Water," 404.
33. H.R. Rep. No. 59-7644, at 1:878; "Bed Saddle for Insane," *Washington Post*, June 22, 1906, 4. White considered himself to be a moderate on the use of mechanical restraint; he objected to legal prohibition but thought that it needed to be regulated, as long as that regulation was done by the profession itself. See William A. White to Henry R. Stedman, March 29, 1911, in Grob, *Inner World of American Psychiatry*, 73; "Semi-Annual Report," April 5, 1910, entry 3, box 2, folder "R, 1908–12," SEH/BOVGC.
34. Joel T. Braslow and Sarah Linsley Starks, "The Making of Contemporary American Psychiatry, Part 2: Therapeutics and Gender before and after World War II," *History of Psychology* 8 (2005): 273. Braslow and Starks refer to this dynamic as "therapeutic discipline." See also Braslow's discussion of "therapeutic rationale" in *Mental Ills and Bodily Cures*.
35. *Book of Rules*, 10.
36. Clinical notes, December 14, 1912, December 22, 1912, January 15, 1914, February 18, 1914, April 15, 1914, and July 15, 1915 entries, in Case File No. 7611, box 89, SEH/CFP.
37. Clinical notes, 1, 3; Ward notes, September 6, 1902, August 10, 1905 entries. All in Case File No. 4535, box 23, SEH/CFP.
38. Ward notes, September 5, 1907, entry, in Case File No. 10191, box 166, SEH/CFP.
39. For a nuanced discussion of hydrotherapy at Saint Elizabeths that acknowledges the different motivations by staff and the different responses by patients, see Gambino, "Mental Health and Ideals of Citizenship," 130–35.
40. *Report of the Government Hospital for the Insane to the Secretary of the Interior* (1905), 14; *Report of the Government Hospital for the Insane to the Secretary of the Interior for the Fiscal Year Ended June 30, 1913*, 31. Both in DOI-LR, box 4.
41. *Report of the St. Elizabeths Hospital to the Secretary of the Interior for the Fiscal Year Ended June 30, 1917*, 28–29, DOI-LR, box 4; *Report of the St. Elizabeths Hospital to the Secretary of the Interior for the Fiscal Year Ended June 30, 1919*, 42.
42. White, *Outlines of Psychiatry*, 10th ed., 151–52, 268–69. For examples of medical thought regarding the rarity of alcohol-related diseases among blacks, see O'Malley, "Psychoses in the Colored Race," 330; Robert Reyburn, comp., *Type of Disease among the Freed People of the United States: Consolidated Reports of Sick and Wounded Freed People and White Refugees under treatment from 1865 to June 30, 1872, by Medical Officers on duty in Bureau of Refugees, Freedmen and Abandoned Lands* (Washington, DC: Gibson Books, 1891), 14.
43. Evelyn Brooks Higginbotham, "African American Women's History and the Metalanguage of Race," *Signs: Journal of Women in Culture and Society* 17 (Winter 1992): 260–62; Emmett J. Scott, *Negro Migration during the War* (New York: Oxford University Press, 1920), 22.
44. On the tendency to negate the existence of gender differentiation among African Americans within late nineteenth- and early twentieth-century racial thought, see Bederman, *Manliness and Civilization*; Stein, *Measuring Manhood*. For a discussion of its manifestation in psychiatric thought, see Doyle, *Psychiatry and Racial Liberalism*, 29–30, 101.
45. Gambino, "Mental Health and Ideals of Citizenship," 133–34.
46. "Report of the St. Elizabeths Hospital to the Secretary of the Interior, 1927," 5–6, in *Government Hospital for the Insane Reports, 1917–1932*, William A. White Collection, Saint Elizabeths Hospital Archives, Saint Elizabeths Hospital Library, Washington, DC; *Investigation of St. Elizabeths Hospital* (Washington, DC: Government Printing Office, 1927), 65–67, entry 48, box 1, folder "A," SEH/White.
47. *Report of the St. Elizabeths Hospital to the Secretary of the Interior for the Fiscal Year Ended June 30, 1921* (Washington, DC: Government Printing Office, 1921), 26. There was scarcely more parity the following year. The 647 male patients were given, on average, 45 treatments, while the 451 female patients were given, on average, 106 treatments. *Report of the St. Elizabeths Hospital to the Secretary of the Interior for the Fiscal Year Ended June 30, 1922* (Washington, DC: Government Printing Office, 1922), 6.

48. *Annual Report of the St. Elizabeths Hospital to the Secretary of the Interior for the Fiscal Year Ended June 30, 1932* (Washington, DC: Government Printing Office, 1932), 2, 14. The report did not give specific statistics for hydrotherapeutic treatments among the male population.
49. Physicians "saw the category 'woman' as a much more discrete, biologically grounded entity than the category 'man,'" Joel Braslow writes. "It was a category in which a whole host of behaviors indicated its 'healthy' existence. Deviation indicated both disease and a breach of a woman's natural state." Braslow, *Mental Ills and Bodily Cures*, 152–62.
50. White, *Outlines of Psychiatry*, 10th ed., 59.
51. White to Members of the Board of Visitors, April 3, 1917, 11–12, entry 3, box 3, folder "R(1), 3/21/16–10/31/19, SEH/BOVGC.
52. For an examination of the history of suggestion as an early form of therapy, see Caplan, *Mind Games*, 80–83.
53. White, *Outlines of Psychiatry*, 10th ed., 59–64.
54. *Report of the St. Elizabeths Hospital to the Secretary of the Interior for the Fiscal Year Ended June 30, 1919* (Washington, DC: Government Printing Office, 1919), offprint, 42, in entry 3, box 3, folder "R(1), 3/21/16–10/31/19," SEH/BOVGC. The diagnostic breakdown of the 111 patients was dementia praecox types (73), manic-depressive types (19), psychoneuroses (8), paranoid states (4), associated with epilepsy (3), compulsion neuroses (2), anxiety neuroses (2).
55. William A. White to Members of the Board of Visitors, April 9, 1919, copy, 15, entry 3, box 3, folder "M–Q, 3/21/16–10/31/19," SEH/BOVGC.
56. Edward W. Lazell, "The Group Treatment of Dementia Praecox," *Psychoanalytic Review* 8 (1921): 169, 174, 176–78. For a history of group therapy during this era, see Gary G. Burlingame and Scott Baldwin, "Group Therapy," in *History of Psychotherapy: Continuity and Change*, ed. John C. Norcross, Gary R. VandenBos, and Donald K. Freedheim, 2nd ed. (Washington, DC: American Psychological Association, 2011), 505–7.
57. Stereotypy was a symptom of psychosis. "In stereotypy," White wrote in his textbook, "the voluntary impulse once set in motion tends to continue or repeat itself in the same way indefinitely, thus we have three forms of stereotypy, viz., stereotypy of *attitude*, of *movement*, and of *speech*." White, *Outlines of Psychiatry*, 10th ed., 90 (italics in the original).
58. Arrah B. Evarts, "The Ontogenetic against the Phylogenetic Elements in the Psychoses of the Colored Race," *Psychoanalytic Review* 3 (July 1916): 274, 277; "Dr. Evarts, Ex-Physician at State Hospital, Dies," *Rochester (MN) Post-Bulletin*, April 4, 1968, 18.
59. Evarts, "Ontogenetic against the Phylogenetic," 278.
60. Conference Report, 1; Clinical notes, October 15, 1909 and January 15, 1910 entries. Both in Case File No. 671, box 2, SEH/CFP.
61. Clinical notes, January 15, 1910, entry, in Case File No. 3985, box 17, SEH/CFP. Judy B. was the patient Evarts referred to as the "little brown woman." Evarts examined Judy from January 1913 to January 1914, and many of the observations she recorded are consistent with her descriptions of the patient she discussed in her article.
62. Clinical notes, April 15, 1920, July 21, 1920, and April 4, 1930, entries, in Case File No. 15105, box 248, SEH/CFP.
63. On the persistence of folk healing practices in African American communities in the twentieth century, see Jeffrey E. Anderson, *Conjure in African American Society* (Baton Rouge: Louisiana State University Press, 2005), esp. 112–49; Carole E. Hill and Holly Mathews, "Traditional Health Beliefs and Practices among Southern Rural Blacks: A Complement to Biomedicine," in *Perspectives on the American South: An Annual Review of Society, Politics, and Culture*, ed. Merle Black and John Shelton Reed (New York: Gordon & Breach, 1981), 307–22; Kirk Anthony Johnson, "The Survival of Traditional Healing in a Contemporary Black Community" (PhD diss., University of Illinois, Urbana-Champaign, 1999); Stephanie Y. Mitchem, *African American Folk Healing* (New York: New York University Press, 2007).
64. SEH/RC, box 1, vol. 2, entry 6103; Clinical notes, June 16, 1906, August 15, 1910, and July 1, 1925, entries, in Case File No. 6103, box 50, SEH/CFP.
65. SEH/RC, box 1, vol. 2, entry 7611; Clinical notes, April 27, 1911, entry, in Case File No. 7611, box 89, SEH/CFP; Case history, 2, in Case File No. 27434, box 389, SEH/CFP. Ada and Ellen are examples of the internalization of a "psychiatry of everyday life." Historian Elizabeth

Lunbeck defines this as "psychiatrists' delineation of a realm of everyday concerns—sex, marriage, womanhood, and manhood; work, ambition, worldly failure; habits, desires, inclinations—as properly psychiatric." Lunbeck, *Psychiatric Persuasion*, 47.

66. SEH/RC, box 1, vol. 2, entry 5071; Case history, 3, in Case File No. 5071, box 31, SEH/CFP; Superintendent to Chief Medical Advisor, via Supervisor, District #4, memorandum copy, May 25, 1921, in Case File No. 27985, box 435, SEH/CFP.
67. Lind, "Diagnostic Pitfalls," 1287; Ward notes, January 6, 1906, August 15, 1906, entries, in Case File No. 15105, box 248, SEH/CFP.
68. As historian Sharla Fett has argued, enslaved African Americans possessed a "relational vision of health," a worldview that was not based on a neat distinction between the sacred and the secular or the spiritual and the natural world. Traditional African and African American folk thought attributed some diseases to physiological imbalances in individual bodies, especially imbalances in bodily fluids such as blood. In addition to their location in biological processes, African and African American folk concepts of illness allowed for the prominence of human and spiritual agency in disease causation. Disease could be the vehicle for divine judgment, an expression of ancestral displeasure, or the result of intracommunity conflict. The health of individuals, in other words, was intimately connected to the social and spiritual relationships that suffused their everyday lives. See Fett, *Working Cures*, 38–40, 56, 75.
69. Anderson, *Conjure in African American Society*, x–xi, 25, 50–74; Fett, *Working Cures*, 85.
70. Evarts, "Ontogenetic against the Phylogenetic," 284.
71. Evarts, "Ontogenetic against the Phylogenetic," 284.
72. SEH/RC, box 1, vol. 2, entry 5140; Clinical notes, September 1, 1909, entry, in Case File No. 5140, box 32, SEH/CFP; Ward notes, September 22, 1913, entry, in Case File No. 10191, box 166, SEH/CFP; SEH/RC, box 1, vol. 2, entry 7870; Clinical notes, April 15, 1913, entry, in Case File No. 7870, box 97, SEH/CFP.
73. Similarly Annie R.'s tendency to rub salt over her body and allow it to cake under her nails may have been linked to the use of salt in conjure. See Mitchem, *African American Folk Healing*, 17. I do not want to overstate my argument here, only seeing rational motivation in acts that, on their face, appear to us as irrational. I merely wish to encourage a more imaginative reading of documents of the official archive that allow for multiple possibilities. On the benefits and challenges of "uncovering the views of mad people in the observations made by others *precisely* by taking their recorded delusions seriously," see Geoffrey Reaume, "Keep Your Labels Off My Mind! or 'Now I Am Going to Pretend I Am Craze but Dont Be a Bit Alarmed': Psychiatric History from the Patient's Perspective," *Canadian Bulletin of Medical History* 11 (1994): 400 (emphasis in the original). Johanna Schoen discusses the need for historians to pay attention to "parallel 'realities,'" or the "reality of a medical history at odds with the self-perception of a historical subject, the reality of a subject's medical narrative at odds with science." Johanna Schoen, *Choice and Coercion: Birth Control, Sterilization, and Abortion in Public Health and Welfare* (Chapel Hill: University of North Carolina Press, 2005), 17.
74. SEH/RC, box 1, vol. 1, entry 2706; Conference report, 2; Clinical notes, July 23, 1910, entry, in Case File No. 2706, box 7, SEH/CFP.
75. Clinical notes, November 17, 1910, entry, in Case File No. 5071, box 31; Clinical notes, January 22, 1912, entry, in Case File No. 8212, box 106, both in SEH/CFP.
76. Clinical notes, October 3, 1913, entry, in Case File No. 4431, box 22, SEH/CFP.
77. Conference report, 1, in Case File No. 5071, box 31, SEH/CFP. It would not have been unusual if Richard had equated medicine with poison. In 1902 Superintendent Alonzo B. Richardson wrote to a friend or relative of Caroline S. to inform her that she had come down with a case of malaria but was resisting treatment. "We have had a great deal of difficulty in getting her to take medicine," Richardson wrote, "as she imagines that it is poison and absolutely refuses to swallow it." See Richardson to Julia King (pseudonym), January 3, 1902, in Case File No. 8206, box 106, SEH/CFP.
78. Case history, 3, in Case File No. 5071, box 31, SEH/CFP.
79. "Maze of unintelligibility" is from John E. Lind, "The Color Complex in the Negro," *Psychoanalytic Review* 1 (October 1914): 414.
80. Clinical notes, November 17, 1910, entry, in Case File No. 5071, box 31, SEH/CFP.

81. Although not the case for every individual patient file, the ward notes generally span from 1900 to the late 1920s. The number of case files for African American patients that serve as the basis of this argument is twenty-two, compared to eleven case files for white patients.
82. Clinical notes, June 3, 1927, in Case File No. 9471, box 141; Clinical notes, January 15, 1916, in Case File No. 9441, box 141; Ward notes, June 23, 1916, in Case File No. 10191, box 166. All in SEH/CFP.
83. See also Gambino, "'These Strangers within Our Gates,'" 400–402.
84. Clinical notes, June 5, 1900, August 2, 1905, and May 5, 1915, entries; Case history, 1, in Case File No. 5343, box 36, SEH/CFP. Although the first name on the 1880 census is different (Orlando), other identifying characteristics, including age and name of wife, match the biographical information in Landro's clinical record. See 1880 US Census (Schedule 1), Washington City, Washington County, District of Columbia, p. 14, family 136, dwelling 118, lines 28–30, accessed June 10, 2010, www.ancestry.com.
85. Clinical notes, May 8, 1911, entry; Conference report, 1, in Case File No. 5343, box 36, SEH/CFP.
86. Special Comm. on Investigation of the Government Hospital for the Insane, H.R. Rep. No. 59-7644, at 1:xxi–xxii, 226–27 (1907). I have chosen not to shield Owsley's identity because his commitment to Saint Elizabeths is part of the public record.
87. H.R. Rep. No. 59-7644, at 1:xxi–xxii. See also "Sustaining Dr. White," *Washington Post*, May 20, 1906, 11.
88. For a discussion of social membership, see Natalia Molina, *Fit to Be Citizens? Public Health and Race in Los Angeles, 1879–1939* (Berkeley: University of California Press, 2006), esp. 1–14.
89. Ward notes, February 7, 1914, entry; Case history, 2; Ward notes, April 6, 1922, entry, all in Case File No. 15105, box 248, SEH/CFP.
90. Clinical notes, July 25, 1914, July 15, 1915, January 15, 1916, entries, in Case File No. 7870, box 97, SEH/CFP.
91. In a study of dementia praecox based on her research on African American female patients, Arrah Evarts remarked on the therapeutic value of work for those patients who had not improved enough to be discharged from the hospital: "Other patients who do not become well enough to leave the hospital, are yet capable of doing a great many of the tasks well to which they have always been accustomed, and are the best workers of the institution on their own or neighboring wards, and in the laundry." Arrah Evarts, "Dementia Precox in the Colored Race," *Psychoanalytic Review* 1 (October 1914): 400.
92. O'Malley, "Psychoses in the Colored Race," 334.
93. Ward notes, October 15, 1906, entry, in Case File No. 4271, box 20, SEH/CFP.
94. Ward notes, October 1, 1913, March 2, 1914, entries, in Case File No. 3985, box 17, SEH/CFP.
95. Ward notes, April 16, 1910, entry, in Case File No. 2706, box 7, SEH/CFP.
96. Evarts, "Dementia Precox in the Colored Race," 388.
97. For two recent critiques of cultural competency by historians of psychiatry, see Metzl, *Protest Psychosis*, 199–212; Gabriel N. Mendes, *Under the Strain of Color: Harlem's Lafargue Clinic and the Promise of an Antiracist Psychiatry* (Ithaca, NY: Cornell University Press, 2015), 157–59.
98. Dowbiggin, *Keeping America Sane*, 66; Lamb, *Pathologist of the Mind*, 167–76.
99. For examples of other institutions that served the African American population in the South, see Noll, "Southern Strategies for Handling the Black Feeble-minded," 140–41; Hughes, "Labeling and Treating Black Mental Illness," 441–42; Susan Burch and Hannah Joyner, *Unspeakable: The Story of Junius Wilson* (Chapel Hill: University of North Carolina Press, 2007), 56–58. This reproduction of racial hierarchies animated the therapeutic regimes in colonial Africa as well. See, for example, Jackson, *Surfacing Up*, 49–50.
100. On prison psychosis, see White, *Outlines of Psychiatry*, 10th ed., 127.
101. Conference Report, August 19, 1922, 4–8, in Case File No. 28129, box 448, SEH/CFP.
102. The following conclusions are based on an examination of the "movement of population" sections of Saint Elizabeths' annual reports from 1921 through 1930. The annual reports used the term *colored*, so this category of patient may have included some people of Asian and indigenous descent. The overwhelming majority of nonwhite patients at Saint Elizabeths in the 1920s, however, were African American.

103. Dowbiggin, *Keeping America Sane*, 111–13.
104. Those years were 1925 (60 percent) and 1926 (65 percent). In 1927, 72 percent of white male patients were discharged as unimproved or as the result of death. However, this was an aberration because close to 500 patients were transferred to US Veterans' Bureau hospitals. See *Report of the St. Elizabeths Hospital to the Secretary of the Interior, 1927* (Washington, DC: Government Printing Office, 1927), 8.
105. This percentage could have been this high because of the transfer of African American soldiers and sailors to Veterans' Bureau hospitals. However, the following year 79 percent of African American male patients were removed from the rolls through unimproved discharges and deaths, and in 1929 the rate was 83 percent. So, unlike in the case of white male patients, the 1927 figure was not anomalous.
106. Conference Report, October 27, 1927, 1–3, in Case File No. 28129, box 448, SEH/CFP.

Chapter 7

1. William A. White, "Mental Hygiene," WMAL, August 29, 1930, published in *Sun Dial* 4 (November 1930): 2–6.
2. White, "Mental Hygiene," 6.
3. Grob, *Mental Illness and American Society*, 236; David J. Rothman, *Conscience and Convenience: The Asylum and Its Alternatives in Progressive America*, rev. ed. (New York: Aldine De Gruyter, 2002), 293–323.
4. National Committee for Mental Hygiene, comp. and ed., *Directory of Psychiatric Clinics in the United States* (New York: Commonwealth Fund, 1932), 29–31; "Applications Swell Agencies in Chest," *Washington Post*, July 4, 1929, 15; White, *Autobiography*, 174; "Church to Inaugurate 'Life Adjustment' Clinic," *Washington Post*, November 10, 1928, 5; Mrs. E. G. Nourse, "Washington Is Well Provided with Mental Hygiene Clinics," *Washington Post*, April 30, 1933, 7; Richardson and Williams, "Hospitals," 675–77.
5. Green, *Secret City*, 155–83, 190–92; Eric S. Yellin, *Racism in the Nation's Service: Government Workers and the Color Line in Woodrow Wilson's America* (Chapel Hill: University of North Carolina Press, 2013), 113–31, 179; David F. Krugler, "A Mob in Uniform: Soldiers and Civilians in Washington's Red Summer, 1919," *Washington History* 21 (2009): 48–77. On the racial limits of Progressivism, see Elisabeth Lasch-Quinn, *Black Neighbors: Race and the Limits of Reform in the American Settlement House Movement, 1890–1945* (Chapel Hill: University of North Carolina Press, 1993).
6. "Act of April 27, 1904," typescript copy, entry 42, Instructions to Staff and Other Records, 1883–1908, box 1, folder 1, SEH/Super; John Koren, *Summaries of State Laws Relating to the Insane* (New York: National Committee for Mental Hygiene, 1917), 44–50.
7. See, for instance, a report on the detention and temporary commitment of an African American man who trespassed on the grounds of the White House, demanding to see President Theodore Roosevelt so that he could deliver God's thoughts about the dishonorable discharge of African American soldiers involved in a riot in Brownsville, Texas, in 1906. "Arrested at White House," *Washington Post*, June 27, 1907, 16.
8. O'Malley, "Psychoses in the Colored Race," 334.
9. *Report of the Government Hospital for the Insane to the Secretary of the Interior* (1904), 16, DOI-LR, box 4.
10. On Progressive reform of commitment laws, see Rothman, *Conscience and Convenience*, 326–28.
11. *Report of the Committee to Consider the Organization and Needs of the Government Hospital for the Insane to the Secretary of the Interior* (Washington, DC: Government Printing Office, 1911), 11–12, in Records Relating to DC, entry 14, box 2, folder "D.C. Lunacy Laws—1939," SEH/Super. On derisive descriptions of the law, see Zigmond M. Lebensohn, "Contributions of Saint Elizabeths Hospital to a Century of Medico-Legal Progress," in Centennial Commission, *Centennial Papers: Saint Elizabeths Hospital, 1855–1955* (Baltimore, MD: Waverly Press, 1956), 45–47.
12. Frederick A. Fenning, "Voluntary Submission to Treatment and Custody in Hospitals for the Insane," *Journal of the American Medical Association* 58 (April 13, 1912): 1104–7.

13. *Report of the St. Elizabeths Hospital to the Secretary of the Interior for the Fiscal Year Ended June 30, 1919* (Washington, DC: Government Printing Office, 1919), 31.
14. Grob, *Mental Illness and American Society*, 135–42.
15. Samuel W. Hamilton, "Psychopathic Building of the Gallinger Municipal Hospital, Washington, D.C.," *Modern Hospital* 22 (February 1924): 134–40. On the increase of segregationist practice in the District in the 1910s and 1920s, see Green, *Washington: Capital City*, 207–33; Yellin, *Racism in the Nation's Service*, 196–203.
16. "1,310 More Treated Here Last Year for Insanity," *Washington Post*, August 3, 1924, 2; Richardson and Williams, "Hospitals," 683; George S. Wilson to H. C. Woolley, January 18, 1930, Records Relating to DC, entry 14, box 1, folder "Bd. of Public Welfare," SEH/Super.
17. "Report Relating to the Modification of Commitment Laws for Mental Patients in the District of Columbia," Records Relating to DC, entry 14, box 2, folder "D.C. Lunacy Laws," SEH/Super; Winfred Overholser, "The Voluntary Admission Law: Certain Legal and Psychiatric Aspects," *American Journal of Psychiatry* 3 (January 1924): 477.
18. *Annual Report of the St. Elizabeths Hospital to the Secretary of the Interior, 1931* (Washington, DC: Government Printing Office, 1931), 10; Copy of Bill S. 5486 and H.R. 15609, enclosure in Secretary of the Interior to Speaker of the House, December 1931; William A. White to Secretary of the Interior, January 2, 1931, both in Records Relating to DC, entry 14, box 2, folder "DC Comm File," SEH/Super.
19. "Committee Hearings," 75 Cong. Rec. 3800 (1932); *Annual Report of the St. Elizabeths Hospital to the Secretary of the Interior for the Fiscal Year Ended June 30, 1932* (Washington, DC: Government Printing Office, 1932), 18.
20. "Made D.C. Alienist," *Evening Star*, May 8, 1914, 17; "Hickling Will Ask Congress to Enact New Lunacy Laws," *Washington Post*, February 14, 1932, 15; "D.C. Congress Plans Speeded," *Washington Post*, October 5, 1934, 13.
21. "Citizens Favor Body to Handle Insanity Cases," *Washington Post*, March 10, 1935; Edwin Melvin Williams, "Closing Chapter," in Proctor, *Washington Past and Present*, 2:907–8; Green, *Washington: Capital City*, 217. The citizens' associations were also at the forefront of creating and maintaining de facto residential segregation through their enforcement of racist restrictive covenants and physical intimidation of prospective black homebuyers. See Yellin, *Racism in the Nation's Service*, 200.
22. "Lunacy Board Wins Support of House Unit," *Washington Post*, March 12, 1936, 13; "Sunday Liquor Bill Is Assailed by Dry Forces," *Washington Post*, December 29, 1936, 15; James D. Secrest, "Senate Votes to Set Site for Art Gallery," *Washington Post*, May 6, 1938, X13; 83 Cong. Rec. 7501 (1938); "Dr. Cohen Is Given Pen That Signed Lunacy Bill," *Washington Post*, June 10, 1938, X17.
23. "New Mental Law Hearings for 14," *Washington Post*, June 28, 1938, X13; Albert E. Marland, "Lunacy Procedure under the New Law," *Medical Annals of the District of Columbia* 8 (January 1939): 6–7. The commission could make one of four recommendations: (1) that an individual was sane and should be discharged immediately; (2) that a clear judgment could not be made and the individual warranted further observation not to exceed thirty days; (3) that the individual was insane and should be committed to Saint Elizabeths or another institution; or (4) that the individual was insane but could remain in the custody of responsible family members or friends.
24. Roger S. Cohen, "The New Law for the Commitment of the Mentally Ill," *Medical Annals of the District of Columbia* 9 (May 1940): 169; Marland, "Lunacy Procedure," 8.
25. William A. White to the Secretary of the Interior, January 2, 1931, 4. Voluntary admission would not become policy at Saint Elizabeths until 1948. See Lebensohn, "Contributions of Saint Elizabeths Hospital," 48.
26. *Report of the Government Hospital for the Insane to the Secretary of the Interior for the Fiscal Year Ended June 30, 1908* (Washington, DC: Government Printing Office, 1908), 7–8; "Insanity Gains Fast," *Washington Post*, January 19, 1908, 7.
27. "Semi-Annual Report of the Superintendent to the Board of Visitors," April 11, 1911, 7, entry 3, box 2, folder "R, 1908–12," SEH/BOVGC; "Money Needed for Insane," *Washington Post*, January 28, 1908, 16.
28. Rothman, *Conscience and Convenience*, 312–13.

29. Conference Report, September 2, 1919; Clinical notes, December 4, 1919, entry; Irene Chappelear to Mary O'Malley, October 26, 1919. All in Case File No. 7611, box 89, SEH/CFP.
30. Clinical notes, December 4, 1919, March 16, 1920, April 3, 1920, entries; Simon D. Tennyson to Dr. O'Malley, October 26, 1919. All in Case File No. 7611, box 89, SEH/CFP.
31. For an insightful study of the role of colonial psychiatry in the policing of African women's mobility, see Jackson, *Surfacing Up*. For a history on black women's activism in early twentieth-century Washington, see Treva B. Lindsey, *Colored No More: Reinventing Black Womanhood in Washington, D.C.* (Urbana: University of Illinois Press, 2017).
32. "In Re Paroled Patients," memorandum copy, March 16, 1904, entry 42, Instructions to Staff and Other Records, 1883–1908, box 1, folder 1, SEH/Super.
33. Case history, 2–4; Conference Report, October 18, 1909, 2–3; Conference Report, January 14, 1910. All in Case File No. 5716, box 41, SEH/CFP.
34. Grob, *Mental Illness and American Society*, 238–58.
35. "Half-Yearly Summary," *American Journal of Insanity* 66 (October 1909): 331–32; Minutes, November 27, 1909, entry 1, box 2, folios 53–54, SEH/BOVM; *Report of the Government Hospital for the Insane to the Secretary of the Interior for the Fiscal Year Ended June 30, 1911* (Washington, DC: Government Printing Office, 1911), 7–8.
36. "Annual Report of the Superintendent to the Board of Visitors," October 3, 1911, 7–8; William A. White to Members of the Board of Visitors, October 1, 1912, 7–8. Both in entry 3, box 2, folder "R, 1908–12," SEH/BOVGC. For a history of the role of eugenics in psychiatric thought and practice, see Dowbiggin, *Keeping America Sane*. On Eugenics Record Office fieldworkers, see Amy Sue Bix, "Experiences and Voices of Eugenics Field-Workers: 'Women's Work' in Biology," *Social Studies of Science* 27 (1997): 625–68.
37. William A. White to Members of the Board of Visitors, March 27, 1912, 7–8, entry 3, box 2, folder "R, 1908–12," SEH/BOVGC.
38. According to historian James Borchert, African Americans made up 93 percent of the District's alley dwellers in 1897. A sociologist conducting a survey of African American housing in Washington in the 1910s and 1920s reported that the 1914 mortality rate for African Americans living in alleys was 372 per 100,000. The mortality rate for African Americans living in houses that fronted the street was slightly better, at 293 per 100,000. Borchert, *Alley Life in Washington*, 42; William Henry Jones, *The Housing of Negroes in Washington, D.C.: A Study in Human Ecology* (Washington, DC: Howard University Press, 1929), 42–43.
39. L.B.T.J., "Our Out-Patient Department," *Sun Dial* 2 (January 1924): 11–14; *Report of the St. Elizabeths Hospital to the Secretary of the Interior for the Fiscal Year Ended June 30, 1920* (Washington, DC: Government Printing Office, 1920), 54; "Cheer Almshouse Inmates," *Washington Post*, January 3, 1920, 8; "Harding Advocates Community Idea," *Washington Post*, October 24, 1919, 18.
40. *Report of the St. Elizabeths Hospital* (1920), 54–55; *Report of the St. Elizabeths Hospital to the Secretary of the Interior for the Fiscal Year Ended June 30, 1921* (Washington, DC: Government Printing Office, 1921), 28–29; *Report of the St. Elizabeths Hospital to the Secretary of the Interior for the Fiscal Year Ended June 30, 1922* (Washington, DC: Government Printing Office, 1922), 13. The social workers were not identified by name in any of the annual reports in the 1920s, nor was the social worker position listed in the "Officers of the Hospital" section that began every annual report. However, as Gerald Grob points out, prior to 1940, the field of psychiatric social work was almost exclusively female. Grob, *Mental Illness and American Society*, 252.
41. *Report of the St. Elizabeths Hospital to the Secretary of the Interior, 1925* (Washington, DC: Government Printing Office, 1925), 9.
42. *Report of the St. Elizabeths Hospital to the Secretary of the Interior, 1926* (Washington, DC: Government Printing Office, 1926), 9.
43. *Report of the St. Elizabeths Hospital to the Secretary of the Interior, 1928* (Washington, DC: Government Printing Office, 1928), 6; *Annual Report of the St. Elizabeths Hospital to the Secretary of the Interior, 1929* (Washington, DC: Government Printing Office, 1929), 8. The demands placed on the social service department, as well as the ever-growing inpatient population, prompted the hospital administration to request more money to hire additional social workers. In doing so, the administration appealed to the cost-cutting mentality growing within

the federal bureaucracy in the early days of the Depression. "Each social worker can care for about 40 patients, which would save the Government approximately $28,000 a year," the administration surmised in 1930, "and with the conditions at the hospital as crowded as they are it would seem that an effort should be made to increase this department." *Annual Report of the St. Elizabeths Hospital to the Secretary of the Interior, 1930* (Washington, DC: Government Printing Office, 1930), 7.

44. Dorothy G. Sproul to Mary L. Stewart, March 29, 1928, copy; Conference Report, November 26, 1927, both in Case File No. 32435, box 508, SEH/CFP.
45. Clinical notes, September 1 and November 10, 1925, entries; Conference Report, November 26, 1927, 1–2; Arthur P. Noyes to Board of Public Welfare, November 28, 1927, copy; Paul L. Kirby to Arthur P. Noyes, November 30, 1927. All in Case File No. 32435, box 508, SEH/CFP.
46. Clinical notes, March 21 and March 31, 1928, entries, Case File No. 32435, box 508, SEH/CFP.
47. Sproul to Stewart, March 29, 1928; Clinical notes, March 21, April 4, April 6, and April 10, 1928, entries. All in Case File No. 32435, box 508, SEH/CFP.
48. Clinical notes, April 10, May 6, July 14, and August 6, 1928, entries, Case File No. 32435, box 508, SEH/CFP.
49. Clinical notes, July 14, October 9, October 10, and November 17, 1928, entries, Case File No. 32435, box 508, SEH/CFP.
50. Clinical notes, April 6, 1929, July 15, 1930, January 15, April 15, and May 22, 1931, entries; Conference Report, June 30, 1932. All in Case File No. 32435, box 508, SEH/CFP. Psychopathic personality was an expansive diagnosis that allowed psychiatrists to broaden the parameters of what constituted abnormality beyond symptoms and signs that were indicative of an actual diseased state. As historian Elizabeth Lunbeck argues, "Many psychiatrists indiscriminately conferred a diagnosis of psychopathic personality on anyone they thought strange or offensive." Lunbeck also suggests psychiatrists—at least at the Boston Psychopathic Hospital—were much more apt to diagnose hypersexual or immoral young white women as psychopaths than they were hypersexual or immoral young black women, given the larger cultural assumptions about black women's "natural" lasciviousness. "Psychiatrists diagnosed as psychopathic only the few black women whose immorality was of such proportions that it offended even the purportedly low standards of their race." Lunbeck, *Psychiatric Persuasion*, 65–71, 204–5 (quotes on 67 and 205). Lunbeck's generalization about the racial dimension of the psychopathic personality diagnosis does not appear to have been the case with Pearl, as nothing in her case record indicated that hospital staff considered her behavior to be particularly revolting or shameless. The final conference report also offers absolutely no clues as to why the clinical staff changed her diagnosis from psychopathic personality without psychosis to psychosis with psychopathic personality.
51. Admission Note, 1–2; Case history, 4; Clinical notes, November 26, December 10, December 19, and December 29, 1930, January 29, 1931, entries. All in Case File No. 36132, box 597, SEH/CFP.
52. Clinical notes, February 25 and August 26, 1931, February 12 and July 22, 1932, March 14 and April 7, 1933, entries; Conference Report, April 13, 1933. All in Case File No. 36132, box 597, SEH/CFP.
53. Case history, 2–4; Clinical notes, September 22, 1930, entry, Case File No. 36290, box 614, SEH/CFP.
54. Conference Report, April 30, 1931, 2; Social Service report, June 24, 1931, 1–2; Clinical notes, February 12, 1932, entry; Conference Report, May 27, 1932, 1–2. All in Case File No. 36290, box 614, SEH/CFP.
55. Conference Report, May 27, 1932, 1–2, Case File No. 36290, box 614, SEH/CFP.
56. The following statements appear in Gilbert's case history: "In giving his family history, however, he did exceedingly well considering the usual reaction for one of his race. . . . General intelligence and knowledge are fairly well in keeping with one of his experience, in spite of his psychotic behavior." By experience, the physician may have been referring to Gilbert's upbringing and personal history. However, its proximity to the physician's racial characterization

makes it difficult to disentangle these. In the end, these kinds of reflections, which are sprinkled throughout Gilbert's case file, as well as others—think of Pearl B.'s and Charles T.'s from the previous chapter—reinforce the idea that the ideological force of race shaped how Saint Elizabeths' psychiatrists approached their African American patients. See Case history, 4, Case File No. 36290, box 614, SEH/CFP.

57. "Church to Inaugurate 'Life Adjustment' Clinic"; Franklin Littell, "The Laboratory Method in Religion," *Washington Post*, May 19, 1929, SM11; *Directory of Psychiatric Clinics*, 30–31. In his article, Littell emphasized how the pastor of the congregation with a number of prominent liberal Washingtonians sought to meld the spiritual power of religion with the secular authority of science.

58. "New Child Clinic Formed in Capital," *Washington Post*, June 18, 1929, 11; "Dr. White Chooses Child Clinic Chief," *Washington Post*, June 27, 1930, 7; *Directory of Psychiatric Clinics*, 30; "Guidance Units to Widen Scope in New Offices," *Washington Post*, February 16, 1936, M16.

59. "229 Cases Treated at Mental Clinic," *Washington Post*, May 30, 1931, 4; "Federal Workers Miss Contacts of Home Town," *Washington Post*, November 13, 1934, 13. According to the latter article, the center's staff saw between four hundred and five hundred clients a year. For every two male clients, there were three females. And among those identifying themselves as Protestant, most were Methodist or Baptist, followed by Episcopalian and Presbyterian. Catholics were the fifth largest confessional group.

60. "Federal Workers Miss Contacts." On the scholarly research on the black psyche under Jim Crow, see Anne C. Rose, *Psychology and Selfhood in the Segregated South* (Chapel Hill: University of North Carolina Press, 2009); Daryl Michael Scott, *Contempt and Pity: Social Policy and the Image of the Damaged Black Psyche, 1880–1996* (Chapel Hill: University of North Carolina Press, 1997), esp. 19–40. The relationship between African Americans and noninstitutional psychiatry is an understudied area that is only beginning to be excavated by historians. For some recent work, see Doyle, *Psychiatry and Racial Liberalism*; Mendes, *Under the Strain of Color*; Martin Summers, "Diagnosing the Ailments of Black Citizenship: African American Physicians and the Politics of Mental Illness, 1895–1940," in *Precarious Prescriptions: Contested Histories of Race and Health in North America*, ed. Laurie B. Green, John Mckiernan-González, and Martin Summers (Minneapolis: University of Minnesota Press, 2014), 91–114.

61. "At Howard," *Baltimore Afro-American*, November 17, 1928, 3; James Monroe, "D.C. Schools," *Baltimore Afro-American*, January 16, 1932, 7; "Hygiene Institute to Discuss Negro," *Washington Post*, May 11, 1936, 4; "To Hold Parley on Mental Ills," *Baltimore Afro-American*, January 21, 1939, 13; "Reduction of Child Crime Pondered," *Baltimore Afro-American*, March 18, 1939, 4; Summers, "Diagnosing the Ailments," 100.

62. "New Child Clinic Formed in Capital"; "Capital Club Women Are Engrossed with Child Welfare Clinic," *Washington Post*, March 8, 1931, A1.

63. "Capital Club Women"; Nourse, "Washington Is Well Provided." See Margo Horn, *Before It's Too Late: The Child Guidance Movement in the United States, 1922–1945* (Philadelphia: Temple University Press, 1989), esp. 9–50. For histories on race and the child guidance movement, see Gerald Markowitz and David Rosner, *Children, Race, and Power: Kenneth and Mamie Clark's Northside Center* (New York: Routledge, 2000); Doyle, *Psychiatry and Racial Liberalism*.

64. Consider, for instance, the following statement by a Catholic University of America graduate student and settlement house worker who conducted a study of black life in one of the District's alleys: "The point that I am making is that almost all these children in the Court may truthfully be termed delinquent, many and various forms of delinquency are constantly in evidence, but some are more delinquent than others." Gladys Sellew, "A Deviant Social Situation: A Court" (PhD diss., Catholic University of America, 1938), 48.

65. *Report of the Government of the District of Columbia for the Year Ended June 20, 1933* (Washington, DC: Government Printing Office, 1934), 85; May-bel, "Career Women of the Capital," *Baltimore Afro-American*, August 2, 1941, 10; "Miss Lenroot Urges Child Aid Increase," *Washington Post*, October 23, 1941, 13.

66. "Guidance Clinics Aid 900 Children Yearly," *Washington Post*, January 29, 1941, 5; "Child Guidance Clinic Sessions Scheduled," *Washington Post*, January 19, 1948, 9. On segregation and integration of the District's playgrounds and schools, see Green, *Secret City*, 290–94, 329–30.

Chapter 8

1. "Patient's Death Will Be Probed," *Washington Evening Star*, July 22, 1936; "Hospital Guards Held for Inquest," *Washington Evening Star*, July 23, 1936; "D.C. Jury Frees Guards in Death," *Washington Herald*, August 13, 1936, all in vertical file, "Hospitals, St. Elizabeths—1946," DCPL; "Aides Freed in Man's Death at St. Elizabeth," *Washington Afro-American*, August 15, 1936.
2. Miriam Ottenberg, "Truman Directive Seen Barring Service Cases at St. Elizabeth's," *Washington Evening Star*, July 22, 1945, in Winfred Overholser Scrapbook, 1944–47, box 25, PWO.
3. For a general discussion of the public criticism—in journalism and popular culture—of the public mental hospital in the postwar US, see Gerald N. Grob, *From Asylum to Community: Mental Health Policy in Modern America* (Princeton, NJ: Princeton University Press, 1991), 70–92. *The Snake Pit*, a 1946 novel by Mary Jane Ward that was made into a film in 1948, epitomized the kind of public criticism that was directed toward a lay audience.
4. The board's 1900 proposal was covered in chapter 4.
5. *Report of the Committee to Consider the Organization and Needs of the Government Hospital for the Insane to the Secretary of the Interior* (Washington, DC: Government Printing Office, 1911), 22–23, in Records Relating to D.C., entry 14, box 2, folder "D.C. Lunacy Laws—1939," SEH/Super.
6. Henry Ladd Stickney, "Report of Formal Inspection of Saint Elizabeth's Hospital (Department of Interior) at Washington, D.C.," April 22–24, 1924, 3, 10, in entry 48, box 2, folder "S," SEH/White.
7. William A. White to G. Lloyd Magruder, December 21, 1907, copy, in entry 3, box 1, folder "M, 1906–08," SEH/BOVGC; "Dr. G. Lloyd Magruder," *New York Times*, January 30, 1914, 9.
8. "Inspection Report for the Bureau of Medicine and Surgery, Navy Department," copy, November 16, 1926, in entry 48, box 1, folder "B," SEH/White.
9. *Annual Report of the St. Elizabeths Hospital to the Secretary of the Interior for the Fiscal Year Ended June 30, 1932* (Washington, DC: Government Printing Office, 1932), 13–14.
10. Grob, *Inner World of American Psychiatry*, 270; "No Separate Lectures," *Washington Bee*, January 21, 1911, 4; "Dr. Wm. A. White Has Weakened," *Baltimore Afro-American*, February 4, 1911, 5.
11. William A. White to Dean Edward A. Balloch, January 14, 1911, in Grob, *Inner World of American Psychiatry*, 270.
12. "No Separate Lectures"; "Color Craze," *Washington Bee*, January 21, 1911, 4.
13. "No Separate Lectures"; Dr. Lucy E. Moten to William A. White, January 20, 1911, and James C. Waters Jr. to William A. White, January 21, 1911, in Grob, *Inner World of American Psychiatry*, 271–72; Sandra Fitzpatrick and Maria R. Goodwin, *The Guide to Black Washington: Places and Events of Historical and Cultural Significance in the Nation's Capital*, rev. ed. (New York: Hippocrene, 1999), 105–6.
14. William C. Borden to William A. White, January 16, 1911; White to Borden, January 19, 1911; White to Borden, February 1, 1911, all in Grob, *Inner World of American Psychiatry*, 271–72; "Dr. Wm. A. White Has Weakened." The *Bee* reported that Thirkield withdrew the Howard students, but it is unclear whether he did it before White proposed the separate lectures. See "Paragraphic News," *Washington Bee*, February 4, 1911, 1.
15. William A. White to William C. Borden, April 8, 1911, and Edward A. Balloch to William A. White, September 20, 1923, in Grob, *Inner World of American Psychiatry*, 272–73.
16. See Yellin, *Racism in the Nation's Service*.
17. "Guards Beat Insane Man to Death," *Washington Tribune*, July 26, 1924, 1.
18. "Grand Jury Orders Probe of Conditions at Hospital," *Washington Tribune*, October 10, 1925, 1.

19. Dianne Dale, "Barry Farm/Hillsdale," in *Washington at Home: An Illustrated History of Neighborhoods in the Nation's Capital*, ed. Kathryn Schneider Smith, 2nd ed. (Baltimore, MD: Johns Hopkins University Press, 2010), 158–64. As discussed in chapter 7, neighborhood associations were segregated, with whites using the term *citizen* and blacks generally using the term *civic* to distinguish their groups. Because Barry Farm was a predominantly black neighborhood, there was no white Barry Farm Citizens' Association, freeing up African American residents to use *citizen* in the name of their association.
20. "Barry Farm Notes," *Washington Tribune*, October 10, 1925, 3; "Barry Farm Notes," *Washington Tribune*, November 21, 1925, 3.
21. "Bill Introduced for Investigation of St. Elizabeth," *Washington Tribune*, December 26, 1925, 1; "Death of Patients Reveals Horrors in D.C. Hospital," *Baltimore Afro-American*, April 24, 1926, 3.
22. Even though de Montis lived in the District, the local press identified her as being a member of the Washington State and Alaska Society and a member of the Women's Legislative Committee of the State of Washington. She developed an interest in habeas corpus and commitment reform after spending six weeks as an inmate in a Washington State insane asylum. See *Washington Evening Star*, October 20, 1934, A-7; *Washington Evening Star*, March 29, 1927, 9; *Tacoma (WA) Times*, August 18, 1917, 8.
23. 67 Cong. Rec. 3074 (1926); E.B.N., "Notes and Comment," *American Journal of Psychiatry* 6 (January 1927): 584.
24. *Report of the St. Elizabeths Hospital to the Secretary of the Interior for the Fiscal Year Ended June 30, 1918* (Washington, DC: Government Printing Office, 1918), 7; *Report of the St. Elizabeths Hospital to the Secretary of the Interior for the Fiscal Year Ended June 30, 1919* (Washington, DC: Government Printing Office, 1919), 7.
25. *Report of the St. Elizabeths Hospital* (1919), 21, 32; *Report of the St. Elizabeths Hospital to the Secretary of the Interior for the Fiscal Year Ended June 30, 1920* (Washington, DC: Government Printing Office, 1920), 39; John Joseph Kindred, "The Neuro-Psychiatric Wards of the United States Government: Their Housing and Other Problems," *American Journal of Psychiatry* 78 (October 1921): 186; William A. White, "The New Saint Elizabeth's Hospital," *American Journal of Psychiatry* 81 (January 1924): 503–5.
26. E.B.N., "Notes and Comment," 579–81. For more on the history of the use of black bodies in white medical schools, see Blakely and Harrington, *Bones in the Basement*.
27. Investigation of St. Elizabeths Hospital, H.R. Doc. 69-605, at 1, 126–27 (1927). Perhaps to preempt further scrutiny of the William Green incident by the comptroller general, Saint Elizabeths' staff published its account of his death. The hospital account attributed Green's injuries to his falling against the barber's chair. It also emphasized the clinical staff's response to Green's injuries and the complete cooperation of hospital officials with law enforcement. See *Memorandum from St. Elizabeths Hospital Regarding the Care and Treatment of Patients and the Fiduciary Relation between the Hospital and Patients, Together with Copies of Correspondence Bearing on These Matters, June 7, 1926* (Washington, DC: Government Printing Office, 1927), 64.
28. "Report of the Special Medical Advisers on St. Elizabeths Hospital," *American Journal of Psychiatry* 6 (January 1927): 545, 559.
29. "Inspection Report for the Bureau of Medicine and Surgery, Navy Department," 7.
30. "Report of the Special Medical Advisers," 557, 564.
31. *Annual Report of the St. Elizabeths Hospital* (1932), 13.
32. "One, 91, 10 Infants in 57 D.C. Deaths," *Baltimore Afro-American*, August 1, 1936, 21.
33. Grob, *From Asylum to Community*, 5–23; Gerald N. Grob and Howard H. Goldman, *The Dilemma of Federal Mental Health Policy: Radical Reform or Incremental Change?* (New Brunswick, NJ: Rutgers University Press, 2006), 18–20.
34. "Dr. Overholser Becomes Superintendent of St. Elizabeth's Hospital," *American Journal of Psychiatry* 94 (September 1937): 480–82.
35. Winfred Overholser, "The Mental Hospital of Yesterday and Today," *Medical Annals of the District of Columbia* 7 (May 1938): 141–44.
36. *Annual Report of St. Elizabeths for the Fiscal Year 1944* (Washington, DC: Government Printing Office, 1944), 1; *Annual Report of the Federal Security Agency: Section Six: St.*

Elizabeths Hospital, 1945 (Washington, DC: Government Printing Office, 1945), 1, 3; Robert J. Lewis, "St. Elizabeth's Hospital Performs Heaviest Task in Vital Wartime Role," *Sunday Star* (Washington, DC), September 24, 1944, in vertical file, "Hospitals, St. Elizabeths—1946," DCPL.
37. 79 Cong. Rec. 4828 (1945), in Overholser Scrapbook 1944–47, box 25, PWO.
38. A similar sentiment was expressed in an article on the crisis of mental illness within black communities that appeared in a 1949 issue of the African American monthly *Ebony*: "If for white patients, the result [of a shortage of mental health resources] has been institutions that are more jails than hospitals, then for Negroes the situation approaches Nazi concentration camp standards—especially in the South where three out of every five colored insane are confined." See "Insanity: Mental Illness among Negroes Exceeds Whites, Overcrowds Already-Jammed 'Snake Pits,'" *Ebony* (April 1949): 19–23.
39. James E. Chinn, "St. Elizabeths Overcrowded and Antiquated, Report Says," *Washington Post*, November 3, 1945, in vertical file, "Hospitals, St. Elizabeths—1946," DCPL.
40. American Psychiatric Association standards recommended one assistant physician for every 150 patients. In 1938 Saint Elizabeths had one assistant physician for every 121 patients. In that same year state mental hospitals had an average of 9.3 patients for every nurse/attendant, while in the District of Columbia, the ratio was 5.1 patients for every nurse/attendant. Saint Elizabeths had an average daily per capita cost of $1.83, as opposed to the state hospital average of $0.80. See Samuel W. Hamilton et al., *A Study of the Public Mental Hospitals of the United States 1937–39: Supplement No. 164 to the Public Health Reports* (Washington, DC: Government Printing Office, 1941), 11, 37–42, 83; Washington Metropolitan Health Council, *Health and Hospital Survey of Metropolitan Washington* (n.p.: 1946), VIII-2–VIII-3, VIII-21.
41. Ottenberg, "Truman Directive"; "Lower Status Seen in Plan for St. Elizabeth's," *Star*, July 9, 1946, in vertical file, "Hospitals, St. Elizabeths—1946," DCPL; Hamilton, *Study of the Public Mental Hospitals*, 7.
42. Ottenberg, "Truman Directive"; "Lower Status Seen in Plan"; "Hospital Head Hits Military Ouster," *Washington News*, May 18, 1946, in Overholser Scrapbook 1944–47, box 25, PWO.
43. "Lower Status Seen in Plan"; *Annual Report of the Federal Security Agency: Section Five: St. Elizabeths Hospital, 1946* (Washington, DC: Government Printing Office, 1946), 399; *Annual Report of the Federal Security Agency: Section Four: St. Elizabeths Hospital, 1947* (Washington, DC: Government Printing Office, 1947), 469, 466; Nate Haseltine, "Woman's Campaign Started St. Elizabeths a Century Ago," *Washington Post and Times-Herald*, March 3, 1955, in entry 62, Scrapbooks, 1953–1957, SEH/Super.
44. "D.C. Officials Will Confer on St. Elizabeth's," *Washington Star*, February 19, 1947, in Overholser Scrapbook 1944–47, box 25, PWO; *Report of the Government of the District of Columbia for the Year Ended June 30, 1944* (Washington, DC: Government Printing Office, 1944), 185; *Report of the Government of the District of Columbia for the Year Ended June 30, 1945* (Washington, DC: Government Printing Office, 1945), 190.
45. "D.C. Officials Will Confer"; "Fowler's Plan to Shift St. Elizabeth's Control Is Hit by Health Council," *Washington Star*, February 28, 1947, in Overholser Scrapbook 1944–47, box 25, PWO; "Our Superintendent," *Elizabethan* 3 (February 26, 1947): 2, in Overholser Scrapbook 1947–49, box 27, PWO.
46. Green, *Washington: Capital City*, 494–95; "3 Oppose D.C. Taking Over 2 Hospitals," *Washington Post*, July 20, 1947, in Overholser Scrapbook 1947–49, box 27, PWO.
47. *Reorganization and Home Rule for the District of Columbia: Hearings before the Subcommittee on Home Rule and Reorganization of the Committee on the District of Columbia, House of Representatives* (Washington, DC: Government Printing Office, 1947), 456–66. The joint subcommittee did work up a bill that reorganized the District's government by eliminating most of the advisory boards. It also extended limited home rule to District residents, allowing them to elect a nonvoting delegate to the House of Representatives and, for the first time since Reconstruction, a city council. The bill was favorably reported out of the House District Committee in the spring of 1948 but died on the House floor shortly thereafter. See Green, *Washington: Capital City*, 495–96.

48. *Annual Report of the Federal Security Agency* (1947), 471; Lewis, "St. Elizabeth's Hospital Performs Heaviest Task."
49. "17% Mental Case Jump Laid to Housing," *Washington Post*, August 1, 1947, in Overholser Scrapbook 1947–49, box 27, PWO; Richard Wolpe, "Tragedy of Old Age: Sane, but Aged, 200 Locked Up at St. Elizabeths," *Washington Daily News*, December 12, 1949, in Overholser Scrapbook 1949–51, box 26, PWO; *Annual Report of the Federal Security Agency, 1948: St. Elizabeths Hospital* (Washington, DC: Government Printing Office, 1948), ix. On postwar therapeutic optimism, see Grob, *From Asylum to Community*, 16.
50. "Voluntary Cases Approved for St. Elizabeths," *Washington Star*, April 20, 1948; N. S. Haseltine, "Voluntary Patients Regaining Mental Health at St. Elizabeths," *Washington Post*, December 19, 1948, both in vertical file, "Hospitals, St. Elizabeths 1947–1949," DCPL.
51. Haseltine, "Voluntary Patients Regaining Mental Health"; "St. Elizabeths Gets 83 Voluntary Cases in First Year of Plan," *Washington Star*, June 2, 1950; "Mental Clinics Urged by St. Elizabeths Officials," *Washington Evening Star*, April 22, 1950, both in vertical file, "Hospitals, St. Elizabeths 1950–1959," DCPL.
52. Green, *Secret City*, 235.
53. Charles Prudhomme and David F. Musto, "Historical Perspectives on Mental Health and Racism in the United States," in *Racism and Mental Health*, ed. Charles V. Willie, Bernard M. Kramer, and Bertram S. Brown (Pittsburgh, PA: University of Pittsburgh Press, 1973), 42–44; "Progress in the Movement to Guarantee Equal Rights for All Citizens in the National Capital," n.d., 4, Series IX, Washington Bureau, 1914–1993, box 226, folder 1, Records of the National Association for the Advancement of Colored People, Manuscript Division, Library of Congress, Washington, DC; Green, *Secret City*, 231. See also Karen Kruse Thomas, *Deluxe Jim Crow: Civil Rights and American Health Policy, 1935–1954* (Athens: University of Georgia Press, 2011), 46–51.
54. Estelle Massey Riddle, "Negro Nurses: The Supply and Demand," *Opportunity: A Journal of Negro Life* 15 (November 1937): 328, box 3, folder 8; "Newsreel," *National News Bulletin* 12 (June 1939): 4, box 3, folder 1. Both in National Association of Colored Graduate Nurses Papers, microfilm, Thomas P. O'Neill Library, Boston College, Chestnut Hill, Massachusetts.
55. Mabel K. Staupers, "The Negro Nurse Advances," typescript, February 1942, 8, box 3, folder 8, National Association of Colored Graduate Nurses Papers; Prudhomme and Musto, "Historical Perspectives," 45; "Nurse Shortage," *Washington Post*, January 1, 1945, 4. For more on the shortage of nurses during World War II and African American nurses' organizational efforts to break the color barrier, see Darlene Clark Hine, "Black Professionals and Race Consciousness: Origins of the Civil Rights Movement, 1890–1950," *Journal of American History* 89 (March 2003): 1279–94.
56. *Annual Report of St. Elizabeths* (1944), 6.
57. "Racial Integration in Nursing," *NAIRO Reporter* 2 (June 1952): 3, box 3, folder 9, National Association of Colored Graduate Nurses Papers.
58. Darlene Clark Hine, *Black Women in White: Racial Conflict and Cooperation in the Nursing Profession, 1890–1950* (Bloomington: Indiana University Press, 1989), 100–102, 183; "Say Negro Nurses Will Be Appointed to Glendale Jobs," *Savannah (GA) Tribune*, August 31, 1939, in Scrapbook, box 4, folder 4, National Association of Colored Graduate Nurses Papers, microfilm; "District of Columbia Votes to Admit Negro Nurses to Membership," *American Journal of Nursing* 51 (September 1951): 36.
59. "Preliminary Report on Interviews with Attendants at St. Elizabeths Hospital," 1; "Conference with Dr. Silk re Saint Elizabeth's," November 17, 1942, both in "Study of Turnover among Attendants of St. Elizabeths Work File 1943"; "The Employment of Negroes as Attendants at St. Elizabeths Hospital," August 1943, 2. All reports in entry 19, box 2, RG 235 Records of the Department of Health, Education, and Welfare, NARA.
60. Arthur B. McLean to George L. P. Weaver, June 12, 1943, copy, enclosed in "Employment of Negroes as Attendants."
61. "Employment of Negroes as Attendants," 1, 3–4; "Preliminary Report on Interviews," 10. On the de facto segregation of government cafeterias during World War II, see Green, *Secret City*, 261.

62. "Employment of Negroes as Attendants," 1; "Final Report," 51, in "Study of Turnover among Attendants."
63. "Employment of Negroes as Attendants," 4. The same African American attendant who suggested there was a natural racial affinity between black employees and patients also pointed out that another dynamic existed on the wards: "But some of them [black patients], of course, hate the colored attendants and would do anything for the whites. It's all in their background. The ones from the South are used to being told what to do by the whites."
64. "Employment of Negroes as Attendants," 2–3.
65. "Employment of Negroes as Attendants," 2–3.
66. "Employment of Negroes as Attendants," 2–3.
67. "Employment of Negroes as Attendants," 4.
68. For an in-depth study of the racial progressivism of New Deal liberals, see Patricia Sullivan, *Days of Hope: Race and Democracy in the New Deal Era* (Chapel Hill: University of North Carolina Press, 1996).
69. Prudhomme and Musto, "Historical Perspectives," 42–43; Lon Tuck, "Dr. Karpman, Psychiatrist," *Washington Post and Times-Herald*, May 18, 1962, C4; "Insanity Threat Greatest at High School Age, M.D. Says," *Baltimore Afro-American*, July 31, 1937, 20; "Dr. John S. Perry Dead; Physician Since 1936," *Washington Post*, November 16, 1962, B6.
70. *Annual Reports Federal Security Agency for the Fiscal Years 1941–1942; 1942–1943* (Washington, DC: Government Printing Office, 1943), 7–8; *Annual Report of the Federal Security Agency 1947: Section 4. St. Elizabeths Hospital* (Washington, DC: Government Printing Office, 1947), 475; *Annual Report of the Federal Security Agency 1949* (Washington, DC: Government Printing Office, 1949), 633.
71. Gillette, *Between Justice and Beauty*, 151–69; Spencer R. Crew, "Melding the Old and the New: The Modern African American Community, 1930–1960," in *Washington Odyssey: A Multicultural History of the Nation's Capital*, ed. Francine Curro Cary (Washington, DC: Smithsonian Books, 1996); *Annual Report of the U.S. Department of Health, Education, and Welfare 1957* (Washington, DC: Government Printing Office, 1957), 7; David Barton Smith, *Health Care Divided: Race and Healing a Nation* (Ann Arbor: University of Michigan Press, 1999), 20–21, 40.
72. Crew, "Melding the Old and the New," 221–25; Green, *Secret City*, 296–98; Asch and Musgrove, *Chocolate City*, 302–3.
73. J.A.K., "Segregation at Gallinger Hospital" and "The Medico-Chirurgical Society Letter of Protest," in *Journal of the National Medical Association* 39 (March 1947): 77–78, 80.
74. J. R. Fuchs, "Oral History Interview with Oscar R. Ewing," May 2, 1969, transcript, Harry S. Truman Library and Museum, accessed June 21, 2014, http://www.trumanlibrary.org/oralhist/ewing4.htm#250; "Race Relations," *Washington Post*, December 16, 1946, 6; Group Relations Committee, *The Social Survey: A Report on Racial Relations* (Washington, DC: Social Agencies of the District of Columbia and Vicinity, 1946); *To Secure These Rights: The Report of the President's Committee on Civil Rights* (Washington, DC: Government Printing Office, 1947), 93.
75. J.A.K., "Segregation at Gallinger Hospital," 77; "Civil Rights Report: D.C. Treatment of Negroes Hit," *Washington Post*, October 30, 1947, 13; "Negro Doctors May Intern at Gallinger," *Washington Post*, November 24, 1947, B2; "League Favors Negro Training at Gallinger," *Washington Post*, December 5, 1947, B1; "Committee to Study Posts at Gallinger," *Washington Post*, May 28, 1939, 12; "Opening Gallinger," *Washington Post*, February 18, 1948, 12.
76. "D.C. Hospital Breaks Color Bar; To Admit Negro Medical Students as Resident Interns with Whites," unidentified newspaper clipping in Scrapbook, box 5, vol. 7, National Association of Colored Graduate Nurses Papers.
77. "N.A.A.C.P. Resolutions in Health Area," *Journal of the National Medical Association* 43 (September 1951): 342–43. On the Hospital Survey and Construction Act, otherwise known as the Hill-Burton Act, see Smith, *Health Care Divided*, 46–47; Thomas, *Deluxe Jim Crow*, 157–81.
78. Louis Lautier, "Eisenhower Studies Powers of Office in Ending Segregation in Washington," *Baltimore Afro-American*, February 14, 1953, 9; W. Montague Cobb, "The National Health

Program of the N.A.A.C.P.," *Journal of the National Medical Association* 45 (September 1953): 338; District of Columbia Branch National Association for the Advancement of Colored People press release, July 14, 1953, Part II, box 30, folder District of Columbia, Records of the National Association for the Advancement of Colored People, Manuscript Division, Library of Congress, Washington, DC.

79. Genevieve Reynolds, "Equality Resolution Passed by Unitarian Church Alliance," *Washington Post*, December 14, 1945, Overholser Scrapbook 1944–47, box 25, PWO; "Unitarian Moderator Sees Liberals in Peril," *Worcester Telegram*, April 26, 1948, Overholser Scrapbook 1947–49, box 27, PWO.
80. W. Montague Cobb, "Solomon Carter Fuller, 1872–1953," *Journal of the National Medical Association* 46 (September 1954): 371; Herbert M. Morais, *The History of the Afro-American in Medicine* (Cornwells Heights, PA: Publishers Agency, 1978), 104–5.
81. Prudhomme and Musto, "Historical Perspectives," 43–44, 47.
82. "Three Washington Hospitals Open Staffs to Negro Physicians" and "D.C. Tuberculosis Hospital Adds First Negro Staff Physicians," *Journal of the National Medical Association* 46 (November 1954): 431, 432; "Medical Society of the District of Columbia Resigns from Citizens Group," *Journal of the National Medical Association* 45 (July 1953): 290.
83. Jeanne Spurlock, "Early and Contemporary Pioneers," in *Black Psychiatrists and American Psychiatry*, ed. Jeanne Spurlock (Washington, DC: American Psychiatric Association, 1999), 9–10; "Brief History of Saint Elizabeths Hospital, Washington, D.C.," 4, vertical file, City Museum of Washington, Washington, DC.
84. Jay L. Hoffman to Winfred Overholser, June 13, 1956, entry 7, Records of the Superintendent, 1855–1967, Administrative Files, ca. 1921–64, box 26, folder "Monthly Reports"; Luther D. Robinson to the Superintendent, July 2, 1957, box 12, folder Annual Reports—June '57, both in SEH/ARSU.

Chapter 9

1. "Centennial Commission, Advance Release," 1955, entry 62, Scrapbooks, 1953–1957, SEH/Super; *Annual Report of the U.S. Department of Health, Education, and Welfare 1955* (Washington, DC: Government Printing Office, 1955), 203–4; Centennial Commission, Centennial Papers.
2. Advertisement for *The March of Medicine*; Bernie Harrison, "March of Medicine Poses a Challenge," *Washington Star*, May 17, 1955. Both in Overholser Scrapbook, June 1954–June 1955, box 30, PWO. See also Richard G. Frank and Sherry A. Glied, *Better but Not Well: Mental Health Policy in the United States Since 1950* (Baltimore, MD: Johns Hopkins University Press, 2006), 29.
3. Dale C. Cameron, "Progress Is Saint Elizabeths' Tradition," *Medical Annals of the District of Columbia* 32 (August 1963): 303; Grob, *From Asylum to Community*, 148–51.
4. Wailoo, *Drawing Blood*, 134–61; UNESCO, "Statement on Race," (1950), in Hammonds and Herzig, *The Nature of Difference*, 313–18; Michelle Brattain, "Race, Racism, and Antiracism: UNESCO and the Politics of Presenting Science to the Postwar Public," *American Historical Review* 112 (December 2007): 1386–413; Jenny Reardon, *Race to the Finish: Identity and Governance in the Age of Genomics* (Princeton, NJ: Princeton University Press, 2005).
5. Grob, *From Asylum to Community*, 5–23; Scott, *Contempt and Pity*.
6. For a recent excellent treatment of the emergence of racially liberal psychiatry in the mid-twentieth century, see Doyle, *Psychiatry and Racial Liberalism*.
7. On the rejection of Lamarckism and recapitulation theory by psychoanalysts in the post–World War I era, see Makari, *Revolution in Mind*, 419–20.
8. Siegfried Fischer, "The Influence of Indian and Negro Blood on the Manic-Depressive Psychosis," *Journal of Nervous and Mental Disease* 97 (April 1943): 409–20.
9. Lauretta Bender, "Behavior Problems in Negro Children," *Psychiatry* 2 (May 1939): 213–28. This is, admittedly, a snapshot of Bender's complex and evolving thought about race and mental development. For more on Bender, see Doyle, "'Racial Differences Have to Be Considered.'"

10. Géza Róheim, "Racial Differences in the Neurosis and Psychosis," *Psychiatry* 2 (August 1939): 389. For other works that sought to explode the reductionist civilized/primitive binary, see Ellen Winston, "The Alleged Lack of Mental Diseases among Primitive Groups," *American Anthropologist* 36 (April–June 1934): 234–38; B. J. F. Laubscher, *Sex, Custom and Psychopathology: A Study of South African Pagan Natives* (London: Routledge, 1937); N. J. Demarath, "Schizophrenia among Primitives: The Present Status of Sociological Research," *American Journal of Psychiatry* 98 (March 1942): 703–7; Erwin H. Ackerknecht, "Psychopathology, Primitive Medicine and Primitive Culture," *Bulletin of the History of Medicine* 14 (June 1943): 30–67.

11. For a recent scholarly treatment of Róheim, see Joy Damousi, "Géza Róheim and the Australian Aborigine: Psychoanalytic Anthropology during the Interwar Years," in *Unconscious Dominions: Psychoanalysis, Colonial Trauma, and Global Sovereignties*, ed. Warwick Anderson, Deborah Jenson, and Richard C. Keller (Durham, NC: Duke University Press, 2011), 75–95.

12. Front matter, *Psychiatry* 3 (February 1940): ii; Otto Allen Will Jr., "D.C. Doctor Pitted Psychiatry against War," *Washington Post*, February 6, 1949, B5. For a history of the foundation, see Robert G. Kvarnes, "The Founding of the William Alanson White Psychiatric Foundation," in D'Amore, *William Alanson White*, 123–26.

13. Ashley Montagu, "Problems and Methods Relating to the Study of Race," *Psychiatry* 3 (November 1940): 494–95.

14. W. M. Krogman, review of *Man's Greatest Myth: The Fallacy of Race*, by M. F. Ashley Montagu, *American Journal of Psychiatry* 102 (July 1946): 843.

15. Ashley Montagu, "Racism and Social Action," *Psychiatry* 9 (May 1946): 145, 147; Ashley Montagu, "Problems and Methods Relating to the Study of Race," 500–502. Montagu was not the only person who equated racism with mental illness. The African American physician and civil rights activist W. Montague Cobb took to labeling antiblack racism, and especially resistance to integration, a "form of mass mental illness" that he called "Confederate disease" or "Confederate sickness." See W. Montague Cobb, "The Washington Scene and the N.A.A.C.P.," 1959, in Part IX, Washington Bureau, 1914–1993, box 227, folder 1, Records of the National Association for the Advancement of Colored People, Manuscript Division, Library of Congress, Washington, DC; W. Montague Cobb, "Modern Recognition of Mental Health," *Journal of the National Medical Association* 50 (September 1958): 323–24. See also Michael E. Staub, *Madness Is Civilization: When the Diagnosis Was Social, 1948–1980* (Chicago: University of Chicago Press, 2011), 23–31, for a discussion of postwar psychiatrists' and social scientists' theorizing of the compensatory nature of racism and anti-Semitism that laid the foundation for authoritarian movements like fascism and Nazism.

16. Albert Deutsch, *The Story of GAP* (New York: Group for the Advancement of Psychiatry, 1959), 6–7, 11, 16–20.

17. Robert J. Lewis, "St. Elizabeth's Hospital Performs Heaviest Task in Vital Wartime Role," *Sunday Star* (Washington, DC), September 24, 1944, in vertical file, "Hospitals, St. Elizabeths—1946," DCPL; "Rising Mental Ills Blamed on Crowding," *Washington Times-Herald*, July 31, 1948, in Overholser Scrapbook 1947–49, box 27, PWO.

18. Rutherford B. Stevens, "Racial Aspects of Emotional Problems of Negro Soldiers," *American Journal of Psychiatry* 103 (January 1947): 493–98. Not all psychiatrists who worked with African American soldiers agreed with the emphasis that Stevens placed on racial discrimination. The same issue in which Stevens's article appeared included an article by Lieutenant Colonel Herbert S. Ripley and Major Stewart Wolf. Based on their observations of black soldiers in the Pacific theater, Ripley and Wolf drew on comparative psychology research of the 1910s and 1920s and invoked a civilizationist argument to explain the prevalence of mental illness within this group. But their work also evinced elements of a psychodynamic interpretation, which made their conclusions amenable to a social psychiatry framework. Herbert S. Ripley and Stewart Wolf, "Mental Illness among Negro Troops Overseas," *American Journal of Psychiatry* 103 (January 1947): 499–512. For more on black psychiatrists' attempts to reckon with mental illness among African American soldiers during the war, see Dwyer, "Psychiatry and Race during World War II."

19. For just a few examples, see Esther Milner, "Some Hypotheses concerning the Influence of Segregation on Negro Personality Development," *Psychiatry* 16 (August 1953): 291–98; Viola W. Bernard, "School Desegregation—Some Psychiatric Implications," *Psychiatry* 21 (May 1958): 149–58; Carl F. Hansen, "Mental Health Aspects of Desegregation," *Journal of the National Medical Association* 51 (November 1959): 450–56. For a more general discussion, see Scott, *Contempt and Pity*, esp. 71–136; Staub, *Madness Is Civilization*, 32–35.
20. Henry J. Myers and Leon Yochelson, "Color Denial in the Negro: A Preliminary Report," *Psychiatry* 11 (February 1948): 39–41.
21. On psychiatric universalism, see Doyle, *Psychiatry and Racial Liberalism*, esp. 35–54.
22. Prudhomme and Musto, "Historical Perspectives," 46–47.
23. Donn Munson, "St. Elizabeths Stands Out as Model Home for Insane," *Washington Times Herald*, September 6, 1952, Overholser Scrapbook 1951–53, box 28, PWO. African American patients were not the only ones who were segregated from whites. Native Americans were too. There had always been a small American Indian population in Saint Elizabeths, but those numbers increased in the mid-1930s, when another federal asylum in South Dakota, dedicated to the care of insane Indians, closed. The Native Americans transferred to Saint Elizabeths were housed separately from white and black patients, and they also participated in "race-exclusive" recreation and leisure programs, mounting, for instance, a show with an all-Indian cast in 1941. *Annual Report of the Department of the Interior 1934* (Washington, DC: Government Printing Office, 1934), 376; *Annual Report of Saint Elizabeths Hospital 1941* (Washington, DC: Government Printing Office, 1941), 7; Putney, "The Canton Asylum for Insane Indians."
24. Arvilla D. Merrill, "Occupational Therapy with Maximum Security Patients: An Adjunct to Group Psychotherapy," *Psychiatric Quarterly Supplement* 23 (1949): 205–23, offprint in container 29, folder 9, BBP.
25. Richard Lyons, "GOP Inherits D.C.'s Problems," *Washington Post*, January 20, 1953, A2; "Ike Urged to Continue Racial Plan," *Washington Post*, November 15, 1952, 4; Don Olesen, "D.C. Orders 23 Agencies to Lower Racial Bars," *Washington Post*, November 26, 1953, 1, 17; David A. Nichols, *A Matter of Justice: Eisenhower and the Beginning of the Civil Rights Revolution* (New York: Simon and Schuster, 2007), 23–40; Robert Fredrick Burk, *The Eisenhower Administration and Black Civil Rights* (Knoxville: University of Tennessee Press, 1984), 61–64.
26. Nichols, *Matter of Justice*, 25, 42–46; "Progress on Integration in Veterans Hospitals," *Journal of the National Medical Association* 45 (November 1953): 437; "Rabb Praises Ikes' [sic] Efforts to Improve Race Relations," *Washington Post*, July 12, 1954, 4.
27. "Progress on Integration in Veterans Hospitals," 437–38. Ward continued, "I have observed many examples of brotherhood in mental hospitals and I don't remember any instances of race prejudice. I think the average white patient regards the average Negro patient as a fellow sufferer." "Insanity," *Ebony* (April 1949): 22.
28. *Annual Report of the Federal Security Agency, 1950, St. Elizabeths Hospital* (Washington, DC: Government Printing Office, 1950), 1–2; *Annual Report of the Federal Security Agency, St. Elizabeths Hospital* (Washington, DC: Government Printing Office, 1951), 2; Francis J. Tartaglino to Winfred Overholser, July 16, 1951, box 9, folder Medical Services Ending June 1951, SEH/ARSU.
29. "Annual Report, Fiscal Year 1952, Registrar Section, July 10, 1952," box 9, folder Annual Report (Administrative)—(Activity) Ending June 1952; O. V. Todd to Sir, July 11, 1950, box 9, folder Annual Report 1949–50. Both in SEH/ARSU.
30. The Detached Service began as a collection of buildings that were separate from the Center building, housing mainly veterans, soldiers and sailors, and civilian men who worked on the hospital's farm. By the 1940s the Detached Service increasingly housed chronically ill military personnel and civilians. See *Report of the Government Hospital for the Insane to the Secretary of the Interior, 1899* (Washington, DC: Government Printing Office, 1899), 23–24; *Annual Report of the Surgeon General of the Public Health Service of the United States for the Fiscal Year 1941* (Washington, DC: Government Printing Office, 1941), 186.
31. "Precis of Activities on West Side Service Fiscal Year 1953," 6–7, container 29, folder 7, BBP.
32. "Report from William G. Cushard to Superintendent," July 1, 1954, 4–6, container 29, folder 7; Cushard to Superintendent, 1955, facsimile of letter, 4, container 29, folder 7. Both in BBP.

33. Jay L. Hoffman to Winfred Overholser, December 14, 1953, box 26, folder "Monthly Reports," SEH/AF; David W. Harris to Superintendent, July 1, 1954, box 11, folder Annual Reports 1954, SEH/ARSU.
34. Jay L. Hoffman to Winfred Overholser, September 23, 1954, box 26, folder "Monthly Reports," SEH/AF; Evelyn B. Reichenbach to Overholser, July 11, 1955, and F. N. Waldrop to Overholser, July 5, 1955, box 11, folder Annual Reports 1955, SEH/ARSU; Hoffman to Overholser, November 9, 1954, and Hoffman to Overholser, December 14, 1954, box 26, folder "Monthly Reports," SEH/AF.
35. Reichenbach to Oversholser, July 11, 1955; Hoffman to Overholser, August 23, 1955, box 26, folder "Monthly Reports," SEH/AF. For other reports of complaining relatives, see F. J. Tartaglino to Overholser, July 9, 1955, box 11, folder Annual Reports 1955; Peter G. Angelos to the Superintendent, July 6, 1956, box 12, folder Annual Reports. Both in SEH/ARSU.
36. Hoffman to Overholser, August 31, 1955, box 11, folder Annual Reports 1955, SEH/ARSU; Hoffman to Overholser, October 11, 1954, box 26, folder "Monthly Reports," SEH/AF.
37. William L. Granatir, "Case Report: The Establishment of a Therapeutic Relationship with a Disturbed Psychotic Patient," *Quarterly Review of Psychiatry and Neurology* 3 (January 1948): 117–22. See also Graven, "Case Study of a Negro."
38. Gambino, "Mental Health and Ideals of Citizenship," 158–61; Grob, *Mental Illness and American Society*, 296–304. Metrazol Treatment schedule; Case no. 35196, March 27, 1938, Metrazol N. N. Both in RG 418 Records of Saint Elizabeths Hospital, Records of the Medical Records Branch, entry 69, Case Files Relating to Metrazoid and Insulin Therapy, 1937–39, box 1, NA.
39. Gambino, "Mental Health and Ideals of Citizenship," 162–67. See also Jonathan Sadowsky, "Beyond the Metaphor of the Pendulum: Electroconvulsive Therapy, Psychoanalysis, and the Styles of American Psychiatry," *Journal of the History of Medicine and Allied Sciences* 61 (January 2006): 1–25.
40. Winfred Overholser, "The New 'Tranquilizing Drugs,'" *Courier of the George Washington University Hospital*, June 1955, 16–17, in Overholser Scrapbook June 1954–June 1955, box 30, PWO; "Nixon Hails New Building Dedicated at St. Elizabeths," *Evening Star*, April 14, 1956, Overholser Scrapbook June 1955–May 1956, box 31, PWO.
41. Henry Allen, "In Saint Elizabeths," *Washington Post*, February 13, 1977, 17. For a critical assessment of the coercive nature of psychopharmacology, see Erick Fabris, *Tranquil Prisons: Chemical Incarceration under Community Treatment Orders* (Toronto: University of Toronto Press, 2011). I thank Anne Parsons for directing me to this source.
42. E. D. Griffin to Overholser, July 10, 1956, box 12, folder Annual Reports 1956, SEH/ARSU; Winfred Overholser, interview by Ann M. Corrick and Bob Nelson, *Washington Viewpoint*, WBC, February 11, 1963, transcript, 8, Writings File, box 7, folder Addresses and Lectures Miscellany 1945–63, PWO. The therapeutic efficacy of the drugs was a central topic of discussion at a symposium held at Saint Elizabeths in 1956. See Francis N. Waldrop, "Reserpine," *Medical Annals of the District of Columbia* 25 (May 1956): 256–58; F. Regis Riesenman, "Chlorpromazine," *Medical Annals of the District of Columbia* 25 (May 1956): 258–60.
43. See Theodore C. C. Fong, "Chlorpromazine and Reserpine in Geriatric Patients," *Medical Annals of the District of Columbia* 25 (May 1956): 260–63; Otis R. Farley, "Complications and Concomitants," *Medical Annals of the District of Columbia* 25 (May 1956): 266.
44. F. J. Tartaglino to Winfred Overholser, July 21, 1953, box 10, folder Annual Reports: Medical Services Ending June, 1953; F. J. Tartaglino to Overholser, July 14, 1954, box 11, folder Annual Reports 1954; Theodore C. C. Fong to Overholser, July 1, 1958, box 13, folder Annual Reports Fiscal June 30, 1958; all in SEH/ARSU. See also White, *Autobiography*; Gambino, "Mental Health and Ideals of Citizenship," 217–18.
45. Joseph Abrahams, "Preliminary Report of an Experience in the Group Psychotherapy of Schizophrenics," *American Journal of Psychiatry* 104 (April 1948): 615.
46. On milieu therapy, see Grob, *From Asylum to Community*, 139–46. In the case of the men of Howard Hall, much to the chagrin of the attendants, the democracy associated with the therapeutic community could be used to subvert the attendants' authority. "At the start," Abrahams

remarked, "some members, when asked to mop the floors, would defer the activity on the plea that they had to refer it to the group." See Abrahams, "Preliminary Report," 615.

47. *Annual Report of the Department of Health, Education, and Welfare, 1954* (Washington, DC: Government Printing Office, 1954), 246–47.

48. "Report from William G. Cushard to Superintendent," July 1, 1958, 4, container 29, folder 7, BBP; Mauris M. Platkin, "Maximum Security with Minimum Seclusion," *Mental Hospitals* 11 (October 1960): 28, 31, in container 29, folder 9, BBP; *Annual Report of the U.S. Department of Health, Education, and Welfare* (Washington, DC: Government Printing Office, 1957), 241; Gambino, "Mental Health and Ideals of Citizenship," 272. Representatives from each service's Patients' Administrative Council formed an institution-wide Hospital Federation of Patients. See Manson B. Pettit to the Superintendent, July 8, 1957, box 12, folder Annual Reports—June '57, SEH/ARSU.

49. "Report from Cushard to Superintendent," July 1, 1958, 4–5; William G. Cushard to Doctor Overholser, July 9, 1960, 4, container 29, folder 7, BBP.

50. Goffman, *Asylums*, 217n67.

51. For an example, see Gambino, "Mental Health and Ideals of Citizenship," 274.

52. Ben Abernathy to Dr. Overholser, March 20, 1957, and Overholser to Abernathy, March 28, 1957, in box 43, folder Saint Elizabeths Hospital, SEH/AF; Gambino, "Mental Health and Ideals of Citizenship," 201–2. According to Matthew Gambino, Overholser's policy allowed for integrated dances as long as white and nonwhite patients refrained from dancing with one another. The letter from the William A. White Service PAG complained of the dances being abolished, but it was likely referring to the ban on interracial dancing.

53. Goffman, *Asylums*, 217 (emphasis mine).

54. To be sure, not all psychiatrists at Saint Elizabeths in the immediate postintegration period were white, but African Americans were underrepresented within the psychiatric profession as a whole, which suggests that their numbers on the Saint Elizabeths staff were not particularly better. As late as 1970, only 1.4 percent of the over seventeen thousand psychiatrists who responded to an American Psychiatric Association survey identified themselves as African American. Franklyn N. Arnhoff and A. H. Kumbar, *The Nation's Psychiatrists—1970 Survey* (Washington, DC: American Psychiatric Association, 1973), 3–5.

55. Harvey R. St. Clair, "Psychiatric Interview Experiences with Negroes," *American Journal of Psychiatry* 108 (August 1951): 113–14; Harold Rosen and Jerome D. Frank, "Negroes in Psychotherapy," *American Journal of Psychiatry* 119 (November 1962): 458. See also Jerome D. Frank, "Adjustment Problems of Selected Negro Soldiers," *Journal of Nervous and Mental Disease* 105 (June 1947): 647–60.

56. St. Clair, "Psychiatric Interview Experiences," 116.

57. Gerald N. Grob, "Origins of *DSM-I*: A Study in Appearance and Reality," *American Journal of Psychiatry* 148 (April 1991): 427–29; Grob, "Psychiatry's Holy Grail," 210–12.

58. For a discussion of the emergence of a post-1945 "psychiatric epidemiology" that emphasized social and environmental factors, see Grob, "Psychiatry's Holy Grail," 212.

59. For a survey of some of this literature, see Alyce C. Gullattee, "The Negro Psyche: Fact, Fiction, and Fantasy," *Journal of the National Medical Association* 61 (March 1969): 119–29 (quote on 123). For a discussion of the black matriarchy discourse among psychologists, psychiatrists, and social scientists, see Raz, *What's Wrong with the Poor?*, esp. 40–44; Ellen Herman, *The Romance of American Psychology: Political Culture in the Age of Experts* (Berkeley: University of California Press, 1995), 199–207.

60. A. J. Prange and M. M. Vitols, "Cultural Aspects of the Relatively Low Incidence of Depression in Southern Negroes," *International Journal of Social Psychiatry* 8 (1962): 104–12. For a critique of Prange and Vitols, see Alexander Thomas and Samuel Sillen, *Racism and Psychiatry* (New York: Brunner/Mazel, 1972), 128–33.

61. D. C. Wilson and E. M. Lantz, "The Effect of Culture Change on the Negro Race in Virginia as Indicated by a Study of State Hospital Admissions," *American Journal of Psychiatry* 114 (1957): 25–32. For a critique of Wilson and Lantz, see Benjamin Pasamanick, "Some Misconceptions concerning Differences in the Racial Prevalence of Mental Disease," *American Journal of Orthopsychiatry* 33 (1963): 72–86.

62. Robert J. Kleiner, Jacob Tuckman, and Martha Lowell, "Mental Disorder and Status Based on Race," *Psychiatry* 23 (August 1960): 271–74. For a good discussion of the racialization of schizophrenia over the course of the twentieth century, see Metzl, *Protest Psychosis*.
63. "Statement by Walter E. Barton, Medical Director, American Psychiatric Association before the Ad Hoc Subcommittee on Saint Elizabeths Hospital of the Education and Labor Committee, U.S. House of Representatives," November 14, 1963, transcript, 12, in General Correspondence, box 3, folder 1963 Nov., PWO.
64. Rosen and Frank, "Negroes in Psychotherapy," 459.
65. For an example, see Thomas Szasz, "The Sane Slave: An Historical Note on the Use of Medical Diagnosis as Justificatory Rhetoric," *American Journal of Psychotherapy* 25 (1971): 228–39. For more on the antipsychiatry movement, see Staub, *Madness Is Civilization*; Grob, *From Asylum to Community*, 279–88; Metzl, *Protest Psychosis*, 133–36.
66. Thomas and Sillen, *Racism and Psychiatry*, 141. See also Paul L. Adams, "The Social Psychiatry of Frantz Fanon," *American Journal of Psychiatry* 127 (December 1970): 809–14.
67. Melvin Sabshin, Herman Diesenhaus, and Raymond Wilkerson, "Dimensions of Institutional Racism in Psychiatry," *American Journal of Psychiatry* 127 (December 1970): 788–89. See also Billy E. Jones et al., "Problems of Black Psychiatric Residents in White Training Institutes," *American Journal of Psychiatry* 127 (December 1970): 798–803.
68. Paul W. Valentine, "Judge Won't Name Psychiatrist to Probe Care at Saint Elizabeths," *Washington Post and Times-Herald*, February 21, 1967, C7; Paul W. Valentine, "St. Elizabeths Called Unfair to the Indigent," *Washington Post and Times-Herald*, May 10, 1967, B5; "Federal Court Clears Hospital of Psychopath's Neglect Charge," *Washington Post and Times-Herald*, August 22, 1967, A18. The case was *Maurice I. Millard, Appellant, v. Dale C. Cameron, Superintendent, Saint Elizabeths Hospital, Appellee*, 373 F.2d 468 (D.C. Cir. 1966).
69. Michael M. Miller to Editor, *Washington Post and Times-Herald*, May 22, 1967, A20; "St. Elizabeths Patient Held Sane, Freed after 26 Years," *Washington Post*, October 14, 1947, 1. Miller was fired from Saint Elizabeths at least twenty years before Millard's suit, so it is unlikely that his characterization of Millard was based on clinical observation.
70. I.B.P., "St. Elizabeths Pioneers Again," *Elizabethan* 11 (June 22, 1955): n.p., Overholser Scrapbook June 1955–May 1956, box 31, PWO.
71. See Smith, *Health Care Divided*, 106–87; W. Michael Byrd and Linda A. Clayton, *An American Health Dilemma: Race, Medicine, and Health Care in the United States, 1900–2000* (New York: Routledge, 2001).

Chapter 10

1. Walter Goodman, "The Constitution v. the Snakepit: How Lawyers Are Proving That Mental Inmates Have a Right to Treatment," *New York Times*, March 17, 1974; Jim Hoagland, "Judge Blasts Juvenile Court 'Blindness and Insensitivity,'" *Washington Post*, April 14, 1967, C4; Grob, *From Asylum to Community*, 290–91.
2. Dale C. Cameron, "Progress Is Saint Elizabeths' Tradition," *Medical Annals of the District of Columbia* 32 (August 1963): 304–5; "Mental Health Project Grant Proposed Plan and Supporting Data," appendix I-i, enclosure in Dale C. Cameron to Winfred Overholser, September 18, 1963, General Correspondence, box 3, folder 1963 Sept., PWO.
3. For other important cases, see Frank and Glied, *Better but Not Well*, 96–98.
4. For a few academic treatments of deinstitutionalization, see Frank and Glied, *Better but Not Well*; Grob, *From Asylum to Community*, 239–72; Grob, *Mad among Us*, 279–311; Grob and Goldman, *Dilemma of Federal Mental Health Policy*; Andrew T. Scull, *Decarceration: Community Treatment and the Deviant—A Radical View*, 2nd ed. (New Brunswick, NJ: Rutgers University Press, 1984); E. Fuller Torrey, *American Psychosis: How the Federal Government Destroyed the Mental Illness Treatment System* (New York: Oxford University Press, 2014).
5. Franklin D. Chu and Sharland Trotter, *The Mental Health Complex Part I: Community Mental Health Centers* (Washington, DC: Center for Study of Responsive Law, 1972), CSA-21.
6. *Annual Report of the U.S. Department of Health, Education, and Welfare* (Washington, DC: Government Printing Office, 1953), 254, 259; *Annual Report of the U.S. Department*

of Health, Education, and Welfare (Washington, DC: Government Printing Office, 1956), 244; *Annual Report of the Department of Health, Education, and Welfare, 1954* (Washington, DC: Government Printing Office, 1954), 248; "Precis of Activities on West Side Service, Fiscal Year 1953," 9–10, container 29, folder 7, BBP.

7. See *Annual Report* (1956), 250–51; *Annual Report of the U.S. Department of Health, Education, and Welfare* (Washington, DC: Government Printing Office, 1957), 240. On the departure of clinical staff for private practice or positions in the academy, see Sherman Kieffer and Francis N. Waldrop, "Attainments and Prospects of Saint Elizabeths Hospital as an Operating Component of NIMH," May 15, 1969, 2, container 31, folder 5, BBP.
8. Grob and Goldman, *Dilemma of Federal Mental Health Policy*, 26–30.
9. *Annual Report of the United States Department of Health, Education, and Welfare* (Washington, DC: Government Printing Office, 1962), 395, 404; Grob, *From Asylum to Community*, 206. For more on psychiatrists' reservations about the JCMIH report, see Grob and Goldman, *Dilemma of Federal Mental Health Policy*, 30–32.
10. Grob and Goldman, *Dilemma of Federal Mental Health Policy*, 32–35; Grob, *From Asylum to Community*, 210–24. This is, admittedly, a very abridged version of a complex history of federal mental health policy in the early 1960s that does not address all of the thorny issues that were debated, such as federalism, funding, and manpower concerns.
11. Grob and Goldman, *Dilemma of Federal Mental Health Policy*, 36; John F. Kennedy to Anthony Celebrezze, February 15, 1963, copy, in Advisory Group on the Future of Saint Elizabeths Hospital, "Final Report of the Advisory Group on the Future of Saint Elizabeths Hospital," May 1964, container 30, folder 4, BBP.
12. Winfred Overholser, interview by Ann M. Corrick and Bob Nelson, *Washington Viewpoint*, WBC, February 11, 1963, transcript, 2–5, Writings File, box 7, folder Addresses and Lectures Miscellany 1945–63, PWO.
13. Grob and Goldman, *Dilemma of Federal Mental Health Policy*, 38–40.
14. "Final Report of the Advisory Group," 2, 4–5.
15. "Final Report of the Advisory Group," 4, 7–8, 11–12; "Mental Health Project Grant," appendix I-i.
16. "Mental Health Project Grant," appendix I-i; "Final Report of the Advisory Group," 6–7, 16–17; Dale C. Cameron to Boisfeuillet Jones, February 18, 1964, in "Final Report of the Advisory Group," 34–35.
17. "Final Report of the Advisory Group," 27–31; Boisfeuillet Jones to Anthony J. Celebrezze, April 27, 1964, copy, container 30, folder 4, BPP.
18. "Final Report of the Advisory Group," 24–25, 27–30; Schuyler Lowe to Boisfeuillet Jones, March 27, 1964, in "Final Report of the Advisory Group," 46. Mention was made of the "relatively small number" of women prisoner patients in the final report, but no concrete proposal for a separate facility was put forward.
19. Allan Beigel, "Planning for the Development of a Community Mental Health Center," *Community Mental Health Journal* 6 (1970): 267–75; Franklin D. Chu and Sharland Trotter, *The Madness Establishment: Ralph Nader's Study Group Report on the National Institute of Mental Health* (New York: Grossman, 1974), 73.
20. Chu and Trotter, *Madness Establishment*, 126; "Reactions to Conclusions and Recommendations of the Final Report of the Advisory Group on the Future of Saint Elizabeths Hospital, February 1964," in "Final Report of the Advisory Group," 38–44. City officials' tepid response to the advisory group was certainly influenced by the frustration that many in the District had with the failure of the federal government to extend home rule to the capital. For more on the politics of home rule in the 1960s, see Gillette, *Between Justice and Beauty*, 170–207.
21. Kieffer and Waldrop, "Attainments and Prospects of Saint Elizabeths," 6–8; *Annual Report of the U.S. Department of Health, Education, and Welfare 1965* (Washington, DC: Government Printing Office, 1965), 403; "Statement by John W. Gardner," August 11, 1967, box 90, folder Saint Elizabeths Hospital, WFP; "NIMH and St. Elizabeths," *Washington Post*, August 16, 1967, A12.
22. "Statement by Stanley F. Yolles," November 8, 1968, 2–3, Entry 13, "Documents/Press Releases Organizations 1968," box 3, RG 511 Records of Alcohol, Drug Abuse and Mental Health Administration, NARA.

23. Chu and Trotter, *Madness Establishment*, 126–44; Stuart Auerbach, "Neighborhood Mental Care Lags, but Help Is Offered," *Washington Post and Times-Herald*, December 4, 1967, B2; Carol Honsa, "2d Area Health Center Opens for D.C. Patients," *Washington Post and Times-Herald*, August 30, 1969, B8.
24. "Area D Mental Health Program," February 27, 1968, enclosure in Stanley Yolles, "Status Report on Planning for Area D Community Mental Health Center at Saint Elizabeths Hospital," memorandum, April 4, 1968; Memorandum for Murray Grant and Stanley F. Yolles, May 13, 1968, 3. Both in Entry 13, "Area D Comm. Mental Health Center, 4/68–8/69," box 6, RG 511 Records of Alcohol, Drug Abuse and Mental Health Administration, NARA. Interestingly, Yolles's status report was sent on the day Martin Luther King Jr. was assassinated. His assassination, of course, sparked civil unrest throughout many American cities, including Washington, DC.
25. "Area D Mental Health Program," 3–4.
26. Memorandum for Murray Grant and Stanley F. Yolles, 4; "Report of the Planning Committee for an Area D Community Mental Health Center," January 7, 1969, 5, 24, 34–35, 38, in Entry 13, "Area D Comm. Mental Health Center, 4/68–8/69," box 6, RG 511 Records of Alcohol, Drug Abuse and Mental Health Administration, NARA. Even though Area D was not a community action program, some of the rhetoric used by the committee, such as "feasible participation" and "community initiative," reflects the dominant paradigm through which policymakers viewed the appropriate relationship between the federal government and local antipoverty efforts in the late 1960s. For more on community action and psychiatry in this period, see Raz, *What's Wrong with the Poor?*
27. Alan I. Levenson, "Potential Problems in the Implementation of the Area D Community Mental Health Center," April 29, 1968, Entry 13, "Area D Comm. Mental Health Center, 4/68–8/69," box 6, RG 511 Records of Alcohol, Drug Abuse and Mental Health Administration, NARA; Kieffer and Waldrop, "Attainments and Prospects of Saint Elizabeths," 10.
28. "Report of the Planning Committee," 26–27, 32–34, 37.
29. "Area D Community Mental Health Center," enclosure in I. A. Tornese to Sherman Kieffer and Francis Waldrop, memorandum, August 6, 1969, Entry 13, "Area D Comm. Mental Health Center, 4/68–8/69," box 6, RG 511 Records of Alcohol, Drug Abuse and Mental Health Administration, NARA; *Programs and Services of the Area D Community Mental Health Center*, DHEW Publication No. (HSM) 72-9011, 1971, 8–9; Roger Peele, "Organizing to Improve Services: The Structuring of Public Mental Health Services," *Medical Annals of the District of Columbia* 41 (August 1972): 495–98. Peele was the first director of Area D CMHC.
30. "Statement by Director, National Institute of Mental Health on Saint Elizabeths," March 29, 1971, n4, container 30, folder 1, BBP; "Report of the Planning Committee," 5–13.
31. Chu and Trotter, *Madness Establishment*, 75.
32. Chu and Trotter, *Mental Health Complex*, CSA-8–CSA-9.
33. Claudia Levy, "Bias against Women Alcoholics Charged," *Washington Post*, September 12, 1971, D1. Some physicians, according to the article, had a patronizing attitude toward female alcoholics, diminishing their disorder by referring to them merely as "drunk women." For his part, Dr. Brown explained that if someone was drunk when coming to the CMHC and refused to sign in (or was incapable of doing so), the staff could not admit the person without violating his or her civil rights.
34. "Administrative/Confidential," n.d., container 31, folder 6; "Statement by Bertram S. Brown, M.D., Director, National Institute of Mental Health Department of Health, Education, and Welfare before the Committee on the District of Columbia United States House of Representatives," April 28, 1975, 15, container 30, folder 2; US Department of Health, Education, and Welfare, Health Services and Mental Health Administration, "Congressional Budget Justification," 1972, 83, container 30, folder 1. All in BBP.
35. "Statement by Stanley F. Yolles," 4; Chu and Trotter, *Mental Health Complex*, CSA-18; *Programs and Services of the Area D Community Mental Health Center*, 11; *Hearings on H.R. 3335, before the Subcommittee on Fiscal and Government Affairs and the Committee on the District of Columbia*, 95th Cong., 44–45 (1977) (statement of Patricia Wells, chairperson,

Citizen Board of Directors, Area D Community Mental Health Center); Luther D. Robinson, "Saint Elizabeths Hospital," *Medical Annals of the District of Columbia* 41 (August 1972): 491.

36. "Congressional Budget Justification," 83; *Departments of Labor, and Health, Education, and Welfare Appropriations for 1970: Hearings before a Subcommittee of the Committee of Appropriations, House of Representatives*, 91st Cong., 628–29 (1969) (statement of Stanley F. Yolles, director of NIMH); Daniel D. Cowell, "Mental Health Training and Research Programs at Saint Elizabeths," *Medical Annals of the District of Columbia* 41 (August 1972): 493–94; *Programs and Services of the Area D Community Mental Health Center*, 18–19; "Statement by Director, National Institute of Mental Health," 2, n7; "This Week in Washington," *Washington Post*, May 14, 1973, A10; "This Week in Washington," *Washington Post*, June 17, 1974, C7; "Coping," *Washington Post*, October 18, 1979, DC7.
37. Chu and Trotter, *Mental Health Complex*, CSA-16, CSA-18.
38. Chu and Trotter, *Madness Establishment*, 150, 129–30.
39. Information on the audit was obtained from handwritten notes in preparation for House hearings on Saint Elizabeths. The author of the notes is not identified. I have not located the audit itself. See "Additional Information on St. Elizabeths Hospital Hearings for DC House Committee," handwritten notes, n.d., box 90, folder Saint Elizabeth Hospital, WFP; Chu and Trotter, *Madness Establishment*, 147.
40. News release of American Federation of State, County, and Municipal Employees, District of Columbia Council 20, n.d.; Walter Taylor, "St. Elizabeths Nurses Ask Hazard Pay," *Washington Star*, n.d. Both in box 81, folder Community Affairs, WFP.
41. Taylor, "St. Elizabeths Nurses Ask Hazard Pay"; "Brief History of Saint Elizabeths, Washington, D.C.," vertical file, City Museum of Washington, Washington, DC.
42. "Additional Information on St. Elizabeths Hospital Hearings" (emphasis in the original); Frank and Glied, *Better but Not Well*, 59–60; Chu and Trotter, *Mental Health Complex*, CSA-17.
43. *Hearings before the Committee on the District of Columbia House of Representatives on Legislative and Oversight Jurisdiction over St. Elizabeths Hospital and Proposals to Transfer St. Elizabeths to the District of Columbia*, 94th Cong., 131–32 (1975) (statement by Dr. Luther Robinson, superintendent of Saint Elizabeths Hospital); "Statement by Bertram S. Brown," 15–16.
44. Edward D. Sargent, "For Former Mental Patients, Their Own Homes," *Washington Post*, January 8, 1981, DC2.
45. Frank and Glied, *Better but Not Well*, 63–64.
46. "Status of Dixon v. Schweiker et al., Civil Action No. 285-74 (D.D.C., filed February 14, 1974); *Dixon v. Weinberger*, 405 F. Supp. 974 (D.D.C. 1975)," in box 153, WFP; Frank and Glied, *Better but Not Well*, 59, 96–97; *William Dixon et al. v. Caspar Weinberger, et al.*, 405 F. Supp. 974, 2 (D.D.C. 1975), in container 30, folder 7, BBP. Caspar Weinberger was the Health, Education, and Welfare secretary.
47. "Statement by Bertram S. Brown," 8–13; Thomas D. Reynolds, "Thinking about Schizophrenia," *Medical Annals of the District of Columbia* 41 (August 1972): 503.
48. *Dixon v. Weinberger*, 405 F. Supp. 974 at 10–11; "Policy Perspective and History of Legislation and Transfer Proposal," n.d., 7, container 30, folder 6, BBP; James F. Dickson, "Issues Analysis Memorandum," April 1977, container 30, folder 5, BBP; "Status of Dixon v. Schweiker."
49. Kenneth Bredemeier, "St. Elizabeths: Hundreds Still Needlessly Kept in Institution," *Washington Post*, March 28, 1982, A1, A14; Frank and Glied, *Better but Not Well*, 94–95, 50; Grob and Goldman, *Dilemma of Federal Mental Health Policy*, 64–67; Kenneth Bredemeier, "A New Life: Returning Mental Patients to the Community," *Washington Post*, March 29, 1982, A1, A4.
50. *Deinstitutionalization of the Mentally Ill, Hearings before the Subcommittee on Fiscal Affairs and Health of the Committee on the District of Columbia House of Representatives*, 97th Cong., vii (1981), in box 167, WFP.
51. *Deinstitutionalization of the Mentally Ill*, 148, 1–2; Bredemeier, "A New Life," A4.
52. Dickson, "Issues Analysis Memorandum," item 1; E. Fuller Torrey, "A Cure for D.C. Psychiatry: Point of View," *Washington Post*, September 4, 1977.
53. Torrey, "Cure for D.C. Psychiatry."

54. Margaret McDonald, "On Losing Accreditation—How a Hospital Reacts," *NASMHPD Info*, March 5, 1976, clipping, box 30, folder 7; Bertram Brown, "Dr. Brown's Statement re Non-Accreditation of Saint Elizabeths Hospital," December 15, 1975, container 30, folder 7. Both in BBP.
55. Dickson, "Issues Analysis Memorandum," item 1; McDonald, "On Losing Accreditation"; "St. Elizabeths—Inside and Out," *Washington Post*, April 3, 1982, A16.
56. "Statement by John W. Gardner," 2; Dickson, "Issues Analysis Memorandum," item 5. Washingtonians had won the right to vote for president and vice president in 1961, but they were largely still disfranchised when it came to city government. President Lyndon Johnson reorganized the District government in 1967 to include a mayor-commissioner and a city council. Residents did not vote for these offices, however; they were appointed by the president. See Gillette, *Between Justice and Beauty*, 179, 190.
57. "A Policy Perspective and History of Legislative and Transfer Proposals from 1963 to Present," n.p., container 30, folder 6, BBP.
58. Stuart Auerbach, "U.S. Help Asked to End St. Elizabeths 'Snake Pit,'" *Washington Post and Times-Herald*, July 10, 1970, C1; Stuart Auerbach, "Independent Agency Asked for D.C. Mental Facilities," *Washington Post and Times-Herald*, July 25, 1970, B1.
59. Bertram Brown to "The Secretary," July 22, 1970, copy, container 31, folder 6; Francis N. Waldrop, "Comments on Report of the 'Rome Committee,'" July 7, 1970, container 31, folder 5; "Position Statements on Questions concerning Transfer of St. Elizabeth's Hospital," 4–5, attachment to Memorandum from Gerald R. Riso, December 21, 1970, container 31, folder 6. All in BBP.
60. "Background on Transfer of St. Elizabeths Hospital to D.C. Health Dept. for Interested Citizens and Organizations," April 30, 1969, 1–3, box 90, folder Saint Elizabeths Hospital, WFP.
61. Dickson, "Issues Analysis Memorandum," item 7; "Policy Perspective and History of Legislative and Transfer Proposals." For more on employees' opposition to the transfer, see Otto, *St. Elizabeths Hospital*, 306–7.
62. *Hearings before the Committee on the District of Columbia*, 94th Cong., 208–9 (1975) (June 2, 1969, letter by William Sheffey and Reverend Shane MacCarthy, cochairs of the Southeast, Far-Southwest Health Steering Committee).
63. "Policy Perspective and History of Legislative and Transfer Proposals"; Dickson, "Issues Analysis Memorandum," item 1; McDonald, "On Losing Accreditation." On the connection between accreditation and Medicare and Medicaid, see Frank and Glied, *Better but Not Well*, 94.
64. *Hearings on H.R. 3335, before the Subcommittee on Fiscal and Government Affairs and the Committee on the District of Columbia*, 95th Cong., 28 (1977).
65. Gillette, *Between Justice and Beauty*, 190–91.
66. *Hearings on H.R. 3335*, 41, 96.
67. Alondra Nelson, *Body and Soul: The Black Panther Party and the Fight against Medical Discrimination* (Minneapolis: University of Minnesota Press, 2011); Jennifer Nelson, *More Than Medicine: A History of the Feminist Women's Health Movement* (New York: New York University Press, 2015).
68. *Hearings on H.R. 3335*, 36–38, 40–42.
69. *Hearings on H.R. 3335*, 44–46. A few months after the subcommittee hearing, E. Fuller Torrey ripped the Washington psychiatric community. Even though the 1,100 psychiatrists in the Washington area made it the top metropolitan area in the world in terms of psychiatrists per capita, these professionals were not "equitably distributed." Of those based in the city, he pointed out, "only three psychiatrists have chosen to practice out of private offices in either northeast or southeast Washington," the less affluent quadrants. See Torrey, "A Cure for D.C. Psychiatry." Chu and Trotter also charged the privatization of psychiatric services in DC—including by black psychiatrists trained at Howard University—with making "mental health care for the District's poor . . . close to catastrophic." See Chu and Trotter, *Mental Health Complex*, CSA-1–CSA-2.
70. *Hearings on H.R. 3335*, 95, 98, 104–5.
71. *Hearings on H.R. 3335*, 105. C. L. Dellums was a prominent leader in the Brotherhood of Sleeping Car Porters and Maids.

72. Alice Bonner, "NIMH's Competence to Monitor Mental Hospitals under Fire," *Washington Post*, March 30, 1977, C3.
73. "St. Elizabeths Cutbacks," *Washington Post*, October 30, 1983, C3; Sandra G. Boodman, "Change Casts a Pall over Mental Hospital," *Washington Post*, October 12, 1986, A1, A10. The overrepresentation of African American male schizophrenics characterized the inpatient populations at other public mental institutions, including Michigan's Ionia State Hospital. See Metzl, *Protest Psychosis*, 11.

Conclusion

1. "Washington: Two Social Levels," *Washington Daily News*, August 25, 1941, in RG 418-P, Records of St. Elizabeth's Hospital, Prints and Negatives: Photographs of Staff, Structures, and Activities, ca. 1920–ca. 1955, box 5, NARA. On Washington's alleys, see Borchert, *Alley Life in Washington*.
2. "Background on Transfer of St. Elizabeths Hospital to D.C. Health Dept. for Interested Citizens and Organizations," April 30, 1969, 1–3, box 90, folder Saint Elizabeths Hospital, WFP.
3. "The politics of decline" is from "A Policy Perspective and History of Legislative and Transfer Proposals from 1963 to Present," n.p., in container 30, folder 6, BBP.
4. Kenneth Bredemeier, "A New Life: Returning Mental Patients to the Community," *Washington Post*, March 29, 1982, A4.
5. US Department of Health and Human Services, *Mental Health: A Report of the Surgeon General* (Rockville, MD: US Department of Health and Human Services, 1999), 80, http://www.surgeongeneral.gov/library/mentalhealth/home.html. For other studies that address the issue of black underutilization of mental health services, see Julian Chun-Chung Chow, Kim Jaffee, and Lonnie Snowden, "Racial/Ethnic Disparities in the Use of Mental Health Services in Poverty Areas," *American Journal of Public Health* 93 (May 2003): 792–97; Harold W. Neighbors, Marc A. Musick, and David R. Williams, "The African American Minister as a Source of Help for Serious Personal Crises: Bridge or Barrier to Mental Health Care?," *Health Education and Behavior* 25 (December 1998): 759–77.

SELECTED BIBLIOGRAPHY

Due to space constraints, this bibliography is limited to secondary sources, excluding PhD dissertations. Not all books and articles that appear in the notes are in this bibliography. I have chosen to include secondary sources that I consider indispensable to understanding the history of Saint Elizabeths and Washington, DC's African American community and sources that have been critical to my thinking about the history of race, mental illness, and psychiatry.

Abbott, Andrew. *The System of Professions: An Essay on the Division of Expert Labor*. Chicago: University of Chicago Press, 1988.

Alfers, Kenneth G. *Law and Order in the Capital City: A History of the Washington Police, 1800–1886*. Washington, DC: George Washington University, 1976.

Anderson, Jeffrey E. *Conjure in African American Society*. Baton Rouge: Louisiana State University Press, 2005.

Anderson, Warwick. "The Case of the Archive." *Critical Inquiry* 39 (Spring 2013): 532–47.

Asch, Chris Meyers, and George Derek Musgrove. *Chocolate City: A History of Race and Democracy in the Nation's Capital*. Chapel Hill: University of North Carolina Press, 2017.

Bederman, Gail. *Manliness and Civilization: A Cultural History of Gender and Race in the United States, 1880–1917*. Chicago: University of Chicago Press, 1995.

Bell, Leland. *Treating the Mentally Ill: From Colonial Times to the Present*. New York: Praeger, 1980.

Berrios, German E., and Roy Porter, eds. *A History of Clinical Psychiatry: The Origin and History of Psychiatric Disorders*. New York: New York University Press, 1995.

Blakely, Robert L., and Judith M. Harrington. *Bones in the Basement: Post-Mortem Racism in Nineteenth-Century Medical Training*. Washington, DC: Smithsonian Institution Press, 1997.

Borchert, James. *Alley Life in Washington: Family, Community, Religion, and Folklife in the City, 1850–1970*. Urbana: University of Illinois Press, 1980.

Boster, Dea H. *African American Slavery and Disability: Bodies, Property, and Power in the Antebellum South, 1800–1860*. New York: Routledge, 2013.

Boster, Dea H. "An 'Epeleptick' Bondswoman: Fits, Slavery, and Power in the Antebellum South." *Bulletin of the History of Medicine* 83 (Summer 2009): 271–301.

Braslow, Joel. *Mental Ills and Bodily Cures: Psychiatric Treatment in the First Half of the Twentieth Century*. Berkeley: University of California Press, 1997.

Braslow, Joel T., and Sarah Linsley Starks. "The Making of Contemporary American Psychiatry, Part 2: Therapeutics and Gender before and after World War II." *History of Psychology* 8 (2005): 271–88.

Brattain, Michelle. "Race, Racism, and Antiracism: UNESCO and the Politics of Presenting Science to the Postwar Public." *American Historical Review* 112 (December 2007): 1386–413.

Brickman, Celia. *Aboriginal Populations in the Mind: Race and Primitivity in Psychoanalysis.* New York: Columbia University Press, 2003.

Brown, Letitia Woods. *Free Negroes in the District of Columbia, 1790–1846.* New York: Oxford University Press, 1972.

Brown, Thomas E. "Dance of the Dialectic? Some Reflections (Polemic and Otherwise) of the Present State of Nineteenth-Century Asylum Studies." *Canadian Bulletin of Medical History* 11 (1994): 267–95.

Brown, Wendy. *States of Injury: Power and Freedom in Late Modernity.* Princeton, NJ: Princeton University Press, 1995.

Burch, Susan, and Hannah Joyner. *Unspeakable: The Story of Junius Wilson.* Chapel Hill: University of North Carolina Press, 2007.

Burk, Robert Fredrick. *The Eisenhower Administration and Black Civil Rights.* Knoxville: University of Tennessee Press, 1984.

Burnham, Donald L. "Orthodoxy and Eclecticism in Psychoanalysis: The Washington-Baltimore Experience." In *American Psychoanalysis: Origins and Development,* edited by Jacques M. Quen and Eric T. Carlson, 87–108. New York: Brunner/Mazel, 1978.

Burnham, John C. *Psychoanalysis and American Medicine, 1894–1918: Medicine, Science, and Culture.* New York: International Universities Press, 1967.

Byrd, W. Michael, and Linda A. Clayton. *An American Health Dilemma: Race, Medicine, and Health Care in the United States, 1900–2000.* New York: Routledge, 2002.

Caplan, Eric. *Mind Games: American Culture and the Birth of Psychotherapy.* Berkeley: University of California Press, 1998.

Carson, John. "Minding Matter/Mattering Mind: Knowledge and the Subject in Nineteenth-Century Psychology." *Studies in History and Philosophy of Biological and Biomedical Sciences* 30 (September 1999): 345–76.

Casper, Stephen T. "The Patient's Pitch: The Neurologist, the Tuning Fork, and Textbook Knowledge." In *The Neurological Patient in History,* edited by L. Stephen Jacyna and Stephen T. Casper, 21–43. Rochester, NY: University of Rochester Press, 2012.

Castel, Robert. "Moral Treatment: Mental Therapy and Social Control in the Nineteenth Century." In *Social Control and the State: Historical and Comparative Essays,* edited by Stanley Cohen and Andrew Scull, 248–66. Oxford: Martin Robinson, 1983.

Centennial Commission. *Centennial Papers: Saint Elizabeths Hospital, 1855–1955.* Baltimore, MD: Waverly Press, 1956.

Cravens, Hamilton, and John C. Burnham. "Psychology and Evolutionary Naturalism in American Thought, 1890–1940." *American Quarterly* 23 (December 1971): 635–57.

Crew, Spencer R. "Melding the Old and the New: The Modern African American Community, 1930–1960." In *Washington Odyssey: A Multicultural History of the Nation's Capital,* edited by Francine Curro Cary, 208–30. Washington, DC: Smithsonian Books, 1996.

Curry, Leonard P. *The Free Black in Urban America, 1800–1850: The Shadow of the Dream.* Chicago: University of Chicago Press, 1981.

Cushman, Philip. *Constructing the Self, Constructing America: A Cultural History of Psychotherapy.* Reading, MA: Addison-Wesley, 1995.

Dain, Norman. *Concepts of Insanity in the United States, 1789–1865.* New Brunswick, NJ: Rutgers University Press, 1964.

Dain, Norman. *Disordered Minds: The First Century of Eastern State Hospital in Williamsburg, Virginia, 1766–1866.* Williamsburg, VA: Colonial Williamsburg Foundation, 1971.

D'Amore, Arcangelo R. T., ed. *William Alanson White: The Washington Years, 1903–1937.* Washington, DC: U.S. Department of Health, Education, and Welfare, 1976.

Damousi, Joy. "Géza Róheim and the Australian Aborigine: Psychoanalytic Anthropology during the Interwar Years." In *Unconscious Dominions: Psychoanalysis, Colonial Trauma, and Global Sovereignties,* edited by Warwick Anderson, Deborah Jenson, and Richard C. Keller, 75–95. Durham, NC: Duke University Press, 2011.

Danziger, Kurt. *Naming the Mind: How Psychology Found Its Language.* London: Sage, 1997.

Deacon, Harriet Jane. "Madness, Race and Moral Treatment: Robben Island Lunatic Asylum, Cape Colony, 1846–1890." *History of Psychiatry* 7 (1996): 287–97.
Deutsch, Albert. *The Mentally Ill in America: A History of Their Care and Treatment from Colonial Times*. 2nd ed. New York: Columbia University Press, 1949.
Deutsch, Albert. *The Story of GAP*. New York: Group for the Advancement of Psychiatry, 1959.
Dowbiggin, Ian Robert. *Keeping America Sane: Psychiatry and Eugenics in the United States and Canada, 1880–1940*. Ithaca, NY: Cornell University Press, 2003.
Downs, Jim. *Sick from Freedom: African-American Illness and Suffering during the Civil War and Reconstruction*. New York: Oxford University Press, 2012.
Doyle, Dennis A. *Psychiatry and Racial Liberalism in Harlem, 1936–1968*. Rochester, NY: University of Rochester Press, 2016.
Doyle, Dennis A. "'Racial Differences Have to Be Considered': Lauretta Bender, Bellevue Hospital, and the African American Psyche, 1936–52." *History of Psychiatry* 21 (2010): 206–23.
Doyle, Dennis A. "'Where the Need Is Greatest': Social Psychiatry and Race-Blind Universalism in Harlem's Lafargue Clinic, 1946–1958." *Bulletin of the History of Medicine* 83 (Winter 2009): 746–74.
Dwyer, Ellen. *Homes for the Mad: Life inside Two Nineteenth-Century Asylums*. New Brunswick, NJ: Rutgers University Press, 1987.
Dwyer, Ellen. "Psychiatry and Race during World War II." *Journal of the History of Medicine and Allied Sciences* 61 (April 2006): 117–43.
Ellenberger, Henri F. *The Discovery of the Unconscious: The History and Evolution of Dynamic Psychiatry*. New York: Basic Books, 1970.
Fett, Sharla M. *Working Cures: Healing, Health, and Power on Southern Slave Plantations*. Chapel Hill: University of North Carolina Press, 2002.
Fields, Barbara Jeanne. *Slavery and Freedom on the Middle Ground: Maryland during the Nineteenth Century*. New Haven, CT: Yale University Press, 1985.
Finnane, Mark. "Asylums, Families and the State." *History Workshop* 20 (Autumn 1985): 134–48.
Foucault, Michel. *Discipline and Punish: The Birth of the Prison*. Translated by Alan Sheridan. New York: Random House, 1977.
Foucault, Michel. *Madness and Civilization: A History of Insanity in the Age of Reason*. Translated by Richard Howard. New York: Random House, 1965.
Fox, Richard W. *So Far Disordered in Mind: Insanity in California, 1870–1930*. Berkeley: University of California Press, 1978.
Frank, Richard G., and Sherry A. Glied. *Better but Not Well: Mental Health Policy in the United States Since 1950*. Baltimore, MD: Johns Hopkins University Press, 2006.
Fredrickson, George M. *The Black Image in the White Mind: The Debate on Afro-American Character and Destiny, 1817–1914* (1971). Reprint, Hanover, NH: Wesleyan University Press, 1987.
Fry, Gladys-Marie. *Night Riders in Black Folk History* (1975). Reprint, Chapel Hill: University of North Carolina Press, 2001.
Gambino, Matthew. "Fevered Decisions: Race, Ethics, and Clinical Vulnerability in the Malarial Treatment of Neurosyphilis, 1922–1953." *Hastings Center Report* 45 (2015): 1–11.
Gambino, Matthew. "'These Strangers within Our Gates': Race, Psychiatry and Mental Illness among Black Americans at St. Elizabeths Hospital in Washington, D.C. 1900–1940." *History of Psychiatry* 19 (2008): 387–408.
Gatewood, Willard B. *Aristocrats of Color: The Black Elite, 1880–1920*. Bloomington: Indiana University Press, 1990.
Gillette, Howard, Jr. *Between Justice and Beauty: Race, Planning, and the Failure of Urban Policy in Washington, D.C.* Philadelphia: University of Pennsylvania Press, 2006.
Goffman, Erving. *Asylums: Essays on the Social Situation of Mental Patients and Other Inmates*. Garden City, NY: Anchor Books, 1961.
Good, Byron J. *Medicine, Rationality, and Experience: An Anthropological Perspective*. Cambridge, UK: Cambridge University Press, 1994.

Green, Constance McLaughlin. *The Secret City: A History of Race Relations in the Nation's Capital.* Princeton, NJ: Princeton University Press, 1967.

Green, Constance McLaughlin. *Washington: Capital City, 1879–1950.* Princeton, NJ: Princeton University Press, 1963.

Green, Constance McLaughlin. *Washington: Village and Capital, 1800–1878.* Princeton, NJ: Princeton University Press, 1962.

Grob, Gerald N. *From Asylum to Community: Mental Health Policy in Modern America.* Princeton, NJ: Princeton University Press, 1991.

Grob, Gerald N. *Mental Illness and American Society, 1875–1940.* Princeton, NJ: Princeton University Press, 1983.

Grob, Gerald N. *Mental Institutions in America: Social Policy to 1875* (1972). Reprint, New Brunswick, NJ: Transaction Publishers, 2008.

Grob, Gerald N. "Psychiatry's Holy Grail: The Search for the Mechanisms of Mental Diseases." *Bulletin of the History of Medicine* 72 (Summer 1998): 189–219.

Grob, Gerald N., and Howard H. Goldman. *The Dilemma of Federal Mental Health Policy: Radical Reform or Incremental Change?* New Brunswick, NJ: Rutgers University Press, 2006.

Hale, Nathan G., Jr. *Freud and the Americans: The Beginnings of Psychoanalysis in the United States, 1876–1917.* New York: Oxford University Press, 1971.

Haller, John S., Jr. "The Physician versus the Negro: Medical and Anthropological Concepts of Race in the Late Nineteenth Century." *Bulletin of the History of Medicine* 44 (March–April 1970): 154–67.

Haller, John S., Jr. "Race and the Concept of Progress in Nineteenth Century American Ethnology." *American Anthropologist* 73 (June 1971): 710–23.

Hammonds, Evelynn M., and Rebecca M. Herzig, eds. *The Nature of Difference: Sciences of Race in the United States from Jefferson to Genomics.* Cambridge, MA: MIT Press, 2008.

Harrison, Robert. "From Biracial Democracy to Direct Rule: The End of Self-Government in the Nation's Capital, 1865–1878." *Journal of Policy History* 18, no. 2 (2006): 241–69.

Healy, David. *Mania: A Short History of Bipolar Disorder.* Baltimore, MD: Johns Hopkins University Press, 2008.

Herman, Ellen. *The Romance of American Psychology: Political Culture in the Age of Experts.* Berkeley: University of California Press, 1995.

Higginbotham, Evelyn Brooks. "African American Women's History and the Metalanguage of Race." *Signs: Journal of Women in Culture and Society* 17 (Winter 1992): 251–74.

Hill, Carole E., and Holly Mathews. "Traditional Health Beliefs and Practices among Southern Rural Blacks: A Complement to Biomedicine." In *Perspectives on the American South: An Annual Review of Society, Politics, and Culture,* edited by Merle Black and John Shelton Reed, 307–22. New York: Gordon & Breach, 1981.

Hine, Darlene Clark. "Black Professionals and Race Consciousness: Origins of the Civil Rights Movement, 1890–1950." *Journal of American History* 89 (March 2003): 1279–94.

Hine, Darlene Clark. *Black Women in White: Racial Conflict and Cooperation in the Nursing Profession, 1890–1950.* Bloomington: Indiana University Press, 1989.

Hoffman, Beatrix. *Health Care for Some: Rights and Rationing in the United States since 1930.* Chicago: University of Chicago Press, 2012.

Holt, Thomas, Cassandra Smith Parker, and Rosalyn Terborg-Penn. *A Special Mission: The Story of Freedmen's Hospital, 1862–1962.* Washington, DC: Howard University Press, 1975.

Horn, Margo. *Before It's Too Late: The Child Guidance Movement in the United States, 1922–1945.* Philadelphia: Temple University Press, 1989.

Hughes, John S. "Labeling and Treating Black Mental Illness in Alabama, 1861–1910." *Journal of Southern History* 58 (August 1992): 435–60.

Huisman, Frank, and John Harley Warner, eds. *Locating Medical History: The Stories and Their Meanings.* Baltimore, MD: Johns Hopkins University Press, 2004.

Hunter, Tera W. *To 'Joy My Freedom: Southern Black Women's Lives and Labors after the Civil War.* Cambridge, MA: Harvard University Press, 1997.

Jackson, Lynette A. *Surfacing Up: Psychiatry and Social Order in Colonial Zimbabwe, 1908–1968.* Ithaca, NY: Cornell University Press, 2005.
Johnston, Allan. *Surviving Freedom: The Black Community of Washington, D.C., 1860–1880.* New York: Garland, 1993.
Kanhouwa, Surya, and Kenneth Gorelick. "A Century of Pathology at Saint Elizabeths Hospital, Washington, DC." *Archives of Pathology and Laboratory Medicine* 121 (January 1997): 84–90.
Kanhouwa, Suryabala, and Jogues R. Prandoni. "The Civil War and St. Elizabeths Hospital: An Untold Story of Services from the First Federal Mental Institution in the United States." *Journal of Civil War Medicine* 9 (January–March 2005): 1–16.
Krugler, David F. "A Mob in Uniform: Soldiers and Civilians in Washington's Red Summer, 1919." *Washington History* 21 (2009): 48–77.
Lamb, S. D. *Pathologist of the Mind: Adolf Meyer and the Origins of American Psychiatry.* Baltimore, MD: Johns Hopkins University Press, 2014.
Laqueur, Thomas W. "Bodies, Details, and the Humanitarian Narrative." In *The New Cultural History*, edited by Lynn Hunt, 176–204. Berkeley: University of California Press, 1989.
Lasch-Quinn, Elisabeth. *Black Neighbors: Race and the Limits of Reform in the American Settlement House Movement, 1890–1945.* Chapel Hill: University of North Carolina Press, 1993.
Leys, Ruth. "Meyer, Jung, and the Limits of Association." *Bulletin of the History of Medicine* 59 (Fall 1985): 345–60.
Lindsey, Treva B. *Colored No More: Reinventing Black Womanhood in Washington, D.C.* Urbana: University of Illinois Press, 2017.
Lunbeck, Elizabeth. *The Psychiatric Persuasion: Knowledge, Gender, and Power in Modern America.* Princeton, NJ: Princeton University Press, 1994.
Makari, George. *Revolution in Mind: The Creation of Psychoanalysis.* New York: HarperCollins, 2008.
Markowitz, Gerald, and David Rosner. *Children, Race, and Power: Kenneth and Mamie Clark's Northside Center.* New York: Routledge, 2000.
Masur, Kate. *An Example for All the Land: Emancipation and the Struggle over Equality in Washington, D.C.* Chapel Hill: University of North Carolina Press, 2010.
McCandless, Peter. *Moonlight, Magnolias, and Madness: Insanity in South Carolina from the Colonial Period to the Progressive Era.* Chapel Hill: University of North Carolina Press, 1996.
McGovern, Constance M. "The Community, the Hospital, and the Working-Class Patient: The Multiple Uses of Asylum in Nineteenth-Century America." *Pennsylvania History* 54 (January 1987): 17–33.
McGovern, Constance M. "The Myths of Social Control and Custodial Oppression: Patterns of Psychiatric Medicine in Late Nineteenth-Century Institutions." *Journal of Social History* 20 (Autumn 1986): 3–23.
Mendes, Gabriel N. *Under the Strain of Color: Harlem's Lafargue Clinic and the Promise of an Antiracist Psychiatry.* Ithaca, NY: Cornell University Press, 2015.
Metzl, Jonathan. *The Protest Psychosis: How Schizophrenia Became a Black Disease.* Boston: Beacon Press, 2009.
Micale, Mark S. *Hysterical Men: The Hidden History of Male Nervous Illness.* Cambridge, MA: Harvard University Press, 2008.
Mitchell, Michele. *Righteous Propagation: African Americans and the Politics of Racial Destiny after Reconstruction.* Chapel Hill: University of North Carolina Press, 2004.
Mitchem, Stephanie Y. *African American Folk Healing.* New York: New York University Press, 2007.
Molina, Natalia. *Fit to Be Citizens? Public Health and Race in Los Angeles, 1879–1939.* Berkeley: University of California Press, 2006.
Morais, Herbert M. *The History of the Afro-American in Medicine.* Cornwells Heights, PA: Publishers Agency, 1978.
Moran, James E. "Asylum in the Community: Managing the Insane in Antebellum America." *History of Psychiatry* 9 (1998): 217–40.
Muhammad, Khalil Gibran. *The Condemnation of Blackness: Race, Crime, and the Making of Modern Urban America.* Cambridge, MA: Harvard University Press, 2011.

Murphy, John P. H. "Progress, Science and the Mind: A History of Saint Elizabeths Hospital." *Medical Annals of the District of Columbia* 7 (October 1938): 313–23.
Nelson, Alondra. *Body and Soul: The Black Panther Party and the Fight against Medical Discrimination.* Minneapolis: University of Minnesota Press, 2011.
Nelson, Jennifer. *More Than Medicine: A History of the Feminist Women's Health Movement.* New York: New York University Press, 2015.
Nichols, David A. *A Matter of Justice: Eisenhower and the Beginning of the Civil Rights Revolution.* New York: Simon and Schuster, 2007.
Noll, Richard. *American Madness: The Rise and Fall of Dementia Praecox.* Cambridge, MA: Harvard University Press, 2011.
Noll, Steven. "Patient Records as Historical Stories: The Case of Caswell Training School." *Bulletin of the History of Medicine* 68 (Fall 1994): 411–28.
Noll, Steven. "Southern Strategies for Handling the Black Feeble-Minded: From Social Control to Profound Indifference." *Journal of Policy History* 3 (April 1991): 130–51.
Oppenheim, Janet. *"Shattered Nerves": Doctors, Patients, and Depression in Victorian England.* New York: Oxford University Press, 1991.
Otto, Thomas. *St. Elizabeths Hospital: A History.* Washington, DC: US General Services Administration, 2013.
Porter, Roy. "The Patient's View: Doing Medical History from Below." *Theory and Society* 14 (March 1985): 175–98.
Prudhomme, Charles, and David F. Musto. "Historical Perspectives on Mental Health and Racism in the United States." In *Racism and Mental Health*, edited by Charles V. Willie, Bernard M. Kramer, and Bertram S. Brown, 25–57. Pittsburgh, PA: University of Pittsburgh Press, 1973.
Raz, Mical. "Between the Ego and the Icepick: Psychosurgery, Psychoanalysis, and Psychiatric Discourse." *Bulletin of the History of Medicine* 82 (Summer 2008): 387–420.
Raz, Mical. *What's Wrong with the Poor? Psychiatry, Race, and the War on Poverty.* Chapel Hill: University of North Carolina Press, 2013.
Reardon, Jenny. *Race to the Finish: Identity and Governance in an Age of Genomics.* Princeton, NJ: Princeton University Press, 2005.
Reaume, Geoffrey. "Keep Your Labels Off My Mind! or 'Now I Am Going to Pretend I Am Craze but Dont Be a Bit Alarmed': Psychiatric History from the Patient's Perspective." *Canadian Bulletin of Medical History* 11 (1994): 397–424.
Reidy, Joseph P. "'Coming from the Shadows of the Past': The Transition from Slavery to Freedom at Freedmen's Village, 1863–1900." *Virginia Magazine of History and Biography* 95 (October 1987): 403–28.
Reiss, Benjamin. *Theaters of Madness: Insane Asylums and Nineteenth-Century American Culture.* Chicago: University of Chicago Press, 2008.
Reverby, Susan M. *Examining Tuskegee: The Infamous Syphilis Study and Its Legacy.* Chapel Hill: University of North Carolina Press, 2009.
Risse, Guenter B., and John Harley Warner. "Reconstructing Clinical Activities: Patient Records in Medical History." *Social History of Medicine* 5 (August 1992): 183–205.
Roberts, Samuel Kelton, Jr. *Infectious Fear: Politics, Disease, and the Health Effects of Segregation.* Chapel Hill: University of North Carolina Press, 2009.
Rose, Anne C. *Psychology and Selfhood in the Segregated South.* Chapel Hill: University of North Carolina Press, 2009.
Rosenberg, Charles E. "The Bitter Fruit: Heredity, Disease, and Social Thought." In *No Other Gods: On Science and American Social Thought*, edited by Charles E. Rosenberg, 25–53. Rev. ed. Baltimore, MD: Johns Hopkins University Press, 1997.
Rosenberg, Charles E. "Body and Mind in Nineteenth-Century Medicine: Some Clinical Origins of the Neurosis Construct." *Bulletin of the History of Medicine* 63 (Summer 1989): 185–97.
Rosenberg, Charles E. *The Trial of the Assassin Guiteau: Psychiatry and the Law in the Gilded Age.* Chicago: University of Chicago Press, 1968.

Rosenberg, Charles E., and Janet Golden, eds. *Framing Disease: Studies in Cultural History*. New Brunswick, NJ: Rutgers University Press, 1992.
Ross, Dorothy. *G. Stanley Hall: The Psychologist as Prophet*. Chicago: University of Chicago Press, 1972.
Rothman, David J. *Conscience and Convenience: The Asylum and Its Alternatives in Progressive America*. Rev. ed. New York: Aldine De Gruyter, 2002.
Rothman, David J. *The Discovery of the Asylum: Social Order and Disorder in the New Republic*. Boston: Little, Brown, 1971.
Sadowsky, Jonathan. "Beyond the Metaphor of the Pendulum: Electroconvulsive Therapy, Psychoanalysis, and the Styles of American Psychiatry." *Journal of the History of Medicine and Allied Sciences* 61 (January 2006): 1–25.
Savitt, Todd L. *Medicine and Slavery: The Diseases and Health Care of Blacks in Antebellum Virginia*. Urbana: University of Illinois Press, 1978.
Savitt, Todd L. "The Use of Blacks for Medical Experimentation and Demonstration in the Old South." *Journal of Southern History* 48 (August 1982): 331–48.
Schoen, Johanna. *Choice and Coercion: Birth Control, Sterilization, and Abortion in Public Health and Welfare*. Chapel Hill: University of North Carolina Press, 2005.
Schweik, Susan M. *The Ugly Laws: Disability in Public*. New York: New York University Press, 2009.
Scott, Daryl Michael. *Contempt and Pity: Social Policy and the Image of the Damaged Black Psyche, 1880–1996*. Chapel Hill: University of North Carolina Press, 1997.
Scull, Andrew T. *Decarceration: Community Treatment and the Deviant—A Radical View*. 2nd ed. New Brunswick, NJ: Rutgers University Press, 1984.
Scull, Andrew T. "Madness and Segregative Control: The Rise of the Insane Asylum." *Social Problems* 24 (February 1977): 337–51.
Scull, Andrew T. "Psychiatry and Social Control in the Nineteenth and Twentieth Centuries." *History of Psychiatry* 2 (1991): 149–69.
Shorter, Edward. *A History of Psychiatry: From the Era of the Asylum to the Age of Prozac*. New York: John Wiley and Sons, 1997.
Shortt, S. E. D. *Victorian Lunacy: Richard M. Bucke and the Practice of Late Nineteenth- Century Psychiatry*. Cambridge, UK: Cambridge University Press, 1986.
Smith, David Barton. *Health Care Divided: Race and Healing a Nation*. Ann Arbor: University of Michigan Press, 1999.
Smith, Mark M. *How Race Is Made: Slavery, Segregation, and the Senses*. Chapel Hill: University of North Carolina Press, 2006.
Smith, Susan L. *Sick and Tired of Being Sick and Tired: Black Women's Health Activism in America, 1890–1950*. Philadelphia: University of Pennsylvania Press, 1995.
Spurlock, Jeanne, ed. *Black Psychiatrists and American Psychiatry*. Washington, DC: American Psychiatric Association, 1999.
Staub, Michael E. *Madness Is Civilization: When the Diagnosis Was Social, 1948–1980*. Chicago: University of Chicago Press, 2011.
Stein, Melissa N. *Measuring Manhood: Race and the Science of Masculinity, 1830–1934*. Minneapolis: University of Minnesota Press, 2015.
Stewart, Larry. "Freud before Oedipus: Race and Heredity in the Origins of Psychoanalysis." *Journal of the History of Biology* 9 (Fall 1976): 215–28.
Stoler, Ann Laura. *Carnal Knowledge and Imperial Power: Race and the Intimate in Colonial Rule*. Rev. ed. Berkeley: University of California Press, 2010.
Stoler, Ann Laura. "Tense and Tender Ties: The Politics of Comparison in North American History and (Post)Colonial Studies." *Journal of American History* 88 (December 2001): 829–65.
Stowe, Steven M. *Doctoring the South: Southern Physicians and Everyday Medicine in the Mid-Nineteenth Century*. Chapel Hill: University of North Carolina Press, 2004.
Sullivan, Patricia. *Days of Hope: Race and Democracy in the New Deal Era*. Chapel Hill: University of North Carolina Press, 1996.

Summers, Martin. "Diagnosing the Ailments of Black Citizenship: African American Physicians and the Politics of Mental Illness, 1895–1940." In *Precarious Prescriptions: Contested Histories of Race and Health in North America*, edited by Laurie B. Green, John Mckiernan-González, and Martin Summers, 91–114. Minneapolis: University of Minnesota Press, 2014.

Swartz, Sally. "Changing Diagnoses in Valkenberg Asylum, Cape Colony, 1891–1920: A Longitudinal View." *History of Psychiatry* 6 (1995): 431–51.

Thielman, Samuel B. "Community Management of Mental Disorders in Antebellum America." *Journal of the History of Medicine and Allied Sciences* 44 (July 1989): 351–74.

Thomas, Karen Kruse. *Deluxe Jim Crow: Civil Rights and American Health Policy, 1935–1954*. Athens: University of Georgia Press, 2011.

Tolman, Charles W. "Theories of Mental Evolution in Comparative Psychology: Darwin to Watson." In *Historical Perspectives and the International Status of Comparative Psychology*, edited by Ethel Tobach, 15–23. Hillsdale, NJ: Lawrence Erlbaum Associates, 1987.

Tomes, Nancy. *A Generous Confidence: Thomas Story Kirkbride and the Art of Asylum-Keeping, 1840–1883*. Cambridge, UK: Cambridge University Press, 1984.

Torrey, E. Fuller. *American Psychosis: How the Federal Government Destroyed the Mental Illness Treatment System*. New York: Oxford University Press, 2014.

Valenčius, Conevery Bolton. *The Health of the Country: How American Settlers Understood Themselves and Their Land*. New York: Basic Books, 2002.

Vaughan, Megan. *Curing Their Ills: Colonial Power and African Illness*. Stanford, CA: Stanford University Press, 1991.

Wailoo, Keith. *Drawing Blood: Technology and Disease Identity in Twentieth-Century America*. Baltimore, MD: Johns Hopkins University Press, 1997.

Warner, John Harley. "The Uses of Patient Records by Historians—Patterns, Possibilities and Perplexities." *Health and History* 1 (1999): 101–11.

Weiner, Marli F., with Mazie Hough. *Sex, Sickness, and Slavery: Illness in the Antebellum South*. Urbana: University of Illinois Press, 2012.

White, Luise. *Speaking with Vampires: Rumor and History in Colonial Africa*. Berkeley: University of California Press, 2000.

Williamson, Joel. *A Rage for Order: Black-White Relations in the American South Since Emancipation*. New York: Oxford University Press, 1986.

Yanni, Carla. *The Architecture of Madness: Insane Asylums in the United States*. Minneapolis: University of Minnesota Press, 2007.

Yellin, Eric S. *Racism in the Nation's Service: Government Workers and the Color Line in Woodrow Wilson's America*. Chapel Hill: University of North Carolina Press, 2013.

INDEX

For the benefit of digital users, indexed terms that span two pages (e.g., 52–53) may, on occasion, appear on only one of those pages.
Note: Figures and tables are indicated by an italic *f* or *t* following the para ID.

Abbott, R. A., 49–50
abolition, 47–48, 51, 320n26. *See also* emancipation; slavery
aborigines, 81. *See also* "primitive peoples"
Abrahams, Joseph, 267, 360–61n46
abuse, 67–68, 127. *See also* assault, of patients
accreditation, 233, 299–301, 302–3
Action for Mental Health (Joint Commission on Mental Illness and Health), 280–81
Adler, Alfred, 337–38n30
admission procedures, 41–45, 50, 85–86, 87, 156–60, 228–29, 342n17. *See also* commitment protocol; voluntary admission
adolescence, 131, 290. *See also* young patients
Advisory Committee on Hospital-Community Relationships, 285
advocacy, 191–92, 287, 302
African American, as term, 12
African American female patients. *See also* women
 hydrotherapy and, 169–70
 integration of wards for, 262
 labor undertaken by, 62, 111, 112*f*, 123–24, 231
 restraint of, 164
 seclusion of, 164–66
 separate lodging for, 58, 106, 326
African American male patients
 as category, 344n466
 housed with criminally insane, 107, 226–27
 hydrotherapy and, 167, 168–69
 lack of facilities for, 167–68
African American patients. *See also* African American female patients; African American male patients; black psyche; family(ies), African American; women
 admission procedures with, 156

conceptions of mental illness, 174–77
discipline of, 161–70
examination of, 157–58
as former slaves, 158
identity construction with, 155–61
increase in proportion of, 235
indifference toward, 157–58
labor and, 180
Lind on, 158
"normal abnormality" of, 146–47, 157–58, 207, 318n13, 340n70
in other asylums, 14–15
population of, 85–86
psychiatrists' rapport with, 270
psychotherapy and, 154–55, 170–79
questions for families of, in assessment, 156–57
relationship to staff, 188–89
restraint of, 164, 166–67
seclusion of, 164–67, 165*t*
separate lodging for, 33–38, 57–59, 102–6, 122–23, 226–27, 326n67
African Americans. *See also* free people of color; slavery
 as attendants, 59–60, 237–39, 240, 241
 in Civil War, 46–47
 Civil War and, 47
 in demographics of Washington, 19–20, 242
 depression and, 271–72
 explaining mental illness among, 74–86
 as having "natural" relationship to labor, 180
 as immune to mental illness, 5–6, 79, 81–82
 increasing focus on insanity in, 73–74, 78–79, 93–94
 as inherently criminal, 107–8
 intellect of, assumptions about, 207

African Americans (*cont.*)
　"mad Negro" stereotype of, 4–5, 6
　malaria and, 29
　in Maryland Hospital, 19
　as medical students, 220–22, 242, 243–44, 352n14
　migration of, to Washington, 48, 51
　as nurses, 238
　as physicians, 242, 243–44, 246
　population growth of, 139–40
　as "primitive," 144–45, 146–47, 173
　as psychiatrists, 361n54
　psychiatry in minds of, 313–14
　recapitulation theory and, 81, 141–43, 250–51
　"relational vision of health" among, 345n68
　as staff, 60, 236–46, 326n72, 356n63
Africans, 78, 318n13
aftercare, 202–4
agriculture, 6, 20, 110
alcohol, 59, 168, 343n42
alcoholism, 53, 287, 291–92, 364n33
Alexandria, Virginia, 21
alleys, living in, 87, 91–92, 204, 309, 349n38, 351n64
almshouse, 15–16, 17, 23
Alzheimer, Alois, 245
American Board of Psychiatry and Neurology, 233
American Hospital Association, 280
American Indians, 5, 141, 176, 316n2, 359n23
American Journal of Insanity, 74–75
American Journal of Psychiatry, 253, 273
American Medical Association (AMA), 228, 247–48, 280
American Medico-Psychological Association, 135, 139
American Missionary Association, 49
American Psychiatric Association (APA), 139, 254–55, 280, 354n40
AMSAII. *See* Association of Medical Superintendents of American Institutions for the Insane (AMSAII)
Anacostia, 27–28, 287–89, 301
Anacostia River, 27–29, 286–87, 288, 331n42
Anderson, L. B., 87
Andrews, Judson, 76, 77
anthropology, 83, 140–41, 252
antipsychiatry movement, 273
APA. *See* American Psychiatric Association (APA)
architecture, asylum, 30–31, 35–38, 107
Area A CMHC, 286–87
Area B CMHC, 286–87, 293, 304, 305–6
Area C CMHC, 286–87, 293
Area D CMHC, 286–90, 305–6, 364n26
Arlington, Virginia, 49, 309, 310
Aryans, in racial thought, 81, 82–83, 330n31
assault, of patients, 10, 217–18, 222–23, 227, 353n27

Associated Charities, 205–6
Association of Medical Superintendents of American Institutions for the Insane (AMSAII), 26, 27–28, 31–32, 53–54, 120–21, 135
atavism, racial, 143–44
attendants, 63f. *See also* staff
　African American, 59–60, 237–39, 240, 241
　employment requirements for, 59
　female, 95–96
　in hydrotherapy, 162–63
　Irish, 59
　race and, 3–4
　racial background of, 59
　racial difference and, 8
　slaves as, 59–60
　white, 240, 241

Babcock, J. W., 83–84
Baillarger, Jules, 330n34
Balloch, Edward A., 220–21
Baltimore, MD, 16, 18–19, 25, 320n18
Barnes, J. K., 99
Barry Farm (neighborhood), 223, 353n19
Barry Farm Citizens' Association, 223, 353n19
Barton, Walter, 272–73
baths, continuous, 162–63. *See also* hydrotherapy
Bazelon, David L., 277
beauty salons, 267
bed saddle, 163–64. *See also* restraints, mechanical
bed straps, 60. *See also* restraints, mechanical
Beers, Clifford, 190–91
Bender, Lauretta, 251, 357n9
benevolent societies, 22–23
Bevis, W. M., 142–43, 146, 256
Binghamton Asylum, 125
biological determinism, 248–49, 251–52, 253
biomedicine, 214–15, 318n10
Blackburn, Isaac W., 98
black matriarchy discourse, 271, 361n59
Black Power, 273, 295
black psyche. *See also* African American patients
　comparative psychology research and, 135–52
　dementia praecox and, 136–37
　deviancy and, 272–73
　as inaccessible, 179
　manic-depressive psychosis and, 136
　mental hygiene and, 192
　white *vs.*, 4–5, 128, 139, 256
Blagden, Thomas, 27–28
Blanton, Thomas, 224–25
Bloomingdale Asylum, 26–27, 131
Blyden, Edward Wilmot, 140–41
Board of Children's Guardians, 205–6
Borchert, James, 349n38
Borden, William C., 221–22
Boston, Thomas, 49–50

Boston Psychopathic Hospital, 350n50
Bradley, Omar, 257
brain anatomy, 84–85, 129
brain morphology, 107–8
brain surgery, 120–21
Braslow, Joel, 344n49
Brickman, Celia, 338n46
Brown, Bertram, 297, 300, 301
Brown, James M., 291–92
Brown, Wendy, 327n97
Brunner, Robert, 217–18
Buchanan, J. M., 77–78, 84–85
Bucke, R. M., 81
Bucknill, John Charles, 54, 60–61
Burnham, John C., 339n62
Butler Hospital for the Insane, 34–35, 59
Buxton, Rex E., 215–16

Caliban (character), 74–75
Cameron, Dale, 277–78
Camp Barker, 48–49
Campbell, C. Macfie, 131
Canton Asylum for Insane Indians, 316n2
Cape Colony, 326n77
Cartwright, Samuel A., 322n56
case files
   as historical sources, 155–56, 341–42n10
   racism and, 341–42n10
   use of, 11, 155–56
   White and, 126–27
Celebrezze, Anthony, 281–82
centennial celebration of Saint
      Elizabeths, 247
chaplains, 41, 153–54, 290
Chappelear, Irene, 200–1
charitable institutions, 97
"charm class," 267
Chicago, IL, 77, 82–83, 242
Child Guidance Clinic, 213–14, 215–16. See also
      young patients
chloral hydrate, 109–10
chlorpromazine, 247–48, 264–66, 279
Chu, Franklin D., 290–91, 293, 294,
      295–96, 366n69
Chubb, E. C. W., 89–90
Citizens' Advisory Council, 198
citizens' associations, 9–10, 96–97, 198, 292, 296–
      97, 348n21, 353n19
citizenship, 9–11, 57, 71–72, 77, 85–86, 91, 94, 97,
      120, 223, 304, 305–6, 313–14, 319n17
civic associations, 10, 198, 223, 227, 244,
      293, 353n19
civil independent patients, 41–43, 66–67, 193
civil indigent patients, 41–42, 43–44,
      199–200, 322n5
"civilization," 5, 6, 72–73, 76, 77, 78–79, 80, 82,
      147–48, 172, 252, 311–12, 336n69, 358n18

civil service employment, 91–92, 236, 302. See
      also federal employment
Civil War, 40, 45–51, 57, 69, 74–75. See also
      Reconstruction
Clinical Branch #3, 261
clinical psychiatry position, 137–38
Clothesline Alley, 309, 310
CMHC. See community mental health
      center (CMHC)
Cobb, W. Montague, 243, 245, 258–60, 358n15
cod-liver oil, 109–10
Cohen, Roger, 198
collective unconscious, 7, 144–45. See also racial
      unconscious
colonial medicine, 338–39n48
colonies, for mentally ill, 15–16, 219–20
colored, as term, 346n102
Commission on Mental Health, 198–99, 348n23
commitment protocol, 11, 43–44, 46–47, 49–50,
      86, 87, 93, 98–99, 191–92, 193–200, 228–
      29, 231–32, 254–55, 323n18, 353n22
Committee of 1,000, 302–3
community mental health care. See also aftercare
   deinstitutionalization and, 277–79
   elderly patients and, 282–83
   family care and, 279
   and inpatient services in Southeast, 284
   Interagency Task Force on Mental Health
      and, 281–82
   Kennedy and, 281–82
   National Institute of Mental Health and, 281
   politics of, 279–86
   race and, 294
   racism in, 294
   young patients and, 282–83
community mental health center (CMHC), 281–
      82, 284–85. See also Area D CMHC
Community Support Program, 296–97
comparative psychology research, 128, 138–39,
      148–49, 152, 251, 312
Congress. See US Congress
conjure, 176–77, 334n45, 345n73
Conser, M. Edith, 174–75
contraband camps, 48–50, 51
"contraband of war" designation, 324n33
contrabands, 48, 71
convicts, 41, 105–7, 334n29. See also prisoner
      patients
convulsive therapies, 126, 342n29. See also
      electroconvulsive therapy
Cook, Samuel Le Count, 89
Cook County Hospital for the Insane, 82–83
Coordinating Committee for the Enforcement of
      the DC Anti-Discrimination Laws, 242–43
cottage system, 99–100, 101
Council of State Governments, 280
Covell, David, 204–5

Coy, Myrtle, 236–37
criminal detention, 43–44, 323n18. *See also* convicts; prisoner patients
criminality, inherent, of African Americans, 107–8
criminally insane, 6–7, 105–7, 260, 334n29. *See also* federal convicts; prisoner patients
Cry of Humanity (play), 247–48
cultural anthropology, 83
culture, 77, 78, 79, 80, 81–83, 251, 270–71, 329n213
Cushard, William G., 261–62, 268

Dabney, David, 274
dances, 269–70, 361n52
Danvers State Hospital, 109–10
Darwinism, 73, 77, 79–80, 328n6. *See also* evolution
Davenport, Charles B., 203–4
Davidson, Eugene, 245
Davies, Gertrude, 173–74
DC General Hospital, 286–87. *See also* Gallinger Municipal Hospital
DC League of Women Voters, 244
DCMHA. *See* District of Columbia Mental Health Association (DCMHA)
D. C. Village, 282–83, 287–89
decentralization, 278
degeneration, 72–73, 80–81, 87–88, 139–40
deinstitutionalization, 277–79, 291–92, 293, 362n4
Dellums, C. L., 306–7, 366n71
Dellums, Ronald, 298–99, 304, 306–7
dementia, 53–54, 85, 129–30, 324n46, 330n38
  paretic, 78, 82–83, 162, 329n19, 330n30, 336n3
dementia praecox, 129–31, 135, 136–37, 140–41, 144–45, 146–47, 150–51, 154–55, 185, 265, 337n16, 340n69, 344n54, 346n91
Democratic Party, 95–96, 222, 281
de Montis, Myrtle, 223–24, 353n22
depression, 136, 271–72. *See also* melancholia
desegregation. *See* integration; segregation
Detached Service, 261, 262, 359n30
determinism. *See* biological determinism
developmentally disabled, 101–3
diagnoses, 53–54, 85, 129–32, 133, 213, 273, 324n46, 330n38
Diagnostic and Statistical Manual: Mental Diseases (DSM-1), 270–71
Dickens, Charles, 2, 309–10
Dickson, James F., 304–5
Diesenhaus, Herman, 273–74
Diggs, Charles, 304
Dillingham, John, 299
discipline, 93, 161–70, 184, 268, 342n17
discrimination. *See* racism
District of Columbia Emancipation Act, 47–48, 51

District of Columbia Mental Health Association (DCMHA), 302–3
District of Columbia v. John R. Thompson Co., 242–43
Dix, Dorothea Lynde, 1, 24–25, 26–28, 33, 36, 247, 248
Dix Building, 287–89
Dix Division, 290–91
Dixon, William, 297
Dixon v. Weinberger, 278, 297, 298, 307
"Don't buy where you can't work" campaign, 242–43
Dooley, Lucille, 213–14
Douglass, Frederick, 56–57, 223
Doyle, Dennis, 317n9, 318n16
dreams, 148–49
drugs. *See* pharmacotherapy/psychopharmacology
DSM-1. *See Diagnostic and Statistical Manual: Mental Diseases* (DSM-1)
Duff Green's Row, 48
Duval, Addison, 235
Dwyer, Ellen, 325n49, 334n33, 335n48
dynamic psychiatry
  emergence of, 129–35
  lunacy laws and, 194
  Meyer and, 132
  military patients and, 227
  promise of, 153
  race and, 125–28
  racial difference and, 135
  White and, 153

Earle, Pliny, 62–63, 325n56
Easby, William, 23–24, 26
Eastern Branch, 27–29, 331n42
Eastern Lunatic Asylum, 14–15, 16, 31
East Lodge, 101–4
East Mississippi Insane Asylum, 84–85
Ebony (magazine), 354n38
economy, regional, of Washington, 20
Eisenhower, Dwight D., 245, 257–59
elderly patients, 104
  community mental health care and, 282–83
  deinstitutionalization and, 284
  families and, 234–35
  as former slaves, 158
  as ill-served, 282–83
  increase in, 234–35
  mental health care parity and, 298–99
electroconvulsive therapy, 126, 248, 254–55, 265, 342n29
Elizabethan (patient-run journal), 233, 275–76
Ellis, Alfred Burdon, 141
emancipation, 6, 71–72, 75, 76, 77–78, 93–94, 328–29n10. *See also* free people of color
employment, 61–62, 63, 91–92, 293, 326n72. *See also* federal employment

endocrinology, 132, 150, 340n78
epilepsy, 20–21, 336n3, 340n81
escapees, 283
ethyl carbamate, 109–10
eugenics, 135, 203–4, 248–49, 329–30n26, 349n36
Evarts, Arrah, 136–37, 140–41, 142–43, 146–48, 164–66, 172–73, 176, 177, 185, 340n69, 344n61, 346n91
evolution, psychiatrists' ideas about, 73, 78, 79–80, 81, 83, 141, 147–48, 173
Ewerhardt, Paul J., 214, 215
Ewing, Oscar, 243–45
exceptionalism, of Saint Elizabeths, 1–3, 9–10

faculty psychology, 81, 129, 330n28
Fair Employment Practices Committee, 238–39, 254
Falret, Jean-Pierre, 330n34
family(ies), African American
　challenges to medical authority by, 117
　economic concerns and, 91–92
　involvement of, 64–67
　mental illness care and, 19–20, 22–23
　moral treatment and, 64
　parole and, 201–2
　questions for, in assessment of patients, 156–57
　reliance of, on Saint Elizabeths, 74
　slavery and, 20
　and stigma of mental illness, 87–88
　in therapeutic experience, 112–20
　and trust in Saint Elizabeths, 88–89
family care program, 279
Fanon, Frantz, 273
farm labor, 110
Fauntroy, Walter E., 299
Federal City College, 293
federal convicts, 41, 283. *See also* convicts; prisoner patients
federal employment, 118–19, 192, 214, 220, 239–40, 258, 302. *See also* civil service employment
Federal Security Agency (FSA), 230, 238–39
Federation of Citizens' Associations, 198
Federation of Civic Associations, 198, 244
Felix, Robert H., 281
Fenning, Frederick A., 195, 224–25
Ferguson, John, 217–18
Fett, Sharla, 345n68
Fillmore, Millard, 1, 26–28
Finch, Robert H., 301
Fischer, Siegfried, 251
Foggy Bottom, 29–30
folder system, 126–27
folk medicine, 176–77, 345n68
　See also conjure

Fong, Theodore, 211, 267
Force, Peter, 18
forced-air ventilation, 58–59, 326n67
forced sterilization, 329–30n26.
　See also eugenics
Ford, Gerald, 300
foster homes, 296, 298–99
Foucault, Michel, 316–17n7, 342n17
Fowler, Walter L., 232–33
Frank, Jerome D., 270, 273
Freedmen's Bureau, 48–49, 51
Freedmen's Hospital, 88, 97, 236–37, 242, 243–44, 246, 332n48
Freedmen's Relief Association, 48
Freedmen's Village, 49, 50
freedpeople. *See also* African Americans; emancipation
　Civil War and, 45–51
　competition with whites, 77
　contraband camps and, 48–50, 51
Freeman, Walter, 161
free people of color, precarious position of, 22
Freud, Sigmund, 7, 134, 137, 144–45, 148–49, 339n62. *See also* psychoanalysis
Fry, Gladys-Marie, 332n48
FSA. *See* Federal Security Agency (FSA)
Fugitive Slave Act, 47
fugitive slave laws, 47, 324n31
fugitive slaves, 90
Fuller, Solomon Carter, 245

Gallinger Municipal Hospital, 191, 196, 210, 243–45. *See also* DC General Hospital
Galt, Alexander D., 31
Galt, John M., 31–33, 54–55, 62, 63–64, 101–3, 241
Gambino, Matthew, 319n17, 342n28, 361n52
GAP. *See* Group for the Advancement of Psychiatry (GAP)
Gardner, John, 285, 301
Garfield, James A., 98, 328n5
gender. *See also* African American female patients; African American male patients
　categorization and, 344n49
　differentiation, 336n69, 343n44
　hydrotherapy and, 168–70
　segregation on basis of, 31, 58, 106, 326n66
general paresis, 78, 82–83, 154, 162, 329n215, 330n30, 336n3
genetic psychology, 142, 144–45
Georgetown, 21, 48, 95, 286–87
Georgetown University, 219–21
George Washington University, 220–21
Georgia State Sanitarium, 135
germ plasm theory, 142
Gilbert, Joseph, 180–81
glands, 131, 340n78

Godding, William Whitney, 1–2, 65–66, 93–94
  on African American mental health, 71
  assumes position of superintendent, 70
  cottage system and, 99–100
  emancipation and, 6, 71–72
  Gray and, 100–1
  on inmate labor, 111
  moral treatment and, 98–99, 120–21
  Nichols vs., 98
  overcrowding and, 105, 108–9, 121
  paternalism of, 98–99
  pharmacotherapy and, 109–10
  philosophy of, 98–99
  racially discriminatory treatment and, 97, 103
  somatic therapies and, 110
  therapeutic pessimism and, 120–21
  women patients and, 111
Goffman, Erving, 269–70, 325n60
gonads, 131
governance, of Washington DC, 9–10, 17–18, 95–97, 233, 258, 304, 354n47, 363n20, 366n56
Grahamstown Asylum (South Africa), 83–84
Granatir, William L., 264–65
Grant, Murray, 284–85
Grant, Ulysses S., 68–69
Graven, Philip, 149, 264
Gray, John P., 100–1, 328n5
Green, E. M., 135–36, 152
Green, William, 222–23, 353n27
Greenlees, T. Duncan, 83–84
Grob, Gerald, 316–17n7, 349n40
ground parole, 202. *See also* parole
Group for the Advancement of Psychiatry (GAP), 254–55, 256–57
group therapy, 171–72, 260–61, 267
Guiteau, Charles, 98, 328n5

Haeckel, Ernst, 141
Hall, G. Stanley, 141–42
Hall, Roscoe, 213
Hammond, William A., 76, 79–80
Harper, Anita, 209–10
Harris, David W., 262
Harris, Elizabeth, 65–67
Harris, Joseph D., 65–67, 103
Hassall, James, 200–1
Hawkins, Howard, 217–18, 227
Hawley, Paul R., 257
Health, Education, and Welfare Department (HEW), 281–82, 283, 284, 285, 301, 302–3. *See also* Health and Human Services (HHS) Department
Health and Human Services (HHS) Department, 298
Health Insurance Portability and Accountability Act (HIPAA), 11
Help Alcoholic Women, 291–92

hereditarianism, 6, 73, 80–81, 142, 328n6
HEW. *See* Health, Education, and Welfare Department (HEW)
HHS. *See* Health and Human Services (HHS)
Hickling, Percy, 197–98
Higley, H. V., 258–59
Hillsdale (neighborhood), 223
HIPAA. *See* Health Insurance Portability and Accountability Act (HIPAA)
Hoch, August, 132
Hoffman, Jay L., 262, 263
Homeopathic Hospital, 332n48
homosexuality, 138–39, 171–72, 270
hoodoo. *See* conjure
Hospital for the Insane (Tennessee), 59
Howard Hall, 107–8, 122–23, 156, 220, 226–27, 257–58, 261, 268, 360–61n46
Howard University, 214–15, 220–22, 224–25, 242, 243–44, 286–87, 352n14
Hubbard, Lois, 140, 173–74, 207, 209–10, 340n81
Hunter, Robert, 26
Hurd, Henry, 78
hydrotherapy, 120–21, 154, 162–64, 167–70, 334n36, 343n39
hyoscine hydrobromide, 109–10

Ickes, Harold, 236, 241
"idiots," 101–3
Illinois Eastern Hospital for the Insane, 100, 132
"imbeciles," 101–3
immunity, to mental illness, 5–6, 79, 81–82
Indianapolis State Hospital, 137
indigents. *See* civil indigent patients
infantilization, of African Americans, 149
insanity. *See* mental illness
insulin shock therapy, 248, 265, 342n29
intake procedure, 156–60, 342n17
integration, 10, 103. *See also* segregation
  aftermath of, 247–50
  of staff, 236–46
  of VA hospitals, 257, 258–60
  of wards, 257–63, 361n52
  in Washington, 258
Interagency Task Force on Mental Health, 281–82
investigation, of Saint Elizabeths, by Congress, 69, 127, 182, 223–26
Ionia State Hospital, 367n73
Irish, 59, 73

Jackson, Andrew, 17–18
JCAH. *See* Joint Commission on Accreditation of Hospitals (JCAH)
JCMIH. *See* Joint Commission on Mental Illness and Health (JCMIH)
Jellife, Smith Ely, 131, 136–37
Jewett, R. W., 45
Jim Crow, 168–69, 220–22, 223, 258, 272, 275

Joe Jefferson Democratic Club, 62–63
John Howard Pavilion, 283
Johnson, John L., 306–7
Johnson, Loren, 204–5, 214
Johnson, Lyndon B., 366n56
Johnson, Mordecai, 215
Joint Commission on Accreditation of Hospitals (JCAH), 299–300
Joint Commission on Mental Illness and Health (JCMIH), 280–81
Jones, S. Preston, 45–46
Jones, William B., 274
Judiciary Square, 19
Jung, Carl, 7, 144–45, 337–38n30, 339n62
Junior Village, 287–89
juries, in commitment proceedings, 194–95, 198–99
Juvenile Protectorate, 205–6

Karpman, Benjamin, 159, 186, 215, 242
Keefe, Frank, 229–30
Kellogg, A. O., 74–75
Kelly, Isaac, 178, 180
Kempf, Edward J., 137–39, 338n46
Kennedy, John F., 281–82, 307–8
Kennedy, Joseph Camp, 328–29n10
Kenney, John A., 243, 244
Kieffer, Sherman, 289–90
Kiernan, James G., 77, 82–83, 98, 330n31
Kirby, George H., 136
Kirkbride, Thomas S., 26–27, 33–34, 99–100
Kraepelin, Emil, 129–32, 133, 134–35, 146–47, 150, 245, 340n69

labor, patient, 61–62, 63, 108–12, 115, 123–24, 180–86, 230–31, 346n91. *See also* occupational therapy
laboratory testing, 156
Lamarckism, 142, 144–45, 250–51, 357n7
Latinos, 286–87, 305–6
Lawrence, Richard, 17–18
Lazell, Edward, 171–72
Lee, Charles A., 325n56
Lee, Robert E., 49
leisure, 62–64. *See also* recreation
Lewis, Nolan D. C., 137, 150–52, 186–87, 340n81
Life Adjustment Center, 191, 213–15
Lincoln, Abraham, 47
Lind, John E., 140, 141, 143–45, 147–49, 157–58, 163–64, 175, 181–82, 186, 212, 242
Littell, Franklin, 351n57
lobotomy, 126, 161, 169
location, of Saint Elizabeths, 13, 27–30
lodging, segregated, 33–38, 57–59, 100, 101, 102, 103–4, 122–23, 220, 226–27, 326n67
Logan Court, 309, 310
Lovell, Moses R., 213–14

Lunacy in Many Lands (Tucker), 71
lunacy laws
 in Maryland, 16
 in Virginia, 16
 in Washington, DC, 41–42, 43–45, 50, 192–99, 235
lunatico inquirendo, 43–44, 92, 193–94
Lunbeck, Elizabeth, 344–45n65, 350n50
Lydston, G. Frank, 107

MacCarthy, Shane, 302
MacDowell, Edith, 178
"mad Negro," 4–5, 6
Magruder, G. Lloyd, 219–20
Makari, George, 341n83
malaria, 28–29
malaria fever inoculation therapy, 126, 154, 162
Manhattan State Hospital, 136
mania, 52, 53–54, 83–85, 129, 167, 324n46, 330n34, 330n38
manic-depressive psychosis, 129–31, 135–36, 251, 337n16
manumission, 20, 21–22, 42
March of Medicine (television series), 247–48
Marland, Albert, 199
Maryland, 16, 42, 47
Maryland Hospital, 18–19, 23–24, 25, 33, 37, 40, 320n18
Massillon State Hospital, 336n6
matriarchy discourse, black, 271, 361n59
Matthews, Eliza, 50
Maudsley, Henry, 53–54
Maul, Herman, 178
Mazique, Edward, 245
McClellan, George, 48
McClelland, Robert, 35–36, 37, 39, 43–44
McFarland, Andrew, 59
McGuire, Hunter, 107
McIntyre, William, 222–23
McKie, Thomas J., 330n35
McKinley, William, 336n6
McKinney, Stewart, 306–7
McLean, Arthur, 238–39
McLean Hospital (Massachusetts), 109–10
McNutt, Paul V., 230, 241
mechanical restraints, 60–61, 163–64, 165t, 166–67, 266, 343n33
Medicaid, 298–99, 302–3
Medical Society of the District of Columbia, 198, 246
medical treatment. *See* pharmacotherapy/ psychopharmacology
Medicare, 298–99, 302–3
medicine. *See* pharmacotherapy/ psychopharmacology
Medico-Chirurgical Society, 10, 243, 245
Medico-Legal Society of Washington, DC, 127

Meharry Medical College, 243–44
melancholia, 53–54, 83–84, 85, 123, 129, 324n46, 330n34, 330n38. *See also* depression
men. *See* African American male patients
Menninger, William C., 254–55
Mental Health Administration, 301
Mental Health Authority, 285
mental health care parity, 298–99
Mental Health Law Project, 297
Mental Health Study Act, 280
mental hygiene
   advocacy and, 191–92
   black psyche and, 192
   local institutions and, 191
   lunacy laws and, 192–99
   outpatient clinics and, 202–3, 204–6, 213–15
   Progressive reform and, 190–91
   racial boundaries of, 199–216
   White and, 126, 190–91, 203
mental illness
   in 17th and 18th centuries, 15–16
   African Americans' presumed immunity to, 5–6, 79, 81–82
   African American vernacular ideas about, 112–13, 174–77
   Civil War and, 47
   contraband camps and, 49–50
   culture and, 77, 271
   as curable, 24–25
   emancipation and, 6, 71, 72–73, 75, 76, 77–78, 93–94, 271–72
   environment and, 30–31
   heredity and, 6, 73, 80
   increase in, 75–76, 93–94
   military service and, 46–47
   modernity and, 5
   neurology and, 73
   race and incidence of, 77, 79
   race neutral approach to, 250, 253, 256, 264
   racialization of, 73–74, 82
   racism and, 253–54, 255–56
   relativist approach to, 252
   as result of maladaptation, 128, 132–33, 150, 187, 190–91, 227, 228, 249, 270–71, 337n22, 340n69
   slavery and, 20–22
   stigma of, 87–88
   in Washington, DC, 9–11
   whites as more susceptible to, 76
Mental Retardation and Community Mental Health Centers Act, 282, 286–87
metrazol shock therapy, 248, 265, 342n29
Metropolitan Police, 86–87, 89, 90–91, 192–93, 196–98, 217, 328n99, 332n54
Metzl, Jonathan, 340n69
Meyer, Adolf, 7, 132, 133–34, 145, 190–91, 337n22

migration, 48, 51, 139–40, 275–76, 287
milieu therapy, 267–68, 269–70, 360–61n46
military patients, 14, 41–42, 43, 45–47, 110–11, 156, 182–83, 187, 218, 223–25, 227, 229, 231–32, 234, 249–50, 323n28, 347n104
Millard, Maurice, 274–75, 362n69
Miller, J. F., 78, 79
Miller, Michael, 274–75, 362n69
Miller, Thomas, 23–24, 25, 26
Millikan, Frank Rives, 325n49
Mills, Charles K., 107–8
minstrelsy, 63–64, 327n86
miscegenation, 143–44
Mitchell, Clarence, 259
mojo. *See* conjure
Moniz, Egas, 161
Montagu, Ashley, 253–55, 358n15
moral treatment/moral management, 39–40
   asylum architecture and, 30–31, 33–34
   defined, 30–31
   employment and, 61–62
   families and, 64
   Godding and, 98–99, 120–21
   labor and, 33, 61–62, 110–11
   leisure and, 62–64
   Nichols and, 30, 33–34, 40, 54–55
   persistence of, 153–54
   and prioritization of white mental health, 32–33, 34
   race and, 31–34, 52–68, 120–24
   White and, 126
Moten, Lucy E., 221–22
Mount Hope Institution, 19, 40
Myers, Henry J., 256–57

NAACP. *See* National Association for the Advancement of Colored People (NAACP)
name, of Saint Elizabeths, 11, 39–40
Nassau, Robert Hamill, 141
National Association for the Advancement of Colored People (NAACP), 10, 223–24, 243, 244–45
National Association of Intergroup Relations Officials, 237–38, 258
National Center for Mental Health Services, Training, and Research (NCMHSTR), 285–86, 289–90
National Committee for Mental Hygiene, 190–91
National Institute of Mental Health (NIMH), 228, 280, 281, 284, 285–86, 289–90, 301, 302–3
National Medical Association (NMA), 243, 244–45
National Mental Health Act of 1946, 228
National Mental Health Advisory Committee, 228
National Urban League, 236–37, 293
Native Americans, 5, 141, 176, 234, 316n2, 359n23

Naval Hospital, 332n48
NCMHSTR. *See* National Center for Mental Health Services, Training, and Research (NCMHSTR)
negro, as term, 12
Negro, as term, 12
"Negro problem," 71–72, 74
neighborhood associations. *See* citizens' associations; civic associations
neurasthenia, 129
neurology, 73, 76, 79–80, 82–83, 101, 107–8, 129, 131, 134–35, 137–38, 227
New Deal, 228, 307–8, 310–11
"New Freedom" era, 192
New Negro Alliance, 242–43
New York Medical Journal, 77–78
New York State Lunatic Asylum, 327n86
Nichols, Charles H., 1–2, 4–5, 14, 26–30, 122–23
  civil indigent patients and, 43–44
  in Civil War, 45–46
  on commitment procedures, 43–44, 50, 323n18
  contraband camps and, 51
  cottage system and, 100
  on diagnoses, 53–54
  diagnoses and, 325n49
  final years as superintendent, 68–70
  Godding *vs.*, 98
  inmate labor and, 61–62
  investigations of, 68–70
  in legislation on hospital operations, 39–40
  moral treatment and, 30, 33–34, 40, 54–55
  and name of hospital, 39–40
  on overcrowding, 99
  paternalism of, 13–14, 55, 57–58
  racism and, 60
  restraints and, 60–61
  segregation and, 57
  and separate living quarters for African Americans, 33–38, 57–59
  transients and, 50
Nichols Avenue, 122, 123
"night doctor," 88–89
NIMH. *See* National Institute of Mental Health (NIMH)
Nixon, Richard M., 300, 301
NMA. *See* National Medical Association (NMA)
Noll, Steven, 336–37n12, 341–42n10
"normal abnormality," 146–47, 157–58, 207, 318n13, 340n70
Northampton Lunatic Hospital, 325n56
North Carolina Medical Journal, 79
Northeast DC, 286–87, 366n69
Northwest DC, 286–87
Noyes, Arthur P., 187–89
nurses, 162–63, 203, 219–20
  African American, 236–38

O'Brien, Joseph, 302, 303*f*
occupational therapy, 153, 257–58, 266. *See also* labor, patient
O'Malley, Mary, 140*f*, 142–43, 144, 146–47, 149, 164–66, 184, 193, 213, 256, 339n59
outpatient clinics, 204–6, 213–15
overcrowding, 38, 99, 101, 105, 107, 108–9, 121, 127, 220, 226, 230–32, 260–61, 277–78
Overholser, Dorothy, 245
Overholser, Winfred
  background of, 228
  on chlorpromazine, 265–66
  demographics changes and, 234–35
  on discharges, 229
  family care and, 279
  and federal status of Saint Elizabeths, 232–33, 234
  integration and, 244–45, 257, 280–81, 361n52
  on mental illness, 255
  military patients and, 232
  segregation and, 245, 257–58
Owsley, Jesse, 182

PAGs. *See* patient administrative groups (PAGs)
Papua New Guinea, 252
paretic dementia, 78, 82–83, 154, 162, 329n19, 330n30, 336n3
parole, 66–67, 116, 200–2. *See also* release
paternalism, 160–61
  emancipation and, 71–72
  of Godding, 98–99
  of Kellogg, 74–75
  of Nichols, 13–14, 55, 57–58
  slavery and, 6
patient administrative groups (PAGs), 268–70, 360–61n46
patient labor, 61–62, 63, 108–12, 115, 123–24, 180–86, 230–31, 346n91. *See also* occupational therapy
patients. *See* African American female patients; civil independent patients; civil indigent patients; criminally insane; elderly patients; military patients; prisoner patients; young patients
patients' rights movement, 278
Peele, Roger, 295–96, 301
pellagra, 336n3
Pennsylvania Hospital for the Insane, 26–27, 33–34, 99–100
Perry, John S., 242
Pettit, Manson, 213
pharmacotherapy/psychopharmacology, 109–10, 247–49, 250, 264–66, 278, 279
Philadelphia, PA, 25
Phyllis Wheatley Young Women's Christian Association, 208–9
phylogeny, 141

physicians, African American, 242, 243–44, 246
Pierce, Franklin, 1, 35–36
police, 86–87, 89, 90–91, 192–93, 196–98, 217, 328n99, 332n54
poverty, 16–17, 91–92, 93, 249–50, 292, 309–10
prefrontal lobotomy, 126, 161, 169
Prettyman, E. Barrett, 197–98
"primitive peoples," 5–6, 78–79, 83, 311–12. See also savages
prisoner patients, 41, 105–6, 156, 234, 260–61, 270, 283, 284. See also convicts; criminally insane; federal convicts
privatization, 366n69. See also community mental health care; deinstitutionalization
Progressive reform, 190–91, 192, 199–200
Providence, RI, 34–35, 59
Prudhomme, Charles, 236, 237, 245, 257
psyche. See also black psyche
  of blacks vs. whites, 4–5, 128, 139, 172, 256
  universalist understanding of, 8, 138–39, 256, 338n46
psychiatric social work, 126, 188–89, 191–92, 202–3, 204–5, 207–8, 210, 213, 236, 241–42, 297, 306–7, 349n40
psychiatrists, African Americans as, 361n54
psychiatry. See dynamic psychiatry; psychodynamic psychiatry; race-neutral psychiatry; social psychiatry
Psychiatry: Journal of the Biology and the Pathology of Interpersonal Relations, 252
"psychiatry of everyday life," 344–45n65
psychoanalysis, 133–35, 137, 154, 170–71, 337–38n30, 339n62. See also Freud, Sigmund; psychotherapy
Psychoanalytic Review, 136–37
psychobiology, 7, 133, 138, 150, 190–91
psychodrama, 229–30, 247, 248, 266
psychodynamic psychiatry, 249, 255, 270–71
psychogenesis, 132, 137–38, 174–75
psychology. See comparative psychology research; faculty psychology; genetic psychology
psychopathic personality, 186, 187–88, 207, 209–10, 350n50
psychophysical parallelism, 132–33, 137–38
psychosexual conflict, 133–34, 139–40. See also sexuality
psychotherapy, 5, 154–55, 170–79, 264, 267, 270, 273. See also psychoanalysis
Public Buildings Administration, 230
public visit days, 98–99
Purvis, Charles B., 67–68, 97

Q Service, 260–61
Quakers, 26–27, 40, 125–26
quinine, 109–10

race. See also African American patients; African Americans; Native Americans; whites
  biological view of, 73, 79–80, 143–44, 248–49, 251, 252, 253
  clinical relationships and, 185
  community mental health care and, 294
  diagnoses and, 54
  discharge rates and, 187, 347n105
  dynamic psychiatry and, 125–28
  eugenics and, 248–49
  hydrotherapy and, 167, 168–70
  and incidence of mental illness, 77, 79
  mania and, 54
  mechanical restraints and, 60–61, 165t
  mental hygiene and, 199–216
  and mission of hospital, 15
  moral treatment and, 52–68, 120–24
  in postwar psychiatric thought, 250–57
  psychotherapy and, 154–55
  seclusion and, 165t
  segregation by, 2–3, 4–5, 14–15, 32–34, 35, 57, 98–109, 122–23, 218–27, 326n67
  site selection and, 29
  social psychiatry and, 250
  staff and, 59
  therapeutic rationale and, 185–86
"race history," 140–41
race-mixing, 143–44
race-neutral psychiatry, 264
race riots, 72, 320n26
"race suicide," 87–88, 138–39, 329–30n26
racial ambivalence, 8, 146, 153–55
racial atavism, 143–44
racial difference, 3–4, 7–8, 15, 101–3, 135, 138–39, 143, 170, 250–51, 253, 312
racialism, 2–3, 8, 318n16
racialization, 3–9, 73–74, 82, 111, 318n10, 319n17
racial topography, 33–34, 321n48
racial unconscious, 144–47, 151, 172–73. See also collective unconscious
racism
  case files and, 341–42n10
  charitable institutions and, 97
  in community mental health care, 294
  confrontation of, in psychiatry, 273–74
  defined, 318n16
  diagnoses and, 213
  institutional, 273–74
  leisure activities and, 62
  as mental illness, 253–54, 358n15
  mental illness and, 249–50, 255–56
  misdiagnoses and, 273
  Nichols and, 60
  persistence of, 264–75
  racialism vs., 318n16
  staff experiences of, 239, 240, 241
"Racism and Social Action" (Montagu), 253–54
Randall, Samuel Jackson, 114
Randolph, A. Philip, 238–39
Randolph, Kirby Ann, 331n44

Ray, Isaac, 34–35
recapitulation theory, 81, 141–43, 250–51, 357n7
Reconstruction, 57, 71–74, 328n9
recordkeeping, 126–27
recreation, 62, 63–64, 153–54, 219, 223, 359n23
recreational therapy, 266
Reichenbach, Evelyn B., 262–63
"relational vision of health," 345n68
relativist approach to mental illness, 252
release, 63–64, 67–68, 118, 186–87, 202, 347n105. *See also* aftercare; deinstitutionalization; parole
religion, 52, 77–78, 80, 84–85, 144, 153–54, 330n35, 351n59. *See also* chaplains
Republican Party, 47, 95–96
reserpine, 248, 264–65, 266, 279
restraints, mechanical, 60–61, 163–64, 165t, 166–67, 266, 343n33
Reverby, Susan, 318n16
Reynolds, Thomas D., 297–98
Richardson, Alonzo, 116, 127, 336n6, 345n77
Richmond, Winifred, 207, 214
rights consciousness, 10–11, 97, 109–20
right-to-treatment, 297
Ripley, Herbert S., 358n18
Risse, Guenter B., 341–42n10
Robben Island Lunatic Asylum (South Africa), 326n77
Roberts, J. D., 85
Robertson, Alexander, 56–57, 60–61, 62–63
Robinson, Aubrey E., Jr., 298
Robinson, Luther D., 246, 295, 296
Robinson, W. A., 134
Róheim, Géza, 252
Rome, Howard P., 301
Rome Committee, 301–2
Roosevelt, Eleanor, 236
Roosevelt, Franklin Delano, 198, 236, 254
Roosevelt, Theodore, 140–41, 347n7
Rosen, Harold, 270, 273
Rouse, Charles H., 277–78
Rouse v. Cameron, 274, 277–78

Sabshin, Melvin, 273–74
Saint Elizabeths
  comparative psychology research at, 128, 138–39, 148–49, 152, 251, 312
  considered as exceptional institution, 1–3, 9–10
  integration of wards of, 257–63, 361n52
  investigations of, 69, 127, 182, 223–26
  overcrowded conditions in, 38, 99, 101, 105, 107, 108–9, 121, 127, 220, 226, 230–32, 260–61, 277–78
  racial segregation in, 2–3, 4–5, 14–15, 32–34, 35, 57, 98–109, 122–23, 326n67
  significance of name, 11, 39–40
salons, beauty, 267
satellite centers, 287–89, 290–91, 295–96

"savages," 74–75, 80–81, 141, 173. *See also* "primitive peoples"
schizophrenia, 130, 265, 270–72, 307, 340n69, 367n73. *See also* dementia praecox
Schoen, Johanna, 345n73
Schroeder, S. F., 212
Schwartz, Lawrence, 305
Schweik, Susan, 12
Scotch douche, 162–63. *See also* hydrotherapy
Scottish commonsense philosophy, 330n28
seclusion, 164–66, 165t, 266
Section 8 housing, 296–97
sedatives, 248, 264–66
segregation, 218–27. *See also* integration; lodging, segregated
  challenges to, 218
  Eisenhower and, 258–59
  gender, 31, 58, 106, 326n66
  hydrotherapy and, 168–69
  informal, of staff, 239
  racial, 2–3, 4–5, 14–15, 32–34, 35, 57, 98–109, 122–23, 326n159
  in Washington, 192, 214–16, 242–43, 258, 348n15
  White and, 127–28, 218–27
senile psychoses, 130. *See also* elderly patients
Serpasil. *See* reserpine
servants' quarters, 33
"sexual furor," 82–83, 107
sexuality, 62–63, 108–9, 138, 147–48, 157–58, 159, 231–32, 251–52, 269–70. *See also* psychosexual conflict
sexually transmitted disease, 72
Shakespeare, William, 74–75
Sheffey, William, 302
Shepherd, Alexander, 96
Sherburn, John P., 49–50
Shipstead, Henrik, 223–24
shock treatments. *See* electroconvulsive therapy; insulin shock therapy; metrazol shock therapy
Shore, Debra, 305
Short, Dewey, 229–30
Silber, K. F., 210–11
single-room occupancy (SROs), 298–99
site selection, 28–30
slavery. *See also* emancipation
  as "benevolent" institution, 80–81
  civil independent patients and, 42–43
  District of Columbia Emancipation Act and, 47–48
  fugitive slave laws and, 47, 324n31
  manumission and, 20, 21–22, 42
  mental illness and, 20–22
  paternalism in, 6
  in patient histories, 158
  patient labor and, 184
  staff and, 60
  in Washington, 20

Snake Pit, The (film), 352n3
Snake Pit, The (Ward), 352n3
social psychiatry, 228, 249–50, 256–57, 272–73, 278, 312
social service department, 206, 209, 210–13, 349n40, 349–50n43
social work, psychiatric, 126, 188–89, 191–92, 202–3, 204–5, 207–8, 210, 213, 236, 241–42, 297, 306–7, 349n40
sodium amytal, 264–65
somatic therapies, 110, 126, 161–70. *See also* electroconvulsive therapy; hydrotherapy; insulin shock therapy; lobotomy; malaria fever inoculation therapy; metrazol shock therapy; restraints, mechanical; seclusion
South Africa, 83–84, 326n77
South Carolina Lunatic Asylum, 14–15, 83–84
South Dakota, 316n2, 359n23
Southeast, Far-Southwest Health Steering Committee, 302
Southeast DC, 27–28, 278–79, 284–85, 290–91, 366n69
Southwest DC, 278–79, 286–87, 290–91. *See also* Tiber Island
Spencer, Samuel, 258
spirituality, 153–54, 351n59. *See also* chaplains; religion
Spitzka, Edward C., 79–80, 81–82, 98, 328n5
Sproul, Dorothy, 207–8, 209, 213–14
SROs. *See* single-room occupancy (SROs)
Stack, Maurice, 127–28
staff. *See also* attendants; nurses; physicians; psychiatric social work
   African Americans as, 60, 236–46, 326n72, 356n63
   assault by, 10, 182, 217–18, 222–23, 227, 353n27
   departures of, to private practice, 279, 363n7
   integration of, 236–46
   moral treatment and, 59–60
   patients' relationship with, 188–89
   racism experienced by, 239, 240, 241
   ratios, 354n40
   reductions, 307
   segregation of, 60, 219–20, 239, 326n72
standards of care, 26
Stanly, Edward, 25–26
Stannard, Amy, 213–14
State Asylum for the Insane (Buffalo), 76
St. Clair, Harvey, 270–71
stereotypy, 172, 175, 177, 344n57
sterilization, forced, 329–30n26
Stevens, Rutherford B., 255–56, 358n18
Stewart, Mary, 208–9
Stowe, Steven M., 325n61
straitjackets, 60, 127. *See also* restraints, mechanical

straps, bed, 60. *See also* restraints, mechanical
Stribling, Francis T., 33
strychnine, 109–10
Stuart, Alexander, 26–29, 36
students, medical, 220–22, 242, 243–44, 352n14
Sullivan, Harry Stack, 252–53
Sullivan, William Van Amberg, 121–22
Sun Dial (in-house newsletter), 153–54, 170
superintendent model, 39
superstition, 144, 172, 173–74. *See also* conjure
surveillance, 33–34, 178, 209
Sweeney, Irwin R., 222–23
Sylvester, Richard, 197–98
syphilis, 72, 154, 156, 240, 329n19, 330n30, 336n3

Tartaglino, Francis, 213, 267
Tempest, The (Shakespeare), 74–75
Tennessee, 59, 76
Tennyson, Simon, 201
terminology, 12
Terrell, Mary Church, 242–43
therapeutic experience, 95–97, 109–20
therapeutic optimism, 153–55, 187
therapeutic pessimism, 121, 130–31, 186–89, 337n17
Thirkield, Wilbur P., 221–22, 352n14
Thomason, Ewing, 229–30
Thorazine. *See* chlorpromazine
Tiber Island (Southwest DC), 29–30. *See also* Southwest DC
Toner, James, 181
Toner, Joseph M., 101, 110
Torrey, E. Fuller, 300, 366n69
toxins, 131
trash, hoarding of, 177
Trinity Community House, 204–6
Trotter, Sharland, 290–91, 293, 294, 295–96, 366n69
Truman, Harry S., 231–32, 236, 243–44, 289–90, 310–11
trust, of families, 88–89
tuberculosis, 72, 93, 204
Tucker, George A., 71, 93–94
Tuke, Daniel Hack, 54, 101–3
Tuke, Samuel, 26–27

unconscious, 5, 133–34, 144–46. *See also* collective unconscious; psychoanalysis; racial unconscious
underutilization, of mental health services by people of color, 313
Uniontown, 27–28
unitary psychosis concept, 336–37n12
universalist understanding of the psyche, 8, 138–39, 263, 338n46
University of the District of Columbia, 293

Index

urban renewal, 287
US Colored Troops, 46–47
US Congress, 303
   in abolition of slavery in Washington, 47–48
   African American citizenship and, 57
   commitment protocol and, 44, 49–50
   in DC governance, 9–10, 95, 96, 233–34, 258, 304
   funding and, 36, 37–38, 58–59, 68–69, 70, 99, 101, 103–4, 224, 300
   integration in Washington and, 258
   investigation by, 69, 127, 182, 223–26
   Joint Commission on Mental Illness and Health and, 280
   lunacy laws and, 196–98
   Maryland Hospital and, 18–19
   transient insane and, 50
   voluntary admission and, 199
U Street, 242–43
Utica Asylum, 125

Valley Green (neighborhood), 289
Valley Green Counseling Center, 289, 290–91
Van Buren, Martin, 18
ventilation, 58–59, 326n67
veterans. *See* military patients; Veterans Administration
Veterans Administration, 8–9, 231–32, 257, 258–60
Vietnam War, 295–96
Virginia, 14–15, 16, 21, 25, 31, 33, 76, 206, 211–12
vocational training, 293
voluntary admission, 195–97, 199, 228–29, 235, 279, 348n25. *See also* admission procedures

Wadsworth, James, 48
Wagner von Jauregg, Julius, 162
Waldrop, Francis N., 262, 301
Wallach, Richard, 47–48, 51
Walter, T. U., 35–36
Ward, Mary Jane, 352n3, 359n27
Warner, John Harley, 341–42n10
Washington, DC, 28
   abolition in, 47–48, 320n26
   African Americans in demographics of, 19–20, 242
   after Reconstruction, 71–74
   consolidation of, 95–96
   effects of District of Columbia Emancipation Act on, 47–48, 51
   Fugitive Slave Act and, 47
   governance of, 9–10, 17–18, 95–97, 233, 258, 304, 354n47, 363n20, 366n56
   home rule in, 304, 363n20
   integration in, 242–45, 246, 258

   lunacy laws in, 41–42, 43–45, 50, 192–99
   migration of African Americans to, 48, 51
   poverty in, 16–17
   slavery in, 20
   transfer of Saint Elizabeths to, 299–308
Washington, Walter, 301, 302
Washington Asylum, 17
Washington Bee (newspaper), 221–22
Washington Board of Trade, 9–10, 96–97
Washington Home Rule Committee, 233
Washington Infirmary, 17
Washington Institute of Mental Hygiene, 191
Washington Metropolitan Health Council, 233
Washington Opportunities for Women, 293
Washington Tribune (newspaper), 222
Waters, George, 42–43
Watt, Howard, 110–11
"We, the Mentally Ill. . ." (television program), 247–48
Weissmann, August, 142
welfare hotels, 298–99
Wells, Patricia, 305–6
Western Lunatic Asylum, 33
West Lodge, 102*f*, 106*f*, 103–4, 105, 230, 260–61, 262–63, 268
West Side Service, 261–62, 268
White, Luise, 338–39n48
White, William Alanson, 1, 140*f*
   assumes position of superintendent, 124, 125
   background of, 125
   dynamic psychiatry and, 133–35, 153
   on faculty psychology, 129, 336n10
   Freud and, 134
   genetic psychology and, 142
   Green and, 136
   hydrotherapy and, 163–64
   investigations and, 127–28
   Jung and, 145
   Kraepelin and, 129–31, 133
   malaria fever inoculation therapy and, 162
   medical student controversy and, 221–22
   mental hygiene and, 190–91, 203–4
   Meyer and, 133
   moral treatment model and, 126
   psychoanalysis and, 134, 170–71
   psychotherapy and, 170
   racial unconscious and, 145
   recapitulation theory and, 142–43
   recordkeeping under, 126–27
   restraint and, 343n33
   on segregation, 127–28
   segregation and, 218–27
   somatic therapies under, 126, 162–64
   on stereotypy, 344n57
   therapeutic pessimism of, 337n17
   vision of, 125–26

whites
- as attendants, 59, 240, 241
- contraband camps and, 48–49
- cultivation of "savage" behavior in, 141
- emancipation and, 71–72
- evolution of, 81
- free people of color competing with, 77
- and integration of staff, 240
- as more susceptible to mental illness, 76
- as nurses, 238
- and policymaking in Washington, 96–97
- privileging of psyche of, 5, 8, 15, 32–33, 139, 172

white supremacy, 184–85, 221
Wilkerson, Raymond, 273–74
Willard Asylum, 100, 334n33
William Alanson White Psychiatric Foundation, 252
William A. White Division, 290–91
Williams, Daniel Hale, 88
Williams, Ernest Y., 215, 242
Williams, Gertrude, 215–16
Williamsburg, VA, 16
Wilson, Anita, 180–81
Wilson, Woodrow, 192
Wilson Park, 121–22
Wines, Frederick, 75
witchcraft, 144, 172. *See also* conjure
Witmer, A. H., 78–79, 93, 123
Wolf, Stewart, 358n18
women. *See also* African American female patients
- alcoholism among, 364n33
- as attendants, 95–96
- as category, 344n49

Woodridge, Annie, 304, 305–6
Woodward, Samuel B., 31–32
Woodworth, John, 67
Woolley, Herbert C., 217–18
Worcester State Lunatic Hospital, 14–15, 31–32, 132, 252
Work, Hubert, 225–26
workshops, 293
World War I, 223–24, 250–51
World War II, 227–35, 237–38
writ de lunatic inquirendo. See lunatico inquirendo

Yochelson, Leon, 256–57
Yolles, Stanley, 281, 285–86, 292, 364n24
York Retreat, 26–27
young patients. *See also* Child Guidance Clinic
- "charm class" for female, 267
- community mental health care and, 282–83, 284
- housed with female patients, 101

www.ingramcontent.com/pod-product-compliance
Ingram Content Group UK Ltd.
Pitfield, Milton Keynes, MK11 3LW, UK
UKHW021252180426
11946UKWH00004B/102